High Praise for

"INSTANT *E.N.E.R.G.Y.*™ is a master guide to the secrets of high level wellness. Dr. Marilyn Joyce has integrated a lifetime of knowledge and experience of body-mind-spirit practices to create an abundance of energy and vitality in our lives."
~ **James Strohecker,** CEO, Co-founder HealthWorld Online, Wellness Inventory. Los Angeles, CA

"Marilyn clearly embraces the principle that your health is the foundation of all wealth, be it material, spiritual, mental, or emotional. But in today's information-rich world, making healthy choices and practicing them can feel overwhelming. Marilyn solves that problem inside the pages of INSTANT *E.N.E.R.G.Y.*™ In clear, practical steps, she condenses her broad base of knowledge, experience, and wisdom into tips, practices, and recommendations that are easy to include in your already busy life. Read it, apply it, and thrive like never before." –
~ **George C. Huang, M.D.,** Freedompreneur Coaching & Consulting. co-author, *Create the Business Breakthrough You Want.* Mount Vernon, WA

In INSTANT *E.N.E.R.G.Y.*™, Marilyn demonstrates, why being healthy in every aspect of life, is not rocket science. She makes what is too often made complex and complicated, easy to understand and apply. And even more importantly, she motivates the reader to *want* to make the changes necessary to live a healthier life. I especially appreciate her emphasis on physical fitness, giving practical advice, and easy-to-apply-solutions that everyone can benefit from.
~ **Dave Hubbard,** Americas Fitness Coach®. author, *If your workout takes longer than 10 Minutes, you're wasting your time!* Kennesaw, GA

In my travels around the US teaching business and financial management, you run into those rare people who set themselves apart from the crowd. Their story exemplifies courage, resolve, achievement, and a level of contribution that is beyond the comprehension of most people. Marilyn is one of those people. She tirelessly works to help people understand how better nutrition can change their lives. Her journey from her death bed to a pillar of health is both inspiring and educational. I have had the distinct pleasure to see her teach and to watch so many of those students leave her training committed to changing their health and the health of others. I am confident her new book will inspire and educate others who seek the path to good health.
~ **Gordon Hester,** Business and Financial Management Expert. Sarasota, FL

With this book, INSTANT *E.N.E.R.G.Y.*™ , The 5 Keys to Unlimited Energy & Vitality!, the first thing you must do is read Dr. Marilyn Joyce's' acknowledgment page for the best story about perseverance ever! As an expert Whine-ologist, I'm here to tell you that this book will change your life. When I got to the chapter, *Conquer Worry*, I substituted Worry with the word Whining and quickly realized that Dr. Joyce's message is a one-size fits all perfect answer to living life as it was meant to be lived.
~ **January Jones,** The Whine Tester. *author, Thou Shalt Not Whine . . . The Eleventh Commandment.* Westlake Village, CA

INSTANT *E.N.E.R.G.Y.*™, is a sure-fire way to ratchet up your resilience and turbo-charge your vitality.
~ **Nannette Oatley, M.A., LPC**. author, *Pain, Power, and Promise.* 2001 U.S. Open Wheelchair Tennis Champion. Prescott, AZ

Dr. Marilyn Joyce was a regular guest on my nationally syndicated health radio talk show, *America Talks Health with Dr. Keith Robinson*. And, in her new book she has once again taken the complicated field of nutrition and lifestyle and made it understandable. She has found the ideal way to motivate us to consume the concepts that we need to have life, and have it abundantly. Her pyramid unlocks the truth that the emotional aspects of life are important determinants of real health. So, I invite you to settle back and prepare for an information feast on really practical and sound nutrition and lifestyle. Hidden in the pages of her book you will also find wonderful pieces of Marilyn's soul that she willingly shares with those who hunger for health and an abundance of energy."
~ **Dr. Keith A. Robinson,** Dental Oncologist, Maxillofacial Prosthodontist, Health Communication Specialist. author, *Growing Older with Your Teeth or Something Like Them! Houston, TX*

Learn from Dr. Joyce's hard-earned wisdom and practical knowledge: HOW to care for yourself and your loved ones, by returning to the vital basics. From breath, to water, to gratitude, to movement and fitness, and the science of powerful nutrition, you will find knowledge and inspiration to make a world of difference in your life. Marilyn is a national (and international) treasure.
~ **Candace Corson, M.D.**, Medical and Nutritional Educator, graduate of Yale School of Medicine, Medical Editor of *Medicinal Plants of North America*, by Jim Meuninck. Grander, IN

Dr. Marilyn Joyce has done it again, INSTANT *E.N.E.R.G.Y.*™ is literally a life saver. I highly recommend this book to all people looking to regain and maintain their health. This outstanding book looks at the needs of the whole person, faced with all of life's daily challenges. Here is a practical book that shows people how they can eat healthy in the real world and how they can actually thrive with increasing energy and vitality. Something of a celebrity in the food and nutritional community, Marilyn Joyce is one of the most sought after speakers in the country, and has finally answered the call to write her latest book. Good health is now at hand.
~ **Stewart Rose**, VP Vegetarians of Washington. author, *The Vegetarian Solution. Portland, OR*

I have had the pleasure to work with Marilyn for years in our pursuit to change the health of people around the world by marketing Juice Plus. Marilyn's success is a testament to her unstoppable resolve to touch and change the lives of people and their health. Her story and courage is an example for others of how you can change your life. Her journey from the depths of a major health challenge to a top author, lecturer, coach and entrepreneur is truly a remarkable story. I am confident her latest book will be another step in her journey to making a difference in the world through better health and nutrition. I am proud to call Marilyn my friend, colleague, and coach.

~ **Jeff Roberti**, National Marketing Director, NSA, LLC. Sarasota, FL (Jeff is a self-made multi-millionaire entrepreneur, an icon within the network marketing industry, and a compassionate philanthropist)

If you're suffering from an *E.N.E.R.G.Y.*™ crisis, just plug into this comprehensive book and TURN ON!

~ **Don Dible,** author, *The Dental Patients Little Book of History, Humor and Trivia,* co-author (Richard H Madow, DDS) *Love is the Best Medicine for Dental Patients and The Dental Team.* Murrieta, CA

Marilyn's book is so inspiringly easy, to help us gain the *E.N.E.R.G.Y.*™ we often lack to live our optimum life. I was just so in awe of her coming from her situation and the illnesses she has overcome, using food, which is today a lost art. Her sharing of her research and life knowledge gives us the skinny on how to navigate the mass marketing propaganda. She even has suggested menus and recipes, as well as a comprehensive shopping list, removing the guess work out of what to prepare to be healthy! How easy is that!

~ **Gloria Martel**, Esthetician, author, *Grow Young by Discovering the Cause of Each Wrinkle and the 10 Steps to Erase Them.* Los Angeles, CA

When Marilyn Joyce, The Vitality Doctor™ talks about maintaining good health and wellness, make sure you listen. After all, what could be simpler than 5 minute programs and what's more important than our health? In her new book INSTANT *E.N.E.R.G.Y.*™, she takes it to the next dimension. I highly recommend it. Thumbs Up MJ!

~ **Alan J. Martin**, Inventor, *The Thumbs Down* method, author, *Thumbs Down, Golf Instruction Made Simple.* East Windsor, NJ

Marilyn's newest publication is truly a gift to us all. Yes the information is compelling, the advice sincere. But it transcends the paper or the binding. It is presented and written in a way that makes the reader feel that Marilyn is personally right there beside them. She writes as a friend, sharing her personal challenges, fears and disappointments. We, the readers, know without any doubt that Marilyn has written this book because she "cares" about our journeys to wellness. We feel her partnership and commitment to truly making a difference. And having that cheerleader beside us, strengthens our resolve to live and be healthier. It is truly a masterful accomplishment.

~ **Carol Ranoa**, National Marketing Director, Wellness Plus, contributing author, *Build It Big.* Temecula, CA

Dr. Marilyn Joyce, RD enthusiastically cuts through the hype to give us what we need to live a more vibrant, useful life. Her unique approach with her 5 simple keys for holistic living encourages us all, to get involved in our own lives more deeply.

~ **Allan Hartley,** Editor/Publisher *New Perspectives* Magazine. Hemet, CA

As a Certified Financial Planner born in 1931, which very few people realize thanks to Dr Joyce's strategies — I now know that financial wealth has little value when not accompanied by good health. Dr Joyce again dissects and explains complex information and lifestyle systems making them incredibly user-friendly. There is no longer an acceptable excuse for not being healthy!
~ **Gordon N. Peay,** CFP, CLU, ChFC, M.A., Advisor & Nutrition Advocate. Playa del Rey, CA

The ideas in Instant E.N.E.R.G.Y.™ are simple, fun and easy to fit into my busy lifestyle. Thank you, Marilyn, for a practical guide that I didn't want to put down! This book is a "must" gift for all your friends and family.
~**Linda Meyers,** National Marketing Director, NSA, LLC, Former Holistic Health Practitioner. Temecula, CA

In a loving approach to life, we would consistently be making choices that move us towards the optimum health, in all areas of our lives—physically, mentally, emotionally and spiritually. Most of us do not live our lives in this manner because we simply don't have a clue where to start. INSTANT E.N.E.R.G.Y.™ eliminates the guesswork and provides the keys to unlock the hidden potential deep within each of us that is just waiting to emerge into flight. You will completely transform your health, on all levels, with this comprehensive, yet simple, guide to a joyfully fulfilled life!
~ **Traci Gaffney,** Founder of *A Loving Way*, A Wellness Advocacy for Children and Parents, creator, *Who I Am* Energy Cards. Temecula, CA

In her book, INSTANT E.N.E.R.G.Y.™, Dr. Marilyn Joyce has created a virtual encyclopedia of self-care, helping readers to gain greater vitality on all levels: physically, emotionally and spiritually. Her wealth of knowledge and the way that she integrates all aspects of health is truly remarkable. She is inspirational and yet practical in her many handy lists. Marilyn's lively and entertaining writing style makes this book an enjoyable read and one that people will want to refer to again and again. I highly recommend it for all who wish to improve their health while increasing their joy in life.
~**Joyce Handler**, Psy.D., Composer, Psychologist. Upland, CA

"Dr. Marilyn Joyce is one of the most knowledgeable Health Professionals I have ever had the pleasure of working with. Her book, "INSTANT E.N.E.R.G.Y.™", is filled with lots of urgently important health information for the whole person (body, mind and spirit), as well as great tasting recipes. She's one of my long-time teachers, so I'm absolutely certain that you can learn a lot from her too."
~**Del Millers**, Ph.D. author, *Simply DELicious & 10—Minute Meals*™, *Dancing with God, 10 Minute Workout*. Los Angeles, CA

INSTANT E.N.E.R.G.Y™ is a must read for anyone who is searching for easy, quick and effective techniques to become healthier and more energetic. Marilyn's 5-minutes strategies to health and vitality are simply amazing and a lot of fun. Being a cancer survivor and a great challenger, Marilyn is one of the world's best experts who can give you a TOTAL health and energy solution that positively impacts every aspect of your being – body, mind, and soul. Follow Marilyn's advice and I guarantee that you will become ultra ALIVE!
~**Mohamed Tohami,** The Success Pharaoh, author, *The Pharaoh's Code*, creator, *The Success Avalanche*. Cairo, Egypt

12/08
with Love + Hugs

Dr. Marilyn

www.marilynjoyce.com

INSTANT *E.N.E.R.G.Y.*™

INSTANT *E.N.E.R.G.Y.*™

The 5 Keys to Unlimited Energy & Vitality!

Dr. Marilyn Joyce, RD
The Vitality Doctor™

Library of Congress Control Number: 2008907533
ISBN: Hardcover   978-1-4363-6537-6
                   Softcover   978-1-4363-6536-9

This book was printed in the United States of America.

To order additional copies of this book, contact:
Xlibris Corporation
1-888-795-4274
www.Xlibris.com
Orders@Xlibris.com
38338

Vibrant Health Academy Unlimited has made **INSTANT** *E.N.E.R.G.Y.*™ available at special quantity discounts for bulk purchase for use as premiums for educational, business, or sales promotional use, fund-raising, or for use in corporate training programs. For more information, please contact our Special Markets Department at: info@marilynjoyce.com, or call us at: 800-352-3443.

Cover Artwork: Xlibris, Karyn Kunst
Pyramid of *E.N.E.R.G.Y.* ™ Artwork: Karyn Kunst
Cover Photography: Art Ranoa
Layout, Design and Illustrations: Xlibris, Grace Kono, Laurie Poel
Editing: Laurie Poel, Xlibris

SEE THE SPECIAL OFFERS AT THE BACK OF THIS BOOK:
The *4-week* **INSTANT** *E.N.E.R.G.Y.*™ teleconference call series, valued at $398.00 for you and a companion, and the *unbelievable* special offer for my *One-On-One* **EXTREME HEALTH** *(Mind-Body-Spirit)* **MAKE-OVER COACHING PACKAGE**, are only available to the purchasers of this book, **INSTANT** *E.N.E.R.G.Y.*™ by Dr Marilyn Joyce. Original proof of purchase is required. The offers are limited to the specific programs outlined in the back of this book and your registration for each is subject to availability of space and/or changes to the program schedules. The teleseminar series, and the one-on-one *Extreme Health Make-Over* coaching package, must be completed by December 2009. While participants will be responsible for any long distance telephone charges, the entire teleseminar series program is 100% complimentary. No more than 2 people from the purchase of one book may attend each of the entire programs outlined. And only the same 2 individuals may attend each, or both, of the programs using the proof of purchase from one book.

Address inquiries and orders to: **Vibrant Health Academy Unlimited**, at:

450 Hillside Drive, Building B, Suite 200, Mesquite, NV 89027
info@marilynjoyce.com
(800) 352-3443 or Fax (951) 461-8283

August 2008 — Copyright © as:
INSTANT *E.N.E.R.G.Y.*™: **The 5 Keys to Unlimited Energy and Vitality!**

First Printing, August 2008

Other Best Selling Books by Dr Marilyn Joyce:

5 Minutes to Health
I Can't Believe It's Tofu!
Laugh at Stress & Love Life
The SoyPal Cookie Weight Loss & Maintenance Program
The Original Hollywood Celebrity Quick Start Diet & Maintenance
Program

Contributing Author:

Walking with the Wise
Walking with the Wise for Health & Vitality
Wake Up, Shape Up . . . Live the Life You Love
Veg-Feasting in the Pacific Northwest
The Veg-Feasting Cookbook
Simply DELicious
Thank God I . . . series (5 titles of the series)

Vibrant Health Academy Unlimited

450 Hillside Dr.
Building B, Suite 200
Mesquite, NV 89027
Phone: 800-352-3443
Email: marilyn@marilynjoyce.com

Websites:
www.MarilynJoyce.com
www.5MinutesToHealth.com
www.ICantBelieveItsTofu.com
www.DrJoyce4Nutrition.com
www.Soy4HealthyWeight.com
www.InspireHealthyEatingDaily.com
www.InstantEnergyToday.com

Dr. Marilyn Joyce, RD, *The Vitality Doctor*™

CONTENTS

A SPECIAL ACKNOWLEDGMENT
For Those Who Trusted That This Book
Would be Written — Even When I Did Not!

There are a few people who have truly been gifts from God during this project and in my life in general. However, before I go into that, I am compelled to express my deepest love and gratitude for the thousands of people who have pre-purchased this book, some of whom waited for the book for more than 2 years. You purchased **INSTANT *E.N.E.R.G.Y.*™** on the faith that it would be of value to you on your journey back to health, or back to better health. And quite frankly, I have pre-sold all of my other books in the past, prior to publication, and met the publication deadlines within the time frames established. This book, however, was another story.

Who knows why things happen in life to hold a project back from completion at the deadlines we unwittingly impose on that project? More than one year ago I thought the book was done and ready to print — and then the worst nightmare possible occurred. As I was about to back up the finished copy on my external hard drive, my whole computer monitor turned gray and began crackling! I stared in disbelief, shock and fear — tremendous fear. Please do not let my worst nightmare become a reality! It did! The crash was due to a hairline fracture in my hard drive! I had gone through this before — but never at such a critical stage of such a major project.

We took action to try to save everything — or at least, to find it again. But, alas, several thousand dollars later, and anxiety beyond compare, the book was gone. You might ask, why had I not backed it up? Well, I was crossing an international border, and thought it not wise to carry a lot of gadgets with me. Mistake! My little memory stick now travels everywhere I go these days. But that is NOW! Back to THEN!

I fell into despair, and was ready to cancel the whole project, refund everyone who had pre-purchased, and count it as a lost cause. However, I am a strong proponent of prayer and meditation. And my loyal and dedicated friend, and assistant, Laurie Poel, who knows me in many ways better than anyone else at this point, encouraged me to just take one day, and go to the one place that completely rejuvenates me — the beach! Can anyone relate? I rebelled at first, stating that I did not have time to just hang out at the beach. She stated a very simple, yet poignant truth. "Well, you're not getting anything done anyway. Just sitting there and feeling bad about the situation is accomplishing nothing. You have no focus, and you're just getting more depressed thinking about the whole situation. Perhaps if you went to the beach you'd experience a different perspective, and gain valuable insights into what the next best step might be. And then come back refreshed and ready to start anew!"

How right she was. Definitely the story for another book! Suffice it to say, I came home and re-watched the movie, *The Secret* (www.thesecret.tv), and then prayed for at least an hour that same night, followed by another hour of meditation. After not sleeping for almost two months, I slept like a baby that night. The next day the phones rang off the hook, and the email boxes were full, with inquiries about the book. Usually we got about one or two inquiries per week. Ironically, I was prepared for the worst on some level — yet the best was the response. Almost everyone said, "I want the book. Just write it!" SO, the next day, I sat down to write, with no agenda, other than to be the messenger of whatever I was meant to write. Unlike the previous book, which was completely planned, this book virtually wrote itself. And there were often stops along the way. As long as I stayed out of the way of frustration, the next chapter would flow. And the next . . . And the next . . .

Several times those stops along the way jumped out of nowhere! I would be so ready to just get on with the book, and then something major would occur to stop the process. Only, of course, for me to learn another valuable lesson that was necessary for, or to meet an incredible person who had something amazing to contribute to, the completion of that particular chapter! It became an awesome journey of self-discovery, as well as a journey of trust in the process and in the belief that I was to include much more of the fundamentals than I had done in the initial book, *5 Minutes to Health*. I am a very driven person by nature, and never want to let people down, so at times I would feel like a terrible and dismal failure. And, daily, the feeling that I was letting a lot of people down truly plagued me, often relegating me a useless vehicle for the flow of this information.

Yet at this point in time, I know with all of my heart, that by following and allowing God's, and the Universe's, plan for this book, it is of far greater value to everyone who reads it than the book I had completed last year. And believe me, there were times when I was not a happy recipient of the lessons I was required to learn in order to write and complete this book from a deeper place!

Would I trade this challenge and experience for the previous outcome? Not in a million years! The personal growth, the developing and deepening connections and relationships with the people who purchased the book, and hung in there, the shared love — WOW, what an incredible journey of growth and understanding. Would I have preferred it to be done a long time ago? Of course! Yet, I do understand that growth comes from the less pleasant circumstances each of us confronts, and hopefully relates to, in ways that bring about win/win solutions. We've all heard that, "You can't always get what you want. And if you try sometime, you find, you get what you need." Who said that? Oh yes, *it was the Rolling Stones!* Well, that was certainly my journey . . .

Words can never express the love and gratitude I have for all of you who have stood by me, with faith, love and, sometimes even some doubt, as this book found its way onto the pages that follow. You are all the wind beneath my sails. I love and cherish you, and I am, forever, deeply committed to your health and wellbeing. May you only ever experience the maximum level of energy and health possible each and every day of your life. And I pray that you really do open this book, read it and use it. Because, after all, my book is like a parachute — IT'S NO GOOD UNLESS IT'S OPEN — AND READ, AND USED — DAILY!

Again:
Thank you so much for your trust and belief in me, and this book. And I would love your feedback, any and all! Email me anytime at: <u>info@marilynjoyce.com</u> or call 800-352-3443.

Love & Hugs Always
Dr Marilyn Joyce
The Vitality Doctor™

ACKNOWLEDGMENTS

When I wrote the acknowledgements for my original book, **"5 Minutes to Health"**, my first book written for the public (versus for libraries, professional associations and magazines, as were my previous written works), I had so many people to thank for each of their specific individual contributions to the various phases of the book's production, from conceptual idea, through to finished product. What a list! And I am, to this day, eternally grateful to everyone previously included in the original book, since this new book might never have made it to print without the efforts and support provided by each of these special individuals in the first book. **"5 Minutes to Health"** went on to become a tremendous success, claiming best-seller status.

It became apparent that, as successful as **"5 Minutes to Health"** was, the time had definitely come for an updated edition. As with everything in life, new information had surfaced on the various subjects covered in the book, and many of the resources had either disappeared or their contact information had changed. Furthermore, since there were so many tools and strategies not included in the original text, that I use daily with my patients and clients, it became evident that the time had arrived to, not only revise the book, but to expand it to include the complete whole person **Extreme Health Make-Over** Programs that I facilitate.

Well that said; no one I know accomplishes a project of this proportion alone! There is no doubt in my mind that, for success in anything, it takes a team of committed individuals working synergistically together for the best possible outcome. Without a doubt, I could write a tremendously long list of people who deserve mention. However, that is not very practical, as that alone could be a book in itself. So I will focus, here, on the individuals who were deeply instrumental in the outcome of this book.

Of all the people who hold an important place in my life and my work, my soul sister, **Ruth Ripley,** right from day 1, almost 40 years ago, has always pushed me beyond my limits. Not necessarily with gentleness, but definitely with unconditional love! She apparently knows better than anyone what buttons to push! Her deep love for me, and total support of my ideas and projects, no matter how outlandish the rest of the world perceives them to be, has been a strong foundation from which I could be creative.

For the past 12 years, I have experienced the most deeply connected love and respect from **Linda and Tim Meyers**, a couple who have not only loved me unconditionally, but believed in me so completely that it has forced me to grow in ways I never thought possible in this lifetime. They opened the door to my extensive global **Juice Plus+®** (www.DrJoyce4Nutrition.com) family, friends and business, and the realization of wonderful and extremely rewarding dreams come true.

Allan Hartley, the publisher of New Perspectives magazine, has definitely been very instrumental in my journey of authorship. He entered into my life, in 1992, at the very moment when I was preparing for the ultimate writing challenge, the writing of my first public book. His faith in my abilities resulted in my position as a featured editor with his magazine. I began writing informative articles about people that I reveled in the opportunity to meet and interview. Today, I continue to contribute to his unique and mind-expanding magazine.

As with everything else in this book, I had a specific vision for a unique, Whole Person Health Pyramid. We needed an *E.N.E.R.G.Y.* ™ pyramid to fully exemplify what I teach. Well, as most of us have come to understand, when that wonderful Universal Power steps in, miracles begin to occur. On a recent trip to Canada to speak, I had the amazing good fortune of reconnecting with a very special young woman who had traversed her own personal health journey. Her career: graphic artist! And she knew exactly what I wanted—and created it! **Karyn Kunst** is, without question, an angel in my life. And a true joy to work with! You can see her valuable contribution to this book in the chapter, The Pyramid of *E.N.E.R.G.Y.* ™, in black and white, as well as the exquisite laminated color version available for sale at my website: www.marilynjoyce.com

And I cannot forget my incredible photographer, **Art Ranoa**. He has an uncanny ability for capturing the true spirit of his subject. I have always dreaded a photo shoot—think of the word "shoot"! Art made the day so much fun! I wanted that playful day to just keep on going! With his tremendous wealth of experience, Art had some unique ideas that I would never have thought of—and was so incredibly open to any suggestions I proposed. The result is an endless assortment of beautiful photos. The challenge: which one to choose! What a wonderful challenge. His work, of course, is apparent on, both, the cover and the back of the book.

Of course, I have to acknowledge my superb publisher, **Xlibris**, for their incredible patience as I went through the many challenges that held up production of the book. I am certain that they are as relieved as I am that we have come to that delicious place of a finished product.

A Special Tribute to a Unique & Outstanding Individual

Even with an outstanding team, there is usually one person who stands out in the group or crowd. In the case of" **INSTANT *E.N.E.R.G.Y.*™"**, that person is **Laurie Poel,** my assistant, confidant, dear friend, and "sister" on so many levels.

I have never before worked with anyone who was as dedicated as I am, and often times more dedicated, to the highest outcome possible for this book, than Laurie. She remained loyal to the production of this book at times when I was ready to throw in the towel. Don't get me wrong. I'm no quitter! Tell me it's not possible, and I'll prove you wrong! Yet, the completion of this book was perhaps one of the greatest challenges I have ever faced. Never have I had so many seemingly apparent setbacks during the process of creating books and resources, as I have with this book. Laurie stood by me continually, many times experiencing the fear of failure, the stress of angry or upset customers doubting this book would ever exist, and the anxiety of all of the setbacks life seemed to dish out along the way.

She, along with me, experienced many sleepless nights, and anxious days, wondering how we would ever get through the tasks ahead of us to make this book a reality. We both knew that this book was not just a book to get written—as in, get it done and over with. No—the writing of **INSTANT *E.N.E.R.G.Y.*™** was definitely directed by a Higher Source. And it had to meet the standards and criteria of this Higher Producer before it could be finished and released. In other words, it was all in God's time—not our time. There were just so many instances that presented themselves along the way that indicated that we had to let go, and let it unfold. Not an easy thing for me, since I like to get into a project and just get it done!

Laurie stood by me during the roughest of times. She so believed in the book and its contents that she would not let me settle for anything that did not convey fully the intended message—it had to express it in a way that people would completely understand it. She questioned everything—sometimes I wanted to scream, STOP! Yet her input was essential to the outcome of what is printed on these pages. When I would reach a point of saturation and lose my ability to really comprehend the disconnect I was creating in my reader's interpretation of what I was recommending, Laurie would challenge me until I eventually determined another, more legible, way of writing the same thing—with her help.

There are truly so many things I could share as far as her actual written contribution to the finished book. Let's just say that she and I did some amazing brainstorming. A lot in fact! I am, without a doubt, and often to a fault, an amazing idea person! Consistent follow through is not always my forte. I need a strong support partner to make sure those ideas get developed and implemented. With Laurie's tenacity for staying on focus and getting even the most challenging work completed, we have this amazing book to offer you, along with the special gifts, outlined at the back of this book. This is our way of expressing our deeply felt gratitude for your undying patience and faith in our commitment to actually complete what we promised. Our goal is, we hope, to give you much more than you expected.

Now let's begin . . .

- FOREWORD -

Why Such a Book by Dr Marilyn Joyce?
The Vitality Doctor™

We've all heard the expression, "Nothing ever remains the same. Change is inevitable!" And that includes all of us — you and me! If we are not changing — in other words, growing — we are stagnant — we're dying. That's right, rotting! Have you ever smelled a stagnant pool of water? If we're not moving — or changing — we're stagnant and rotting, or dying!

So, when I first wrote my original book, *5 Minutes to Health*, the place I was coming from, in the process of creating and writing that book, was a far different place than where I am at today. **INSTANT *E.N.E.R.G.Y.*™** reflects my own shift, or growth, from a focus on the physical perspectives of health, primarily nutrition, to a focus on the whole person perspectives of health: physical, mental, emotional and spiritual. Being optimally healthy depends on being wholly healthy — every aspect of our entire being is in balance.

A tall order, you say. Absolutely! Is it possible, or even feasible, to believe that each of us can achieve this balance? Well, why not? Remember the expression — and you'll read it again in this book, since repetition is the mother of learning — "For things to change first I must change?" And another important expression you'll likely stumble upon in this book is: "Change your mind to change your life." And you can change your life in an instant, by changing your mind — or your thought — in that instant. These are not simply expressions. They are proven facts, proven by many folks who have applied them to their own lives! And yes, it does take consistent practice at first like anything else. There's that word again: Repetition!

Well, all of that said, I have decidedly changed — or expanded — my mind about almost everything since I wrote *5 Minutes to Health*. And my life is completely different today than it was when I traveled the continent promoting my baby (that book) — yes, it actually took *9 months* to write *5 Minutes to Health*! And I absolutely referred to it, upon completion, as my baby. As with all babies, it grew up. And, as all of us who have raised children know, the growing up process takes a lot longer than the original 9 months of gestation! Hence, over the past almost 14 years, my baby grew up into a very well rounded, multi-faceted, young adult.

No longer simply satisfied or fulfilled with meeting only the physical (nutritional) needs, **5 *Minutes to Health*** morphed into **INSTANT E.N.E.R.G.Y.™**, a book that addresses the depth and breadth of the various dimensions of the *human being-spirit*. All of the basic elements from **5 *Minutes to Health*** are still here, though completely revised to reflect the wealth of new information, and expanded learning and experience, I have undergone since that book was originally written. However, **INSTANT *E.N.E.R.G.Y.*™** includes, and expands on, all of the various aspects of the work I do with my patients and clients today. A whole new, and extremely comprehensive, section has been added, with more than 20 new chapters addressing all four dimensions of whole person health—again, those are physical, mental, emotional and spiritual—that need to be in balance and harmony in order for us to enjoy a completely fulfilling, healthy and vibrant life.

And that's not all! The, already thorough, References and Resources section (now dubbed *The Library)* has been completely revised and updated, as well as tremendously expanded to include a wide variety of new resources, while eliminating those that have bitten the dust since the mid-90's. The best part is that all of the information in this section is compiled in a much more comprehensive and organized format than previously provided in *5 Minutes to Health*, thanks to the persistence and genuine commitment of my amazing editor, Laurie Poel, to make it the most valuable tool possible for the reader—You!

Wait, there's even more value added to this new book, **INSTANT *E.N.E.R.G.Y.*™**, than ever provided by **5 *Minutes to Health***. Remember: **5 *Minutes to Health*** grew up! So the focus in this new book is not on overcoming illness, although all of the strategies and information included here will prove to be valuable tools in anyone's journey back to health from a life challenging illness. However, the focus of **INSTANT *E.N.E.R.G.Y.*™**, is on *prevention* of illness—and on creating and maximizing your energy and vitality, anywhere, anytime, using innovative, easy, quick, and healthy 5-minute strategies, that can be done by anyone! What more could you ask for? And who better than *The Vitality Doctor*™ to provide this information for you?

Well, let me first state that I was not always *The Vitality Doctor*™! The person you go to for simple, quick solutions for *creating energy surges in an instant* when you're experiencing a *"personal"* energy crisis! And we're not talking about lack of fuel in your car! So, please allow me to take you on a journey—my journey—that led me to where I am today, and to the writing of this book . . .

In 1984, I, Marilyn Joyce, had the world by the tail! Or so it seemed! On the surface, everything looked like it was working. I had my own nutrition consulting business, demanding a high fee for my services. I was living in a beautiful home which I owned, driving the car of my dreams, traveling extensively, dating very successful, and generally interesting, men in the business world, and was basically writing my own ticket in every aspect of my life.

My peers, my employers, my clients and my audiences alike, had only great things to say about my work and my pleasant, friendly, accommodating (people pleasing) nature! I would bend over backwards to make sure that I had covered every possible detail, and more, in the name of my work. It was not uncommon for me to work around the clock for days on end in order to meet unrealistic deadlines. My resume was full of letters from satisfied clients stating that, "Marilyn always gives at least 130% to every challenge she is faced with." But, after all, this business was my baby, and that's what one had to do to get ahead! Or so I thought!

For about two years I rode the crest of that wave, and *believed* on some level that I loved every moment of it. Though, quite frankly, I did spend a lot of time marveling at my seemingly great success. And spent many sleepless nights wondering how I had managed to pull this off, and how long it would last before something would bring it to a crashing halt. You see, I did not really enjoy the feeling of success! I was too busy worrying about it coming to an end!

And, end it did! Suddenly my world shattered around me. In other words, I was so focused on what I did not want (everything good coming to an end) versus what I did want (joyful and continued progress and success)! Guess what I created. My business contracts, which were primarily government-based, ended overnight, with sudden cutbacks in spending in the particular arena of my focus. My car was totaled in the first major accident of my driving career. Somehow, I and my friends, who were in my car at the time, were only slightly bruised, if at all. Yet that did not deter a lawsuit by one of my passengers. A nasty ending to a so-called friendship!

There's more! One of my closest friends, for reasons unknown at the time, committed suicide a week later. Her business was at its greatest height of success at the time! And we, her closest friends, all envied her wonderful marriage to one of the most loving, demonstrative men we had ever known! Something in this picture did not fit!

What appeared to be unfolding into the relationship of my dreams, ended about the same time as the suicide occurred. One day we were speaking about marriage. The next day, without any explanation, "the love of my life", called the whole thing off!

And, of course, as a result of this whole sequence of events, I was faced with a monthly mortgage that was now beyond my means. So I began the process of selling my beautiful home with all of the amenities I had come to enjoy and cherish. I knew it couldn't get worse than this! After all, nothing that I had worked so long and so hard for, was still available to me. My world seemed to be disintegrating around me.

Wrong! To coin a phrase, what happened next was, literally, the straw that broke the camel's back!! An unusual looking, hard, shiny black mole appeared on my face. My vanity took me to the doctor. The shock of the diagnosis sent me spinning. Melanoma! I'm sure you could have, literally, knocked me over with a feather. Though I had no idea, at the time, how serious this diagnosis could be, it represented the "C" word — the word we all whispered about when someone we knew was marked by it.

However, I was assured that we got it early, and that there was probably no cause for concern. Out of hospital a week, I was rushed back into the hospital, with tremendous pain in my uterus. You can probably guess by now what the diagnosis was.

Here I was 36 years old, and given a death sentence. After all, in every hospital or nursing home I worked in, the moment a patient or resident was diagnosed with any kind of cancer, we began preparing him or her for "the end," in other words, DEATH! It is not uncommon to hear a doctor or a nurse state that "It's only a matter of time!" And, at the time, I bought into that belief, hook, line and sinker, so to speak. Who was I to believe that my odds were any better than anyone else's?

Was I depressed? You're darn right I was! Did I show it? Not a chance! The world was only going to see me at my best. By this point in my life, it was ingrained in me that I must never let anyone see my vulnerabilities, my weaknesses. I was known, by most people who knew me, as a survivor. And furthermore, I was a Dietitian, who talked about health and how to achieve it. So, it was critical that I put up a good front, until the bitter end. If people were aware of my condition, I would lose my credibility! At least that was my belief at the time.

Several years into my struggle with cancer, someone in a nowhere town in mid-somewhere USA, really summed up the entire story of my life, at least until that point in time: "Lookin' good! That's all you care about, Marilyn! Your only concern is what you and your life look like to the onlooker! Make sure you don't let anyone get too close now, just in case they get to know who you really are." So you might say that I was at an impasse in my life and with my illness.

Without going into the gory details of my illness, suffice it to say I went progressively down hill. At the point at which I was given only a short amount of time, the realization that "Lookin' good!" was not cutting it, hit like a lightning bolt! I was not looking good! And the myriad of excuses I used to explain my tremendous weight loss and extreme fatigue were growing old, and not very believable.

I had tried everything! Every diet and every program I could find or stumble upon. Every idea anyone suggested. Every vitamin and mineral supplement ever written about, whether in scientific or popular lay publications. Every herb and every tea anyone talked about. My own personal library of books and information filled every shelf in my home and covered every available space on my floors. And let's not forget that I was a trained dietitian with a major emphasis on biochemistry. If anyone should have the answers, I should! Right? Wrong!

Well, if I had remembered my biochemistry, I might have had some answers sooner. However, cancer, like all illnesses, is a teacher. And my lesson was about learning to listen. It was obvious that I did not have all of the answers. Yet, in my effort to hide my own challenge, I would attempt to find a solution for everyone else's challenge or health crisis, as a way of avoiding dealing with my own situation. Of course, the day of reckoning always arrives! And fortunately it saved my life!

A Home Show, a Vita-Mix machine, a young man knowledgeable about things I had forgotten about, and a Bernie Siegel workshop. *Love, Enzymes and Miracles!* (My own summation of this cumulative set of events.) As I began to research and remember about enzymes in food, and the need for that food to be alive and wholesome, filled with all the nutrients necessary for the biochemical functions of my body, I saw the need for a drastic change from foods that simply provided calories, to foods that had a lot more than calories and fat to offer.

With a lot of help from a couple of devoted and true friends, and the implementation of very basic and quick-to-prepare recipes, my health began to improve. The focus was mainly on raw foods in more bioavailable forms. A wide variety of fresh vegetables and whole grains formed the basis of my diet, with the addition of a little fruit and a small portion of fish every day. I added green things, such as spirulina, barley grass, chlorella, various seaweeds, and GMO-free (no genetic engineering) protein powders.

To begin with, however, I had almost no energy to even eat. Sucking on ice chips was, initially, the extent to which I was able to ingest anything. However, little by little, I was able to consume more foods in this ice chip form, and later, foods in liquid forms. Using a Vita Mix-Machine, which is a high-powered blender, food processor, grinder, grater, chopper and mixer all rolled into one machine, I got all of my foods in the whole food state, but in a much more bioavailable and digestible form. Within a few months, I was able to tolerate more solid foods. Just for the record, I have continued to use my Vita-Mix machine (see Equipment, in The Library Section of this book) simply because of the speed with which a delicious, wholesome meal can be prepared, and because of the amazing taste and consistency it provides.

As well, I realized throughout my own healing process, that the most productive practices I employed were also generally the simplest, least time-consuming practices! Whether they involved the physical, mental, emotional or spiritual aspects of getting well again, *simplicity* was, and is, always the key.

Since my recovery, I have continued to incorporate the 80-20 principle in all areas of my life. In my diet, that principle translates into the foods I eat being predominantly free of over-processing and over-preparation. Once in a while, when I go out with friends, I may indulge in foods that are not as close to natural as the foods I eat at home. But "fast food" is never an option! It is simply not on my menu! And left to my own devices, I will choose a restaurant that serves a variety of healthy food choices, versus the opposite. I steer clear of the rich desserts and items prepared with heavy cream sauces. In this day and age, you just never know what might be lurking in those "fancy" foods!

In my work with patients and clients, it became evident to me that those who incorporated a similar pattern of simple healthy eating and lifestyle habits began to see major improvements in their health. Their energy and vitality, within a short period of time, were dramatically improved. Getting back to basics in all aspects of our life seems to be the key to outstanding health, and boundless vitality, regardless of age! The minute we move away from a simple, somewhat basic, lifestyle, we begin to complicate our lives and to create tremendous stress on our bodies, which in time, leads to a breakdown of the overall efficiency of our immune function. And then our bodies, in turn, become susceptible to, and fall prey to, an attacking illness.

So you see, this book is the result of my own journey back to wellness from a life challenging illness, as well as the results of my extensive work with a wide variety of degenerative illnesses in my nutrition and lifestyle practice. It is at the request of my patients and clients, to put all of the basics and strategies I teach them, into a form they can refer to at any time, that this expanded book, became a reality! And it is written, as I previously stated, as much if not more, with prevention of illness, versus overcoming an illness, in mind!

It is important to state here, that when it comes to creating, maintaining, and optimizing whole person wellness, there are no magic bullets. There is no one thing that will be the answer for everyone. Yet a simple, high quality diet together with a balanced, harmonious lifestyle program, fully addressing the physical, mental, emotional, and spiritual aspects of wellness, will, at least, give a person a solid foundation for the creation of the highest degree of health and vitality possible. For a more individualized program, designed specifically for you, it is important to seek out reliable, credible professionals to work with you. Do take a moment to check out my *One on One Coaching Programs* at www.marilynjoyce.com; and why not give yourself the gift of a life changing experience with my one of a kind, personal *Extreme Health (Mind-Body-Spirit) Make-Over*.

Furthermore, be assertive! Take nothing at face value. Ask questions. Become involved, and be a participant in your healing process — or in your illness prevention program. Choose health and wellness over illness! Choose quality over quantity. Choose natural, whole foods over processed, denatured foods. Choose simplicity over complexity. Choose to be self-reliant, taking responsibility for your own health and vitality, versus depending on your doctor or other healthcare providers to "make" or "keep" you well. Seek out the kind of support you need, and use it! If you are ill, or not quite up to par, see your illness or malady as your teacher, not your friend or enemy, and pay attention to what it is trying to teach you. In other words, be proactive (the stance of a responsible (response-able, self-determined individual), versus reactive (the stance of a victim) in all areas of your life!

Most importantly, think of this road that you are about to travel on, as an adventure. It is an opportunity to explore your options and to try new approaches to the way you live your life. It is your chance to fully take charge of your body and your life.

With love, I offer this book, to assist you in making some of the changes necessary to insure your continued health, as well as renewal and expansion of your energy and vitality. Or, perhaps the strategies and tools provided here will assist you in overcoming a life-challenging illness, should that be the journey you happen to find yourself on at this time.

I will leave you, at this point, with two statements that I have internalized over the years, and now embody in my own consciousness, as a result of my personal journey back to wellness and vitality. And yes, you may be very surprised by their absolute simplicity!

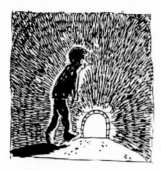

"If it doesn't flow, it doesn't go!"
    However, it is important to remember that, from time to time, there may be rapids along the way!

And remember:
    "It ain't over `till it's over!" (& it ain't over, 'till you're 6 feet under!)

Dr Marilyn Joyce, RD
The Vitality Doctor™

Vibrant Health Academy Unlimited
800-352-3443
www.marilynjoyce.com
info@marilynjoyce.com

OUR CRAVING FOR SIMPLICITY
personal
HAS COST US OUR ^ E.N.E.R.G.Y.™

In our modern existence, we bend over backwards to create a simpler, more convenient and efficient environment, in which the flow of our lives is unencumbered by a series of monotonous tasks and activities, such as housework and cooking, walking the same route day after day, answering the phone, or phones, every time they ring, bouncing up and down to change the channels on our TV's, and even, actually leaving our homes to shop for 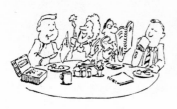 the essentials of life. We have machines for every task! And, in fact, for every activity in our lives!

Of course the thought of the upkeep, maintenance and cleaning of the equipment is enough to have us running out to the nearest fast food establishment for most of our meals! Or we're ready to chuck a machine, or gadget, at the slightest sign of dysfunction. For that matter, many of us are so completely "technologically challenged," that we have no idea how to use most of it efficiently anyway. In an effort to simplify our lives we have in fact complicated them!

And with a gadget for every job, we hardly know where to start or what to use for any given task, or activity. So, the confusion halts us in our tracks. The fear of cleanup alone stops the equipment from making it out of the cupboard and onto the shelf, or wherever it is needed for use. The common lament that I hear from my patients and clients, and the population in general, is that it takes just too much time and effort to prepare healthy food, and to practice consistent healthy lifestyle strategies. This thought alone stops the process of doing what we know we need to do to get and stay healthy! So, we have all of this equipment "just in case" (we might use it), and the attitude of "why bother?" (because it will take too much time and effort anyway).

As if that thought by itself was not enough of a deterrent to the implementation of healthy habits, the other most common reason expressed for continuing to purchase, for example, convenience foods and fast food meals, is the supposed expense of buying healthy foods, such as fresh fruits and vegetables and natural unprocessed grains and protein sources.

Working in the field of health and fitness for the past 40 plus years, the latter 25 plus years as a dietitian, primarily in private practice, and working in conjunction with a variety of health and fitness centers, as well as institutions for the care of the ill or infirmed populations, it became clear to me that most people do not have a clue as to how simple it can be to create overall health in their lives on a consistent basis. In their frustration, weeding through text, after complicated text, most of which address the *why* instead of the *how-to,* they give up and return to, or continue their old, generally unhealthy nutrition and lifestyle patterns. Their excuse: *It is just too complicated to figure out what to do to be healthy!*

In my work with my patients and clients, I outline the various strategies and techniques required to effectively reach, and maintain, optimum health and vitality. In the past, at their request, I used to go into their homes and, literally, empty out their refrigerators and cupboards of all of the health-robbing processed items taking up the space required for nutritious and life-supporting foods. We would then shop together (The only way to learn is by doing!), and stock their kitchens with the highest quality foods and condiments available, purchased from the best sources in their area.

We then evaluated and simplified the amounts and types of equipment used for every task and activity performed in their home, including each of the methods incorporated for food preparation, personal care, and home care. And finally, I provided a variety of easy, quick recipes and food lists to get started with, as well as lists of simple necessities, equipment, tools, and strategies required for efficiency and ease of use in each of the areas of their lives that we had evaluated.

Within weeks, even days, I received calls telling me how much better, not only my patient was feeling, but also the rest of the family or household members!

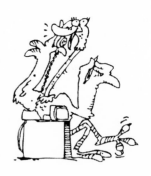

Over the years, my clients, patients, and even friends, have asked me to put all of these recipes, food and equipments lists, guidelines, efficiency lists and systems, references and resources, and quick and easy strategies, into a form that they can refer to at any time, instead of having to call me every other day for ideas or confirmation that what they were doing was health-promoting, or appropriate to their needs. Today, since my own schedule, at this point in my life, is so full with the demands of my work, travel, and speaking commitments, I am no longer able to respond to all of the individual demands that come pouring in. Hence, another reason for this book!

Special Note: *Do not miss your opportunity to participate in the accompanying 4-week teleseminar series that supports and assists anyone who acquires a copy of this book, in achieving their own personal health goals and unlimited energy to boot! See the coupon at the back of this book which allows you to participate in this valuable program, valued at $398.00, for free.*

INSTANT *E.N.E.R.G.Y.*™ is going to show you, the reader, that being healthy in every aspect of your life, and eating nutritious foods, is absolutely no more expensive or time-consuming, if even as expensive and time-consuming, as all of those unhealthy lifestyle practices you now engage in, and all of those convenience foods you eat, which are so, unfortunately, readily available. And all of which seem so appealing, thanks to the efforts of diligent advertising agents who have little or no knowledge of, or interest in, nutrition and healthy lifestyle strategies. But who have a tremendous vested interest in a wide profit margin! *Remember, advertisements are for profit only, not for your health!*

And let's not forget the cost of being sick! Just add that injury to the insult of all of the unhealthy foods and unhealthy activities most of us engage in every day! Because, the fact is that this wonderful machine of ours can only withstand so much abuse — and it certainly seems to withstand a lot — before it finally breaks down.

Well, here's the great news! This book will show you how simple, quick and easy, good nutrition, and whole person lifestyle, practices and strategies, leading to sound health, can be. Though there is a lot of supporting information as to the why's for doing the recommended steps, activities and strategies, this is primarily a *How-To* manual! There are no tricks to being healthy. Just simple, straight-forward techniques, which take little or no effort or time to incorporate into your life on a consistent daily basis. *The goal here is to dispel the myths that you have to be rich to be healthy, and that only those who have the luxury of time can achieve optimum whole person health.*

With only a few minutes a day, throughout the day, and a well setup kitchen, and home, with only the most necessary utensils and appliances, the most appropriately stocked pantry and refrigerator, the most efficient and user-friendly tools and equipment, anyone can achieve enviable health and vitality! Physically, mentally, emotionally and spiritually!

Every effort has been made to put the information in this guide, as I choose to refer to this book, into a simple format, which is easy-to-follow and incorporate. Lists and charts are used whenever feasible, so that the reader may easily make copies of these to place in appropriate places for reference, such as a refrigerator, cupboard or closet door, bathroom mirror, home gym wall or corkboard, and even, an office corkboard or wall.

As much as possible, choice — your choice — has been an important aspect of this book's contents. Choice of specific meals consumed. Choice of the foods selected. Choice of the amount and types of seasonings used. Choice of the physical activities you prefer to experience. Choice of the methods of inner exploration you adopt. Time and again, it has been proven that, when people make their own choices, they are more likely to stick with them. Because most of us feel, very often, that we have so little control over the various aspects of our lives, it is very important for us to have a sense of control and choice with respect to what we put into our bodies, and how we care for our overall health on all levels. Generally, we just need the facts, the directions, and some useful ideas, to get started on the exciting and adventurous, and sometimes challenging, journey towards optimum health and unlimited vitality. My deepest desire is that this book will entice you into joining me on this wonderful trip through life, joyfully and energetically skipping along, on the road to fun and adventure, in the abundant world of tasty and appetizing delights, and in the creation of unlimited energy and vitality!

Human

It is my mission to conquer the global, epidemic ∧ Energy Crisis with innovative, quick and easy, 5-minute healthy strategies anyone can do, anywhere, anytime!

So, are you ready to begin? Okay, let's hit the road!

INSTANT *E.N.E.R.G.Y.*™ — 5 Minutes At A Time

Have you ever felt that it was just impossible to be healthy, fit and full of energy every day of your life? And that there is just no time at all left in the day for YOU? How many times have you promised yourself that you would eat healthier foods, only to feel that it was too time-consuming to prepare them? Or made a promise to yourself that this was the year that you would exercise regularly, paid a good chunk of change for a gym membership, and then never got back there after the first couple of workouts?

The fact is that being truly healthy and fit is the sum total of all that we do each and every day: mentally, physically, emotionally and spiritually. Your daily habits must nourish your body, mind, heart and soul. For example, when your body and mind are relaxed, and you are at peace, in a state of pleasure, your metabolism and digestion function at their peak levels of efficiency.

We have all heard the expression: You are what you eat! Well, yes, and no . . .

Yes, we do need nutrient dense foods, packed with all of the essential nutrients necessary for optimum efficiency of the thousands of metabolic functions going on simultaneously, 24/7, throughout our bodies. However, there's much more to it than that!

How many of us have known someone who has eaten what seems to be the perfect diet — lots of raw, organic fruits and vegetables, meats that are hormone and antibiotic-free, only 100% whole grain products, no fast foods, avoidance of sweets and processed oils, and on and on . . . And on top of all of that, they have exercised regularly, and even attended yoga classes (usually for the wrong reasons — for exercise and weight loss versus breathing, relaxation and meditation!). One day this person is diagnosed with cancer, or some other major illness, and soon after, they are dead. And we are all mystified. How could this happen? They do everything perfectly and they die!

Well, it is not that simple. It is not simply about what you eat. And not all exercise is created equal! What's more, if you are continually stressed out with work, especially if it is work you dislike, and you lie awake night after night worrying about your job, kids, marriage, unpaid bills, etc., how do you think all of those negative thoughts and sleepless nights are going to impact your health? If you don't take time out to just be still and breathe, you develop a lack of oxygen flow, which is essential for the maximum utilization of all of those nutrients in your healthy diet. Furthermore, if you don't take time out to relax, your body will always be in a constant state of tension. And this tension creates constriction of blood flow, of airflow, of cellular uptake of water and nutrients, and of efficient elimination of toxins and other metabolic waste byproducts. Whew!

Many years ago, during my very early 20's, I decided to more fully explore the field of yoga in the country of its origin, India. Well, after all, I am a product of the 60's, and the Beatles, our revolutionary rock band of the time, did open the doorway to deeper inner exploration of oneself, and reflection of our individual and unique purpose for being here now. Many of us even read the book, "Remember, Be Here Now," by Ram Dass. And the slogans of the day were: "I have to find myself," or, "I am going _____ (fill in the blank with where) to find myself." As if we were somewhere other than where we were in that moment! It took me a very long time to realize the truth that, wherever I am, there I am. There was just no way to get away from myself! That's the subject of another book . . .

So what did I learn during my India experience. Far more than I can share here, that is for certain. However, a set of five principles for maximum health and longevity were set forth and taught—and those five principles have remained the corner stone of much of my life. When I veered away from those principles, the price I paid was very high. When I live those five principles, incorporating them into my daily life, I am filled with energy, vitality, joy, and a love of, and for, life.

How many of you believe that there are no accidents, no coincidences? I, for one, am a total advocate of this philosophy. So, let me share with you an epiphany I had very recently. After a year of fires (The 2007 fires will always be remembered by those of us who reside in Southern California!), a packed schedule of travel for work, seeming setbacks at every turn with the production of this book, and absolutely no down time to just be still by myself (which is truly the only way that I for one can regenerate), I opted to stay home alone on Thanksgiving. I was so looking forward to this day of peace, quiet and personal reflection of thanksgiving for all the wonderful people, things, events and experiences in my life.

Prior to this special day, I shopped for healthy food, purchased deliciously scented aromatherapy candles, and even bought a new luxurious fluffy towel to wrap myself in following my first lengthy bath of the year! Can you believe it? I teach my patients and my clients how important it is to take time out and just luxuriate in a warm bubble bath, unwinding and releasing all of their built up tensions, while peaceful meditation music carries them far beyond the constrictions of their three dimensional physical environment. And I had not even done it myself—in my own home!

Well, you know what happens to the best-laid plans of mice and men? They often go awry—but are replaced with something better—much better! I awoke early on the morning of Thanksgiving, bounced out of bed, absolutely full of energy. Something was racing through my mind, making my heart flutter with excitement and anticipation. The title of this book is "**INSTANT E.N.E.R.G.Y.**™" Was it possible that the word, **ENERGY,** could be an acronym for the five key principles I teach? Feverishly, I clicked away on the keyboard of my ever-present Mac. There it was. In amazement, I stared at the page. Thank you God! And, "All in God's time," took on a whole new meaning for me that glorious morning.

Before I go into **ENERGY** as the acronym for my program, let's first look at the five age-old principles that have guided yoga practitioners for thousands of years. These principles incorporate the health of the whole person, not just the physical, or the emotional, or the mental, or the spiritual part—but the mind-body-spirit concept. There is only true health when all the parts of you are functioning synergistically in balance—and in harmony—with each other.

The 5 Key Principles

From the day we are born until the day we leave this fair planet, the 5 essential principles for optimum health and vitality are the same:

- Deep, Slow, Rhythmic Breathing
- Healthy, Natural, Whole Food Nutrition
- Regular, Cell-Regenerating Exercise
- Relax, Rejuvenate and Meditate (Daily Restorative Relaxation & Communication with God or your Higher Power or your Higher Self)
- Attitude of Gratitude (Optimistic Thinking & Meditation)

Let's expand on thought patterns that will support you in developing and maintaining your daily practice of the 5 essential Principles.

- Deep, Slow, Rhythmic Breathing
  - *Think:* Oxygen for protection against cancer, heart disease, diabetes, MS, fibromyalgia, lupus, etc, and premature aging

- Healthy, Natural, Whole Food Nutrition
  - *Think:* Vitamins, minerals, antioxidants, phytochemicals, bioflavonoids, enzymes, probiotics, and calcium-rich foods (for bone regeneration as we age)
- Regular, Cell-Regenerating Exercise
  - *Think:* Develop strong, healthy, firm muscles for support, nourishment and development of strong bones
- Daily Restorative Relaxation, Rejuvenation, and Meditation
  - *Think:* Time out for nervous system regeneration, tension and stress release, total body balance and harmony, & inner peace and calm
- Optimistic Thinking & Meditation . . . *includes an Attitude of Gratitude*
  - *Think:* Self-acceptance, self-love, self determination, self esteem & the power of your words, thoughts & intentions in the creation and realization of your deepest desires and visions for your life

And now for the piés de resistânce, the tool that will make it easy to keep your focus when everything else in your life is distracting you from your commitment to get, and stay, healthy once and for all! Let's start with the first word in the title of my book:

INSTANT, just when everyone has you convinced that there is no such thing as Instant Gratification; I'm here to tell you they're wrong! That's right. You read that correctly. **INSTANT ENERGY = INSTANT GRATIFICATION!** The pages that follow are filled with quick and easy things you can do, that take only a few minutes, and instantly create a delicious feeling of energy — right at the moment you thought the only solution was to take a nap! Save your naps for when you hit the pillow at night. You'll sleep a whole lot better at night if you don't nap during the day — and instead do something that will invigorate you and get your blood and oxygen flowing.

Napping is a cop out! And it just leaves you feeling sluggish and bleary eyed when you need to feel alert and full of life. You have no doubt heard the expression: "A change is better than a rest." Well, there's a lot of truth to that statement. Think about how tired and fed-up you have felt just before a vacation. All you could think about was vegging out on the beach, or luxuriating in a comfy bed until late in the morning. But is that what happened? Maybe for the first day, if at all! But just being in a different place, seeing and doing different things created an energy surge within you that you had not previously thought possible.

So, change what you are doing, make it a healthy change (read this book from back to front for all of the amazing ideas and strategies), do it for a few minutes — and watch out.! The fabulous results will amaze you.

Remember your new mantra: **INSTANT ENERGY = INSTANT GRATIFICATION!**

We're not done yet! Remember what I shared with you about my revelation on Thanksgiving morning? Gosh, I get all goose bumpy when I come to this part. Definitely *Higher Intervention*! By the way, that was the name of my company years ago, following my survival of cancer. The acronym for *Higher Intervention* is the **H** and the **I**. So I decided that I wanted to get **H I** (High) with a little help from my friends, God and the angels. Well, that's just what happened here! Why did I have that thought on that very special day of the year? And who would have thought that **ENERGY** would so perfectly summarize what I learned so long ago, that has formed the basis of everything I teach today? Are you ready?

E — Exhale First
N — Nutrition Excellence Daily
E — Exercise for Cell Rejuvenation
R — Relax, Rejuvenate Your Soul
G — Gratitude Attitude
Y — *Your* 5 Keys to Unlimited Energy & Vitality

So, are you ready for some of that INSTANT E.N.E.R.G.Y. ™? Get ready! Get set! Go!

You are about to open your parachute — and fly through the rest of your life. You see my book is your parachute. And as the saying goes, "It's no good (the parachute) unless it's open!"

1. KEY PRINCIPLES TO LIVE BY

For INSTANT *E.N.E.R.G.Y.*™

MASTER YOUR BREATH – MASTER YOUR LIFE!
A Precious Tool for Your Spiritual Adventure

Life depends on breathing, our most primal of all functions. We require oxygen coming in, and carbon dioxide going out, in order to survive. You can live a long time without food, a few days without water – but not more than a minute or two without breathing! Breathing is totally automatic, yet completely within our control. As such, it is a bridge between the conscious and the unconscious. Yet most of us have no clue how to breathe!

You read that right! Most of us breathe only from the neck up – and complain of fatigue, and experience a general lethargy towards living. Full body breathing is the only way to experience true vitality and unlimited energy. In yoga, we refer to that as the Complete Breath. Oxygen is life force enhancing. And it is not about buying oxygen at an Oxygen Bar, or in a bottle! It is about learning to breathe deeply so that your body can absorb more oxygen from the air you breathe. The chemistry of your body can virtually be changed, by improving your breathing. All of your bodily functions will become much more efficient, your mental acuity will be enhanced, and your emotional disposition will be more adaptable, harmonious, content, and balanced.

On a physiological level, proper breathing is essential for the following reasons:

- It carries oxygen to the trillions of cells that make up your body (some research indicates that deep breathing carries 10 times more oxygen throughout your body compared to fragmented or shallow breathing).
- It increases blood circulation.
- It rids your lungs of impurities and waste (carbon monoxide, lactic acid etc.).
- It combats fatigue.
- It increases energy and vitality, leading to a feeling of well-being.
- It leads to better, more refreshing sleep.
- It calms the nerves, and relaxes us.
- It can prevent illness, such as bronchitis and other bronchial conditions, colds, flu, coughing, etc.
- It improves our complexion, prevents acne, and gives us rosy cheeks and a healthy glow.
- It improves your vocal abilities, whether you are a singer, speaker, or an actor.

> It enhances your physical performance, whether you are an athlete, dancer or stage performer.

But that's only the beginning, the tip of the iceberg. Conscious breathing, where you are aware of each breath you take, as you take it, is learned by regular, consistent, daily practice. And breathing consciously expands our consciousness. It is a direct path to our deepest, innermost place — to our Higher Self — that place within us that is completely one with God, and therefore, one with all of the answers to all of the questions for which we seek answers. It is the place where we realize our wholeness of body, mind and spirit, and where only our Oneness with the Creator and the Universe exists. From this place we can experience a level of energy and vitality that is never possible when strictly living at the physical level. Here, we connect to our Prana, or vital life force, the source from which we can fully realize and express our true whole person nature, and our unique Divine purpose for being here now.

Swami Vivekananda, in his paper on Hinduism, in the late 1890's, explained beautifully in this succinct thought-provoking story, the progression towards ultimately controlling our Prana:

"<u>From gross to subtle:</u> *There was once a minister to a great king. He fell into disgrace. The king, as a punishment, ordered him to be shut up in the top of a very high tower. This was done, and the minister was left there to perish. He had a faithful wife, however, who came to the tower at night and called to her husband at the top to know what she could do to help him. He told her to return to the tower the following night and bring with her a long rope, some stout twine, pack thread, silken thread, a beetle, and a little honey . . . The good wife obeyed her husband, and brought him the desired articles. The husband directed her to attach the silken thread firmly to the beetle, then to smear its horns with a drop of honey, and to set it free on the wall of the tower, with its head pointing upwards. She obeyed all these instructions, and the beetle started on its long journey. Smelling the honey ahead it slowly crept onwards, in the hope of reaching the honey, until at last it reached the top of the tower, when the minister grasped the beetle, and got possession of the silken thread. He told his wife to tie the other end to the pack thread, and after he had drawn up the pack thread, he repeated the process with the stout twine, and lastly with the rope. Then the rest was easy. The minister descended from the tower by means of the rope, and made his escape. In this body of ours the breath motion is the silken thread; by laying hold of and learning to control it we grasp the pack thread of the nerve currents, and from these the stout twine of our thoughts, and lastly the rope of Prana, controlling which we reach freedom.*"

Breath Awareness Exercise

Our world today is full of stressed out folks who do absolutely nothing to reduce stress during a demanding day, or even at the end of a long over-taxing day. They drive home from a trying day at work, compounded by a long drive home, stuck in traffic. Or perhaps their whole day was spent dealing with some not so nice folks on the phone, or in long boring meetings with some fairly intolerable individuals. Once home, they head for the cupboard, the refrigerator or the liquor cabinet, with a strong impulse to just drown their sorrows, and / or stress, in the bottle or food, or both.

Wait! Is that you? Well, that just won't work. Unless you unwind first, all of your body's energy is going to the handling of the stress, which means it is arming itself for *fight or flight* — neither of which you plan to do. The problem is that you will not digest anything under those conditions. When the body is preparing to deal with the stress, most of the body's blood supply is gong to your extremities, not to your digestive organs! So, oops — *indigestion / heartburn* . . .

And then you feel like you know what, for the rest of the evening — unless you resort to some disgusting form of antacid. Before you know it, this has become a nasty habit — and you just never feel well, ever. Life becomes one long dull roar of a headache, and constant indigestion, burping, flatulence (that thing we call gas!), and heartburn. You resign yourself to this discomfort, and the *"magic pills"* for relief. But there is another way!

So, would you like to know what it is? And would you believe that it only takes "5" minutes? No, I am not kidding! Just 5 minutes! This strategy has been tested by thousands of people just like you, globally, who have attended my seminars, or who have been my patient, not to mention all of my friends and family who have had the good fortune of trying it as well. It can literally transform your life if you actually do it everyday — for just 5 minutes.

Warning: After you have experienced the amazing results in just 5 minutes a day for a few weeks, you may find yourself wanting to spend 10, or even 15 — or, *oh my gosh*, even 20 minutes — doing this. Just thought I should prepare you.

<u>*Okay, here's the breathing technique*</u> *that I teach my patients, clients and seminar attendees. It is a simple breath counting system, and it is of the utmost importance to focus the mind entirely upon the action of breathing! Keep in mind that the way*

we breathe is a reflection, and an expression, of the way we live. Shallow breathing, from the top of our lungs, is that of a stressed out, anxious, restless, even angry, individual. Abdominal deep breathing is used to breathe through high tension states, and stressful situations. By changing the way you breathe, you can literally change the way you live.

The Process:

How do you keep time?

First, get a timer and set it for 5 (or more) minutes. Put it where you can reach it easily to start it when you are ready to begin. It can also be as simple as wearing a watch, with a built-in timer (These are readily available, and generally very inexpensive, these days!), especially if you are always on the road with your work, or even when traveling for pleasure.

What sounds inspire relaxation and peace?

Put a great meditation CD into your CD player, or have one programmed onto your iPod, or on your computer. It should be one with gentle calming music, or nature sounds. I enjoy *The 5 Minute Hour* (A series of five 5-minute meditations, available at the products section of: www.marilynjoyce.com), or something from Steven Halpern (His life's purpose has been producing amazing music for the soul, available at: www.innerpeacemusic.com). If you are at home with all of your equipment, put the remote next to where you will be sitting or lying. Otherwise, have your iPod or computer close to where you will be relaxing and breathing.

Where do I do it?

Find a quiet place where you won't be distracted. Remember, this is only for 5 minutes! So stop making excuses for why you can't take time out! Your life depends on it! I'm sure your family can live without you for *5 minutes*! 5 minutes now may prevent a lifetime without you later! Get real with yourself, and your family. Take it from someone who learned the hard way!

You can do any of the following:

lie down on a comfortable couch, or the floor (on a comfortable mat) with your feet up
or sit in a comfortable cross-legged position on the floor,
or sit in a comfortable straight-backed chair.

How do I do it?

➤ Do this breathing process on an empty stomach. You don't need any of your blood and energy supply going to digestion, instead of your brain, where it is needed for the optimal concentration.

➤ Wear loose, comfortable clothing, with nothing that constricts your breathing or blood flow—no elastic bands, belts, corsets, or tight-fitting bras.

➤ Keep your back completely straight, yet relaxed (imagine a thread from the top of your head pulling you gently in straight line up to the sky).

➤ Make sure your arms, legs, wrists, and ankles are all uncrossed unless you are sitting on the floor in a cross-legged position.

➤ Start the music (with that remote you placed in a handy location) and the timer.

➤ Close your eyes. Allow yourself to feel the sounds of the music.

➤ Now begin breathing, first by exhaling every ounce of air, forcefully, through your mouth with a vocal whoosh sound.

➤ Slowly inhale (breathe in) deeply, through your nose, while fully, but comfortably extending your abdomen, and as you are inhaling count to 4 in your head.

➤ Then hold your breath for a count of 4, and just be with the music as you count.

➤ And then slowly release your breath to a count of 4, as you exhale through your nose.

➤ Continue to inhale, hold, and exhale, each to a count of 4, until the 5-minute timer alerts you that you are done. It will come sooner than you think! And remember always to breathe deeply and slowly without strain.

How do you feel? Amazing, isn't it, what just 5 short minutes can do for you body, mind and spirit, with focused energy and intention? Now, go ahead and enjoy your snacks, or dinner, or that cocktail. *What was that you said? You don't crave that drink, or those quick snacks that you thought you wanted before you took that 5 minutes out just to be still and breathe?* Well, you see, those endorphins you produced during your little break have appeased you in a way that junk food never could. Just another wonderful benefit that you have derived from this simple little process! So, whenever you feel tired, depressed, stressed out, or discouraged, just do 5 minutes of this breathing process; and watch your fatigue or undesired emotion, just magically disappear. Your mental balance will be re-established, and you'll feel like a new person, ready to tackle anything that comes your way — well, almost anything.

NOTE: *As you practice this, you may eventually, after a few weeks or a few months, decide that you want to try a longer breath-count. In fact, I absolutely recommend this. Think about what happens when a weight, stretch, or yoga posture becomes very comfortable. We know, that in order to improve our strength, our flexibility and our performance, it becomes necessary for us to increase the weight used, the length of the stretch, or the length of time we hold a yoga pose.*

The same is true of breath-work. *If we want to expand our capacity for the intake of life-giving oxygen, and release more carbon dioxide and lactic acid, the build up of which can leave us feeling tired and lethargic, then we must push ourselves just a little farther with our breath-count. That expansion of our limits and possibilities, in whatever area of our life we achieve it, brings rewards far beyond our ego-centered comprehension. Like the Law of Diminishing Returns – The longer you do the same old thing, the worse the results. No change, no gain! Change one thing, and watch what happens!*

So go ahead . . .
Add just one more second to the inhalation/holding/exhalation pattern, e.g. 5-5-5.

WATER: THE MIRACLE ELIXIR OF LIFE!

It is important to remember the theme of this book: *Instant Energy—5 minutes at a time!* How does water fit into this? Well, nothing is much easier or faster to fit into your day than water. Just fill two clean "glass" 1-liter jugs or bottles in the morning, and place them in a convenient location or locations so that they are always within eyeshot. Don't wait until you are thirsty to drink the water. Aim to complete drinking, one full jug in the morning, and one in the afternoon. We'll talk more about the types of water containers that are best in just a minute. For now, you are probably asking . . .

Why a Chapter on Water?

Well that is a very good question and simple to answer. Water is life. You can live a long time without food. But you will probably not make it past 10 days without water! And major damage will likely occur to your brain (Dying cells from dehydration occurs in as few as 3 days!), and other organs, from this fluid depletion in a far shorter time frame. You can lose 50% of your fat, your protein, and your glucose, and still survive. But the most water you can lose from your body and still be alive is 20%!

As you can see from the information on the following page, the largest single component of your body is water. And that applies to all living matter! Nothing in the body can occur without water. And the body has no way to store water; it needs a fresh supply everyday. Digestion, assimilation, circulation, building, repair, and elimination depend on movement throughout the body, and that cannot happen without fluids! The average adult loses about 2.5 to 3 liters of water each day, with more being lost during strenuous or prolonged exercise, or during hot weather, or the combination of both heat and exercise. And if you are a frequent flyer, like me, you can lose up to 1.5 liters of water during a 3-hour flight. This water loss must be replaced. You can get a portion of your water from the foods you eat. See the detailed list of foods, and their composition of water, at the end of this chapter.

A body made up of 60-80 % water (depending on who authored the article or book), living on the typical Western diet of about 10-15 % water-rich foods, is destined to die a slow and very uncomfortable death. I personally believe that a very healthy body is about 80-85% water, and that the bulk of the diet of a healthy individual is made up of foods that are between 75-95% water. Again, see the list at the end of this chapter for the water content of a variety of foods.

I think a word on aging is in order here, even though I don't, personally, believe it should have the impact that it, apparently, does have on our western culture today. It is important to understand that as we age, we may lose our thirst sensation, to a large degree, due to impaired bodily functions. Medications, such as diuretics and laxatives, used liberally among all ages, especially the elderly, can also result in dehydration. Conditions, including chronic illness, reduced mobility (either from lack of exercise, from an illness, or both), hormonal changes, decline in kidney function, and diabetes, just to mention a few, can also lead to dehydration. My grandparents both lived well into their 90's in Scotland, with no illnesses to speak of, and each of them selected the day that they passed on to meet "their Maker" (good Scottish term for God!). Why did they live so long and healthfully, while all around them were dying before their time? A healthy diet of fresh produce, picked, as needed, directly from their own extensive garden, which was planted and harvested with amazing love and daily attention, along with a lot of water, from the break of dawn through to bedtime, plus a long walk every day (15-20 miles—and I'm not exaggerating—after all they had no TV or computer to veg in front of!), combined with an excellent work ethic, were just a few of their secrets.

Facts about the Water Composition of Your Body:

65%-75% of our body is water
83% of our blood is water
75% of our brain is water
76% of our muscle tissue is water
90% of our lungs are water
98% of our blood plasma is water
90% of the world's population is dehydrated
75% of the US population is dehydrated

(See the image to the right for more details.)

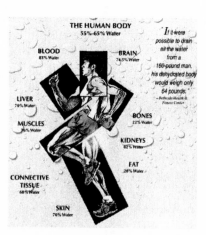

Signs of Dehydration:

> ➤ No urination for 6 or more hours
> ➤ Dry mouth—the last outward sign of dehydration
> ➤ Yellow urine—mildly dehydrated

- Orange or dark colored, strong smelling urine — severely dehydrated
- Constipation, intestinal cramps
- Cavities in teeth — a major result of dry mouth
- Excessive thirst
- Nausea
- Headaches and feeling stressed — sense that you are overwhelmed or can't cope
- Nosebleeds — due to dry mucosal membranes in the nose, mouth and throat
- Crinkled / wrinkled skin
- Lethargy and weakness of muscles — Every metabolic function, including energy production must have water; enzymes, the catalysts must have water to be activated.
- Daytime fatigue and tiredness — Lack of hydration is the number one trigger.
- Foggy brain — difficulty with concentration and focus, inability to focus on printed material and the computer screen. Only a 2 % drop in body water can cause any of these symptoms.
- Mood swings, irrational behavior, and slow responses
- Confusion, disorientation, hallucinations — Brain function diminishes significantly with just mild dehydration (see foggy brain above.)
- Metabolism slowed down — result of only minimal dehydration
- Weight gain — due to impaired metabolism
- Chronic hunger, especially for sweet foods and other snack items
- Allergies and asthma — due to impaired lubrication, lymphatic flow, digestion and elimination
- High blood pressure / low blood pressure — due to imbalance of fluids throughout your body. Your body will respond according to its own predisposition.
- Heartburn — shortage of water in the upper part of the gastrointestinal tract
- Back and joint pain — research so far, indicates the possibility that the equivalent of 8 to 10 glasses of water per day could ease these conditions for up to 80% of sufferers.
- Bladder cancer — 5 glasses of water each day reduces risk by 50%.
- Breast cancer — that same 5 glasses each day reduces the risk by 79%.
- Colon cancer — 5 glasses of water every day decreases the risk by 45%.
- Alzheimer's Disease & Senility — 75%-85% of the brain is water, so even just mild chronic dehydration over time leads to major cell death within the brain tissue.
- Kidney failure with chronic long-term dehydration — which may result in death

The Many Functions of Water in Your Body:

➢ Aids in digestion and assimilation of the food we eat

➢ Carries your digestive juices to where they are needed in your body

➢ Lubricates and cushions your joints

➢ Lubricates and moistens your nasal passages, eyeballs, and intestines — in fact, all of your mucosal membranes, including your mouth and lungs

➢ Maintains the health and integrity of the trillions of cells that make up our body

➢ Transports oxygen, vitamins, minerals, phytochemicals, bioflavonoids, amino acids, glucose, enzymes, hormones, and a multitude of other substances and chemicals needed by the body, throughout the body

➢ Balances the electrolytes (positive cat-ions: sodium, potassium, magnesium, calcium; and negative anions: bicarbonate, chloride, phosphate, sulfate, organic acids, and protein compounds) — substances that disassociate into positively and negatively charged ions when in water, and are crucial to our body's water distribution, absorption, diffusion, acid-base balance, and muscle and nerve reaction.

➢ Creates shiny hair, clear eyes, and glowing moist skin — from adequate fluids moving continuously through your body

➢ Acts as a shock absorber for the spine, joints, eyes, and amniotic sac enveloping the fetus during pregnancy

➢ Regulates and balances your body temperature through sweating — retains body warmth in the winter and cools the body when the temperature is hot, by evaporation from the skin and lungs

➢ Assists in the burning of glucose and in the breakdown of fat for energy

➢ Removes and helps to eliminate waste byproducts (including excess electrolytes and urea) of metabolism, through the kidneys, and through the intestines

➢ Regulates the continual movement and flow of the lymphatic system (the body's sewer system) for detoxification of your body

➢ Reduces the risk of cystitis (along with a diet high in alkaline ash producing fruits and vegetables — see the chapter on Help for Indigestion) by clearing the bladder of bacteria

➢ Relieves constipation — especially if you get enough fiber from fresh produce, whole grains and legumes (beans, peas, lentils)

➢ Relieves and reduces fluid retention in ankles, feet, legs, and hands — less water intake causes the body to go into survival mode, holding onto water in the extracellular spaces (outside the cells)

> ➢ Improves endocrine function — so the endocrine glands more efficiently produce, control and coordinate all of the activities of the hormones (messengers) throughout your body

Optimal Times to Drink Water:

Note: If you have not been a water drinker until now, DO NOT SUDDENLY DRINK A LOT OF WATER. Increase in water consumption should be slow and deliberate — add 8 oz per week until you have reached the recommended amount for your body weight. See the Rules of Thumb below for how to calculate this.

> ➢ First thing in the morning when you arise — 8-12 oz, room temperature
> ➢ ½ hour before meals if possible, but at least 10 minutes prior
> ➢ 1-2 hours after a meal
> ➢ 1 ½ to 2 hours before going to bed
> ➢ When the temperature is hot — an extra 2 glasses of water daily for every 5°F above 85°F
> ➢ When exercising — add more, especially if the temperature is hot. Remember: even light exercise uses at least half a gallon of water in a day, which is eliminated in sweat, urine and simply breathing! So — Hydrate! Hydrate! Hydrate!!

WATER MUST BE REPLACED EVERY 24 HOURS!

Two wonderful resources that I recommend, include: *Your Body's Many Cries for Water*, and *ABC of Asthma, Allergies and Lupus*, both by the late Dr. F. Batmanghelidj, MD. The website, which is full of very mind-provoking and useful information, is www.watercure.com. The doctor's message to the world was, "You are not sick, you are thirsty. Don't treat thirst with medication." And further more, Dr. Batmanghelidj stated, "In my professional and scientific view, it is dehydration that is the biggest killer, more than any other condition you could imagine. The different aspects and 'chemical idiosyncrasies' of each individual's body reaction to the same pattern of dehydration, have received different professional labels and have been treated differently and ineffectively."

Rules of Thumb For Water Intake:

> ➢ Drink ½ your body weight of water in ounces, daily. Example 180 lb = 90 oz. of water daily. Divide that into 8 or 10 oz. glasses and that's 9-10 glasses of water per day.

> ➢ Use ¼ tsp. of salt—only sea salt i.e. Celtic Sea Salt, Real Salt or raw salt for every quart of water you drink. DO NOT use commercial processed salt—the grocery store varieties!
> ➢ Use salt (only the above listed salts) as needed, and minimally, with food. As long as you drink adequate clean, filtered water, you can use the salt. Your brain cells, and your entire body of trillions of cells, require salt and water to survive.
> ➢ Avoid or limit caffeinated and alcoholic drinks. These are diuretics and will dehydrate you. For every 6 oz. of caffeine or alcohol, you require an additional 10 to 12 oz. of water to re-hydrate.

Can I Drink Too Much Water?

Yes! Though dehydration, overall, is by far the more prevalent condition. The condition of water intoxication, which is very rare, is known as hyponatremia. We see this most commonly in people with eating disorders, such as anorexia nervosa and bulimia, who drink water in place of food. This has also been observed in individuals experiencing mental disorders, such as schizophrenia. Sodium, which is necessary for muscle contraction and sending nerve impulses, drops to very dangerously low levels in the blood, due to the high concentration of fluids. So, the kidneys (muscles themselves) can't eliminate enough of these fluids. In my client practice, I have seen hyponatremia lead to a coma, and eventual death, following a variety of symptoms including headaches, cramps, depression, blurred vision, and convulsions. Again, this condition is very rare—you do need to drink water everyday!

The Big Question—What Water Can I Drink?

Without fail, I am continually asked, what water is safe? Should I drink bottled water? Should I avoid tap water? What bottled water is the best—or safest? Is distilled water okay—or the best? Are the plastic bottles that water comes in, safe? Do I need oxygenated water? What's all the hoop-la about molecular structure of water?

A quick answer on distilled water and tap water:

Avoid distilled water—it is dead water. Remember: You are residing in a magnificent living organism that needs vibrantly alive foods and water, with the life force intact, in order to thrive. Distilled water is like processed, denatured foods—DEAD!

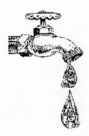

So what about tap water? Is it safe? Our water supply is contaminated with the many waste products of today's modern industrial and agricultural practices. Heavy metal toxicity in our water is rampant, and increasing daily! Among them are: arsenic (from industrial run-off and pesticide residues), chlorine (carcinogenic disinfectant and bleaching agent), fluoride (disrupts enzyme function in the body), hydrogen sulfide (byproduct of decayed underground organic matter), lead (leads to damage to the brain, nervous system and kidneys), methyl tertiary butylated ether — MTBE — (gasoline additive that may be carcinogenic), chromium VI (byproduct of

industrial processes and is carcinogenic), nitrates and nitrites (from fertilizers and livestock waste, and become carcinogenic nitrosamines in the stomach), radon (radioactive gas, can cause death due to cancer), and nuclear waste (deadly radioactive materials). Even the pipes carrying the water to your residence or business are sources of contamination! So what do you think? Sound safe?

To protect yourself, have your water checked at least annually for pollutants, and don't wait for the government, or anyone else, to take care of your water for you. Take responsibility for your own health — no one else will! One of the most valuable steps I took, when I purchased my new home, was to have a whole house water filtration system installed. Prior to having this system installed, however, I had become nauseous and lethargic. Somehow, I sensed that the water might be the problem. Sure enough . . . And now, two years later, all is well, my water tastes great and I feel protected. You have to make this decision for yourself. Even if you choose to believe that your tap water is safe, the very least you must do, is to find a way to remove the chlorine, which is necessary in order to kill harmful bacteria in our water supplies. The problem is that it is one of the most carcinogenic chemicals on the planet as well!

Here are my thoughts on bottled water:

More and more, I am convinced that plastic bottles of water are not the answer, if you care about either your health, or the environment. The fact is that it is difficult to clean the narrow mouth of most plastic water bottles by normal washing. Therefore, bacteria grow easily and quickly around the mouth of the bottle, in just a few hours, leading to contamination of the water in the bottle. I have actually observed green algae growing in bottles of water, after only a couple of days of drinking from the bottle, without cleaning it between uses. That, alone, is enough to convince me to change to glass, ceramic, and stainless steel.

Let's face it! Drinks from non-plastic containers always taste better anyway! And think about the day you left that plastic bottle in your car in the direct sunlight. Then you took a swig—Yuk! All you could taste was plastic. And then you'll tell me that the compounds of that plastic bottle did not leach into the water? Sorry, I don't believe it! Personally I don't care how safe the government, or anyone else, tries to tell me those plastic bottles are; I'm not convinced!

Also, as an environmentalist, I have to say a few words about the polyvinyl-chloride (PVC: the name alone is scary—think VINYL flooring!) manufacturing of plastics. PVC releases dioxins into the environment, during both the manufacturing and incineration of plastics, and is a known carcinogenic agent. Plastic is a non-renewable resource, and the toxic production process is extremely resource and energy intensive. So, my recommendation is to use glass wherever possible, at home, at the office, even in your car if you have a good holder. Ceramic is my next choice. Both, it and glass are non-harmful and great renewable resources. Failing either of those options, select a good quality, stainless steel (inside and out), wide-mouth container, and remember to wash it daily. Make sure it is not lined with an epoxy finish. Finally, for those times when nothing but plastic is an option, based on the research I have done to date, I would suggest using only bottles, marked on the bottom, with the #2, #4, or #5. And without question, it is imperative that you recycle the plastic bottles! For updates on water bottles, check out our *Special Reports* at www.marilynjoyce.com

So a Word About Bottled Penta Water . . .

All of the above said, when I do drink bottled water on the road, I look for the Penta brand of water. Ultra-purified, Penta, which is comprised of the smallest and most absorbable liquid molecule, the 5 H2O, or pentamer (The Penta-hydrate process reduces the large molecular clusters of H2O-based water into single pentamer clusters.), is created using a 13-step purification process. The objective of this process is to eliminate every possible impurity found in water, including chlorine, arsenic, pesticides, bacteria, chromium 6, lead, fluoride, and MTBE. Results from research with Penta water indicates faster gastric emptying, faster hydration, faster nerve firing, and increased muscle power. This water also got more oxygen to the cells significantly faster and more efficiently than any other water.

The Perfect Beverage of Choice for the Athlete or Weekend Warrior ...

Another fact, observed in research on carbohydrate-based drinks, is that water leaves the stomach faster than any beverage with added sugar, such as Gatorade and other commercial sports drinks. Over the years, clients of mine have asked what they can drink, while in a race, or a sports activity that demands a good source of fluids and electrolytes. Not being an expert in sports nutrition, I turned to my healthiest clients, some of who are world-class athletes, and asked for their input. Their recommendation that follows, works extremely well. A few years ago I had the opportunity to personally test it out. I signed up for a 3-day walk/run for cancer research. Being someone who likes to get things done, I decided to play full out, doing whatever it took to get through the experience with grace and ease. I incorporated the healthy athlete's beverage of choice:

1 gallon of Penta water
Juice of 1 large orange
Juice of 1 large lemon
Juice of 1 large lime
Juice of 1 pink grapefruit (optional)

If you have an allergy to any one of these fruits, just skip it and use the others. Use an citrus squeezer (electric if conditions permit) to juice the fruits, collecting as much of the pulp as possible, and adding it to the water. Drink as needed throughout the race, competition, or run. Make more as required.

My 3-day experience was a joy. Not only was I well hydrated, due to the enzymes, electrolytes, and a little natural sugar, I had energy to burn, felt great each day, and was able to complete each day quickly and more efficiently than most of the other participants. *This really works!*

For more information on Penta-hydrate and Penta water, you can call 800-531-5088, or visit:
www.hydrateforlife.com or www.pentawater.com.

Where Else is Water Found?

Approximately 80% of our water intake comes from drinking water and other beverages, and the other 20% comes from food. Of course, that percentage is based on consumption of a healthy diet versus the SAD (Standard American Diet) eating pattern of most people in the Western hemisphere! Assuming these percentages are accurate for some of us, the recommended amount of fluids, including water, and fluids from foods, would be approximately 9-10 cups for women, and about 12-13.5 cups for men.

While 20% may seem like a lot of fluid to get from food, many common food items are mostly water. On the following page, you will find a list of some foods with high water content, followed by foods that are relatively low in water content. You will notice that the foods that are high in water content are the foods we are continuously hearing about every day in the news—recommended for the thousands of health building nutrients they contain! Plant foods! Fruits and vegetables! So start chewing . . .

NOTE: If you lightly steam your veggies, *do not add salt* to the cooking water. Salt will draw the water out of the produce during the cooking process, so you will significantly reduce the amount of water that would normally be available in the raw food. I rarely eat cooked produce, so it had not occurred to me to mention this fact. Thanks to my wonderful and efficient assistant, Laurie, I was reminded that most people do cook their veggies, or at least some of them!

Percentage of Water Found in Commonly Consumed Foods

FOOD	% of WATER	FOOD	% of WATER
Cucumber	96%	Acorn Squash	88%
Chinese Cabbage, Bok Choy	95%	Oranges	88%
Celery	95%	Peaches	88%
Lettuce	95%	Carrots	87%
Zucchini	95%	Beets	87%
Tomatoes	94%	Raspberries	87%
Spaghetti Squash	94%	Brussels Sprouts	86%
Yellow Squash	94%	Blackberries	86%
Asparagus	92%	Dandelion Greens	86%
Bell Peppers, red, green, yellow	92%	Apples	85%
		Yogurt (1 cup)	85%
Cabbage	92%	Kale	84%
Cauliflower	92%	Pears	84%
Cilantro/Coriander	92%	Mango	82%
Escarole	92%	Grapes	81%
Mushrooms	92%	Parsnip	80%
Pumpkin	92%	Bananas	75%
Spinach	92%	Sweet Potato	73%
Strawberries	92%	Pasta, cooked	69%
Watercress	92%	Fish, baked	68%
Watermelon	92%	Rice, cooked	68%
Broccoli	91%	Lentils	67%
Grapefruit	91%	Cassava/Yucca Root	60%
Mustard Greens	91%	Beef	50%
Turnip Greens	91%	Cheese	40%
Cantaloupe	90%	Whole Grain Bread	38%
Green Beans	90%	Butter	16%
Honeydew Melon	90%	Nuts	5%
Okra	90%	Soda Crackers	4%
Rutabaga	90%	White Sugar	Trace
Milk (1 cup)	89%	Oils	0%
Papaya	89%		

DETOX FOR LIFE:
CLEANSE AND HEAL YOUR BODY

A sign I saw recently at a gas station really impacted me. "A clean engine always delivers power." Of course it reminded me of the fact that most of us take much better care of our cars than the vehicle we live in and use everyday to move through our lives. Perfect health requires proper nutrition, a healthy and active lifestyle, time for relaxation, reflection and prayer, and efficient detoxification practices.

Overtax your liver, the primary organ of detoxification, and you will overtax every organ in your body responsible for balancing your hormones! (For more information on hormones, check out our *Special Reports* at www. MarilynJoyce.com. Out of balance hormones lead to a build up of residual waste by-products of metabolism. When the liver is overtaxed, it can't do its job of:

> ➢ Removing these waste by-products
> ➢ Cleansing the blood of harmful chemicals, viruses, and bacteria
> ➢ Storage of essential nutrients and blood
> ➢ Production of bile which is vital for digestion of fats
> ➢ It's critical role of metabolizing proteins, fats and carbohydrates

Are you one of the vast numbers of people in this developed nation who suffer from chronic constipation—and believe that one or two bowel movements in a week are normal? Do you suffer with chronic fatigue on an ongoing basis? Do you often experience gas and bloating or stomach pain—in general, poor digestion—after eating? Or worse, do you suffer with acid reflux or severe heartburn following a meal? Or perhaps you suffer with IBS (Irritable Bowel Syndrome) or diverticulitis. Is bad breath a cause of constant embarrassment? Has your libido completely flagged? Do you suffer with headaches and depression? Or have you noticed that indescribable "brain fog" no one wants to talk about for fear of the development of a senility disease being implicated? Or perhaps persistent diarrhea is interfering with your daily life! Or maybe you are experiencing unexplainable excess weight gain, or severe PMS?

We are all so caught up in looking good—on the outside! We spend fortunes on our hair, nails, skin, teeth, and clothes to cover all of our flaws. But our colon, on the inside, which serves as the sewer system for our entire body, along with our lymphatic system, is ignored, forgotten about, taken for granted, and left to function on its own—until that fateful day when we are diagnosed with a major illness, such as colon cancer. Or for that matter, any kind of cancer or other degenerative illness!

Everyday, we are exposed to thousands of chemicals and toxins — at home, at work, through our food (processed packaged foods, a multitude of simple sugars, and those pesky trans fatty acids and hydrogenated fats), our water, and the air we breath, not to mention the various over-the-counter and prescription drugs we take. There is a saying that death begins in the colon. According to Vegetarian Times in March of 1998, "autopsies often reveal colons that are plugged up to 80% with waste material."

You should be eliminating the equivalent of what you are taking in — *everyday*! If not, the remainder accumulates and hardens, sticking to the colon walls. This is turn inhibits the proper function of absorbing the nutrients from the fecal matter. Instead the colon is forced to absorb the various toxins from the accumulated wastes that also provide a perfect breeding ground for unhealthy parasites.

So what's the solution? — a good and simple detox program that contains a lot of plant fibers and healthy oils, along with lots of water. The program I use with my clients, as well as myself, is a very simple 7-day system that prepares you, cleans you from the inside out, and starts you on the road to consistent maintenance. And the first step is to make sure you have time to just relax and take some very warm baths throughout the duration of the program. It is important to keep activity to a minimum while going through the process. Colonics are also a valuable tool for removal of the hardened accumulated fecal debris attached to the colon wall. I recommend at least 3 colonics during this week.

First of all, let's look at the health benefits you will gain from an overall detoxification program. We could fill a page or two with the beneficial outcomes, but for now, let's focus on the primary benefits that are very far-reaching with respect to your overall health and longevity. They are as follows:

➢ Release of toxins / poisons throughout your body
➢ Clear skin of eruptions, hives, pimples, and rashes, as well as a sallow coloring
➢ Promote shiny, healthy, vibrant and strong hair
➢ Protect your nervous system and enhance brain function and mental acuity
➢ Reduce risk for cancer, heart disease, PMS, fibromyalgia, chronic fatigue syndrome, MS, Alzheimer's, lupus, fibroid tumors, endometriosis, and perhaps type 2 diabetes
➢ Loss of excess weight, leading to increased energy and vitality

➢ Feel better than you have in years with a renewed vigor for life and glowing skin!
➢ Enhance sexual performance and libido

And you will just plain LOOK GREAT without even thinking about it!

What Exactly Is The Detox / Cleanse Designed To Do?

This Plan — and all of that which is included in this book — is designed to:

➢ Provide a jump-start to your new or renewed health and wellness program — a quick and easy method which starts the process of creating, in your life, new 5-minute health habits and strategies, and helps to motivate you to stay on the program in this book.
➢ Maintain your initial commitment to gaining or regaining your health, and help you continue to stay on a healthy program for life.
➢ Assist you in making healthier, more wholesome, food and lifestyle choices.

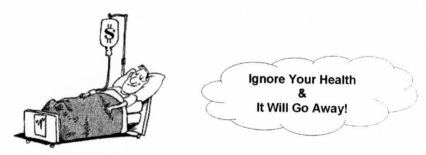

Ignore Your Health
&
It Will Go Away!

➢ Educate you in healthy lifestyle choices: recommending appropriate exercise guidelines, encouraging relaxation and self-nurturing, motivating shifts in attitudes about food, exercise, substances and oneself. This is the purpose of this entire book — the detox just starts the process!
➢ Provide a simple, delicious easy-to-follow 7-Day **Detoxification Diet.**
➢ Make available the right products and information necessary to help you adhere to the program.

The Detoxification Plan is broken down into 3 distinct phases, each of which has a very definite and specific purpose.

■ *Phase 1* **Preparing for the Detoxification / Cleanse**
■ *Phase 2* **7-day Detox Diet**
■ *Phase 3* **Transition into Lifetime Healthy Habits**

Phase 1 — Preparing for and Enjoying the Detox Program

Prior to beginning the program:

> ➢ Throw out or give away all foods that are triggers for you when your temptation is low: bread, crackers, baked products, potato chips, nuts, snacks, cookies, cakes, pies, ice cream, dairy products, chocolate, and other candies and sweets.

> ➢ Sit down with a pen and paper, and a cup of green tea with lemon, and write a list of all of the benefits of having a slim, healthy and fit physique. And then list the consequences of being unhealthy, out-of-shape, and possibly overweight. Now put all of this on an index card and carry it with you at all times. Refer to these lists often. Make several copies and place them in conspicuous areas where you can't miss them.

> ➢ Program yourself for a week at home relaxing and rejuvenating your body. Stock up on your favorite videos, music CD's, magazines, books, candles, flowers, perfumes, bath oils or salts, essential oils (I personally love the Young Living Oils!), lotions, etc.

> ➢ Consider turning off your phones, including your cell phone(s), and let your VM systems or answering machines take the calls.

> ➢ Pamper your inner self, your quiet self — that part of you that rarely gets the care and attention it deserves — by soaking in a bathtub or treating yourself to a massage. Add some Epsom Salts to the bath water, as the salts will draw out the toxins that have accumulated and are about to be released during the detox program. *It is recommended that you add this step (daily bathing with Epsom Salts) to your daily regime throughout the 7 days.*

> ➢ Plan the start of the program at a time when you do not have heavy or pressing work or personal commitments.

> ➢ Call a friend who is supportive of your desire and efforts to cleanse and rejuvenate your body, if you find yourself weakening — maybe they will even want to join you on your journey! *And you can do this step any time throughout the week as well.*

> ➢ Acquire the necessary equipment and incidentals for ease of following through with each step of the program — even if you have to borrow from someone who has these items. You will need:

> > ✓ Vita-Mix machine
> > ✓ Rebounder (mini-trampoline)
> > ✓ Bathtub
> > ✓ Timer

- ✓ Yoga mat
- ✓ Candles
- ✓ Epsom Salts
- ✓ Essential Oils
- ✓ Lotions, facial scrubs and masks
- ✓ Dry Brush Kit
- ✓ Calming music CD's (see the *5 Minute Hour* CD at my website under audio products — www.marilynjoyce.com)
- ✓ DVD comedies
- ✓ Flowers for several rooms in your home — very relaxing
- ✓ Work-out clothes that you feel good wearing
- ✓ Satin bed sheets — or something similar — makes you feel pampered

Phase 2 — 7 Day Detox Diet

So, in a nutshell, here is my 7-day plan . . .

Strategies for Success throughout the program:

- ➤ Drink lots of water between meals to flush out the toxins. Always have a minimum of 8-8 oz glasses, preferably 10-12 glasses, each day of the program.
- ➤ Drink no water with meals — only ½ hour before or 1 hour after.
- ➤ Make sure all produce is organic. No point attempting to clean out our insides while adding more toxins is there?
- ➤ Avoid all alcohol, caffeine, tobacco, and soft drinks — no recreational drugs of any kind!
- ➤ Eat / drink meals slowly, chewing your food and beverages (that's right, even your beverages) well, and savor every morsel.
- ➤ Dry brush your entire body every morning before you shower. There are many sizes, shapes, and styles of body brushes to fit your individual needs. Proponents of dry brushing, including me, believe that by dry brushing you get rid of dead skin cells and surface toxins on the skin, allowing the skin, which is the body's largest organ of elimination, to breathe and to detox more efficiently. This, in turn, energizes your skin to improve lymph and blood flow, and decreases puffiness. Like a light acupressure treatment, the gentle brushing also has a calming effect.

How to Dry Brush:

- ✓ Allow 5-10 minutes
- ✓ Get into the shower

- ✓ Use a brush with soft bristles, a loofah sponge, or a silk mitten
- ✓ Brush in small circles, moving towards the heart, applying very light pressure
- ✓ Avoid skin rashes, broken skin, the face and inner thighs (areas of thin skin), varicose veins, broken blood vessels
- ✓ Start with your feet, work up each leg, then each arm, brushing from fingertips towards your heart
- ✓ Reach round to your back, brushing towards your stomach
- ✓ When finished enjoy your shower

➢ Light stretching should be done in the morning before you start your day, and in the evening to end your day. See the exercise chapter, *Fit in Fitness*, for the Sun Salutation. This is a very effective way to stretch every part if your body. Do one complete cycle just before, and right after, your time on the Rebounder, to prevent any stiffness.

➢ Bounce on your Rebounder — mini-trampoline — for 1 minute the first day, 2 minutes on the 2nd and 3rd days, 3 minutes on the 4th and 5th days, and 4 minutes on the 6th and 7th days. Use a timer to insure that you fulfill the time commitment. See the chapter, *Fit in Fitness*, for details on the importance of the Rebounder (www.reboundair.com). It is imperative that you clear the lymphatic system as you detox your entire body, releasing the accumulated toxins into the sewer system of the body for release.

➢ Treat yourself daily to one of: a massage, a sauna with steam, a Tai Chi class, a yoga class, or any other relaxing program available to you. And it is imperative for rejuvenation, to take time to be still and meditate or pray, or preferably do both.

➢ Go for a 15-minute walk after your evening "meal" to release any tension and to enjoy the evening air. Walk with a supportive buddy.

➢ Visualize yourself at optimal health, completely cleansed and rejuvenated. Do this 3 times during the day — first thing in the morning, midday, and last thing in the evening. The very best time to do this is just as you are awakening, and just before you go to sleep. That is when your brain is most receptive to receiving and assimilating this new information. Remember: all successful people, including world-class athletes, claim that this is their secret weapon in achieving their goals. However, you must do it with the intensity of feeling that you would experience as if you have already achieved your desired health goals.

➢ At the end of the week reward yourself with a non-food gift. Determine this reward in advance. What do you deeply desire that would assist you in keeping your commitment to complete the entire week of self-care? Maybe it is new clothes, a concert, a new CD set, a day at a spa, a trip to a special resort, a sexy pair of shoes you've had your eyes on for a while . . . *Make it something you personally consider very special.*

"To lose one's health renders science null, art inglorious, strength unavailing, wealth useless, and eloquence powerless." Herophilus, c. 300 B.C.

Day One:

- Begins with the evening meal. Drink an 8 oz glass of water first with 2 Juice Plus+® Garden Blend capsules.
- Salad only — lots of raw greens, sprouts, celery, carrots, cherry tomatoes, parsley, watercress, green and red peppers, and cucumbers.
- Add small amounts of Udo's Oil Blend (a combination of oils in one bottle, combining the correct balance of omega 3, 6, and 9 fatty acids, together with the other essential fatty acids — distributed by Flora, Inc.), apple cider vinegar or balsamic vinegar, hummus, sesame, pumpkin and sunflower seeds, and pine nuts.
- Enjoy as you chew very slowly and with intention. Follow about ½ hour later with a very warm bath, with or without Epsom salts.

Day Two:

- Water first. Drink 8 oz with 2 Juice Plus+® Orchard Blend capsules.
- Fruit next — a variety of fruits in season (slices or chunks of cantaloupe, watermelon, strawberries, tangerines, oranges, various berries, etc.).
- Follow with a small green salad (using the same ingredients as the evening before).

Lunch & Dinner:

- Water first — 8 oz with 2 Juice Plus+® Garden Blend capsules before Dinner.
- Then have a salad (see the evening of Day One for details).

Days Three & Four:

- Water first — Always 8 oz with 2 Juice Plus+® Orchard Blend Capsules in the morning.
- Fresh processed (in Vita-Mix if possible) whole fruit juice — one fruit only.

Every two hours after that you need to have each of the following in this order:

- ✓ 1 oz of Udo's Oil
- ✓ 1-2 oz of wheat grass juice or Perfect Food by Garden of Life (green powder mixed into 8 oz of water)
- ✓ 1 cup of fresh watermelon Juice (make in Vita-Mix machine so that nothing is thrown out)
- ✓ Another shot of Udo's Oil
- ✓ Another shot of wheatgrass juice or glass of Perfect Food & 2 Juice Plus+® Garden Blend capsules
- ✓ A cup of fresh processed (in Vita-Mix if possible) whole food vegetable juice (include some carrots, celery, cucumbers, watercress and parsley, any one of or combination of these.

Days Five & Six:

The same as Days Three and Four with one exception:

Add a smoothie midday, of one of the following combinations (processed in a Vita-Mix for best consistency):

a) ½ avocado, about 10 almonds (soaked overnight), ½ fresh green apple with skin on, and a drop of liquid stevia to sweeten. You can add one of the 1 oz shots of Udo's Oil to this smoothie.

b) ½ avocado, 1 fresh peach, a handful of sunflower, pumpkin and sesame seeds (all soaked overnight), and a drop of stevia to sweeten if necessary. Udo's Oil can be added to this.

c) ½ avocado, about 10 almonds (soaked overnight), and 2 fresh carrots. Add a drop of stevia if necessary.

Day Seven:

Repeat the program outlined for Day Two.

And After Day 7 — Now What . . .

Remember to come off the cleanse slowly — no animal proteins at all for the first 3-5 days, if at all. And keep soy protein and legumes (beans, peas, and lentils) to a minimum for the initial 3 days following the cleanse. Take a good bifidus supplement (I strongly recommend BB536 probiotic by Morinaga Nutritionals — www.morinu.com — and see the chapter, **Dr. Joyce Recommends** . . . for more on probiotics and BB536) after you have completed the detox. This is especially important after you have completed a series of colonics, should you choose to incorporate colonics over the week. The minimum recommended is 3 colonics over the 7 days.

Cheers to your renewed health and vitality!! And who knows — you may even drop a few of those unwanted pounds that have snuck up on you lately! You will definitely feel a lot lighter and cleaner from the inside out, and your increased alertness, focus and concentration may just astound you. Your life may never be the same again!

A Note on Toxic Emotions:

Not many people can look and feel vibrant and fully alive while feeling anxious depressed or stressed. It is critical to address the problems in your life that may be prematurely aging you. Many times we are carrying suppressed feelings in our subconscious mind that we are not even aware of on a conscious level. It is crucial to uncover these feelings because there is also an emotional aspect to detoxifying the body. And often, when we are going through a detox program, feelings of grief, sadness, or anger may surface during your cleanse. This is perfectly normal. If you experience "toxic emotions," let them come to the surface, acknowledge them, and then let them go. That way you can rid your body of any negative suppressed feelings.

It's important to plan your cleanse when you have time to rejuvenate. Plan to incorporate time for reflection, meditation, or a quiet hobby like reading. Stretching or yoga will help calm emotional upsets and help keep you from reabsorbing toxins in your tissues. And remember to reflect on your experiences and make a decision, in advance of beginning the program, to fully enjoy every step of the journey. As with everything in life, and especially during a cleanse, it is not the end that is important, but rather, the journey and all of the unique experiences you will have along this 7 day path.

Phase 3 — Transition into Lifetime Healthy Habits

Here are some general guidelines and suggestions for continued success in keeping your newly cleansed and rejuvenated body functioning optimally, while efficiently balancing your immune system. Read ALL guidelines before beginning. And have fun with this flexible, adaptable program! It is a *choice-based system*, designed to fit into your lifestyle/pattern of eating. You will find everything you need too succeed throughout the pages of this book.

➢ Use attractive plates and bowls. This lifts your spirits when eating.

- ➢ Take small bites, chew food slowly and thoroughly; savor every bite.
- ➢ Drink non-caffeinated herbal teas without sweeteners of any kind and natural unsweetened mineral waters, as desired throughout the day. Other alternatives: Pero or Postum (coffee substitutes), seltzer water, organic Swiss water-processed, or water-processed, decaffeinated coffee, if drinking coffee at all.
- ➢ If you drink caffeinated coffee, limit your intake to a maximum of one to two cups per day, and again, only organic.
- ➢ Drink eight 8-12 oz glasses of water throughout the day. The herbal teas and natural mineral waters can be substituted for the water. It is also OK to add fresh squeezed lemon juice or lime juice to teas and waters.
- ➢ Drink no water or other liquids with meals; only 15-30 minutes before, or 1 hour after.
- ➢ Drink green tea at least once per day, preferably young loose leaves. A good brand is Dragonwell from China.
- ➢ Avoid tobacco and soft drinks, and limit caffeine from any source.
- ➢ Limit alcohol consumption to a maximum of 1 drink per day, preferably wine or beer. It is high in empty calories that turn quickly to sugar in your body (cancer feeds on sugar), low in nutrition.
- ➢ Increase activity any way you can. Include aerobics, stretching and outdoor activities. Recommend at least a 15-30-minute walk / run every morning and / or evening.

Other strategies:

- Walk or run upstairs whenever possible
- Park car a farther distance from destination
- Put some music on and move to it
- Take a walk during lunch break / Go for a swim
- Jump rope — the new rage / Find a buddy to stretch with
- Bounce for 5 Minutes on a Rebounder (www.reboundair.com)

- ➢ For a meal on the run fresh fruit with an 8 oz carton of nonfat yogurt or soymilk, or 1-½ oz of organic low fat cheese. Best brands of yogurt, organic milk and soymilk: Trader Joe's, Alta Dena, Mountain High, Continental, Brown Cow, Nancy's, Silk, Horizon.
- ➢ For an evening snack the best choices are fresh fruit or fruit sorbet (blend fruit with ice).
- ➢ Limit pasta intake to a maximum of 2 times per week, *only whole grain*, i.e. quinoa, spelt.
- ➢ Limit red meats, including beef, pork and lamb, to a maximum of 2 servings per month, free-range, organic (no hormones/

antibiotics). 1 serving of any meat is equal to 4-5 oz for women, 5-6 oz for men.

➢ Buy nothing with more than *3 grams fat per serving* listed on the label (see Chapter on *Get the Skinny on Fats*).

➢ Choose meats, including fish, which are baked, broiled, roasted, grilled, steamed, or stir-fried without oils or fats.

➢ Sauté or stir-fry foods in stock or water instead of oil.

➢ Marinate meat, chicken, turkey, fish, tofu, or tempeh in broth, lemon juice, flavored vinegars (avoid distilled), nonfat yogurt, tomato or vegetable juice, instead of oil.

➢ Determine your unhealthy trigger foods, if you have any, such as ice cream, chocolate, chips, nuts, cheese, cookies, etc. And do not buy them or keep them in your home.

➢ If dessert is a must, finish your meal with fresh fruit, ½ cup fruit sorbet (blend fruit with ice), ½ cup nonfat frozen yogurt, plain kefir, or a fruity iced tea lightly sweetened with 1 tsp pure maple syrup, or Organic Sucanat, or Stevia.

➢ When eating out, follow the guidelines and suggestions in the Eating on the Run Chapter.

➢ If you indulge beyond the recommended proportions or range of foods recommended, enjoy that meal or that snack, and get back on track with the next meal. *One meal or snack will not destroy all of your previous efforts or your health!*

Always, Always . . .

Visualize and _feel_ yourself reaching and maintaining your goal of being clean from the inside out and optimally healthy.

Now, go to the 30-Day menu plans to choose the healthy breakfast, lunch and dinner choices that will inspire you to stay on track every day. And then email us (marilyn@marilynjoyce.com) or call us (800-352-3443) to tell us about your experiences during and after your detoxification program. Plan a cleanse at least once a year!

A WORD ABOUT SUPPLEMENTS

As this is a book focused on real, predominantly living foods, healthy eating, and healthy lifestyle and attitude practices, I do not plan to devote much space to a discussion on supplements. However, because the question of whether or not to incorporate their use into a healthy nutritionally fit program always comes up, along with the question, *if so, what and how much,* it is apparently an important enough issue to at least provide a few basic guidelines.

The truth is that everyone's body is different, with varying requirements for each of the multitude of nutrients. And when an individual follows a dietary regime that is predominantly made up of living foods, such as fresh fruits and vegetables, whole, unprocessed or minimally processed grains, and cultured foods, e.g. tempeh, miso and yogurt, not only are most, if not all, of their needs met, but the body becomes so tuned into its own needs that it signals deficiencies through cravings for certain healthy foods, or reacts negatively to the intake of others. To determine the specific requirements of an individual, the services of a qualified health professional, such as a Registered Dietitian, or an MD who specializes in nutrition, or a related health practitioner with a background in biochemistry and human nutrition, and perhaps a strong working knowledge of herbs, should be employed.

In my practice, I believe that it is often necessary to incorporate *some* additional supplemental therapy, and generally only for a specific period of time, depending on the individual's unique health situation. Therefore, I regularly recommend a variety of basic supplements, along with a whole food-based nutritional support system, and the fairly radical shift in nutritional intake outlined in *CULINARY STRATEGIES AND TOOLS FOR SUCCESS*. Some reasons for implementing such guidelines are as follows:

1. Almost everyone I see in my own practice has been on a nutritionally deficient dietary regime for years prior to our work together.
2. There is a need for a reduced caloric intake below the recommended level for optimum nutritional support, in order to reduce and balance the individual's weight.

3. The client has just been diagnosed with moderate to severe symptoms of a degenerative illness, such as heart disease, stroke, cancer, diabetes, chronic fatigue syndrome, arthritis, or AIDS.
4. Any combination of the above listed factors.

I will stress here, however, that under no circumstances should nutritional supplements replace a balanced intake of healthy, wholesome, and simply prepared foods. The word **supplement** means just that, a "desirable addition" (as defined by Webster's dictionary) to whatever else you are including. Supplement does not mean, "on its own!" *It is to be taken with something.*

Furthermore, supplements are made up of micronutrients, including vitamins, minerals, antioxidants, and phytochemicals, which are so small they can only be seen by the eye under a microscope. These tiny molecules require macronutrients, the proteins, carbohydrates and fats in our foods, which are visible to the eye, to carry them throughout the body to the places where they are needed. In other words, they are carried to the body's many cellular factories, for breakdown into even more microscopic molecules, to be used for the millions of bodily metabolic processes.

So you see, **if you wake up and swallow a handful of supplements with a cup of coffee every morning, you are as good as flushing those nutrients down the toilet!** They have nothing to work with. I cannot begin to count the number of clients who, after only one month of incorporating this change into their morning regime, i.e. taking their supplements with food instead of on an empty stomach, report increased energy and a greater sense of well-being! Why not try it and see for yourself?

As far as what supplements to take, why, and when, see the chapter, **Dr Joyce Recommends** . . . As you will notice with almost everything I recommend, there is an emphasis on whole-food based products. You will understand why when you read the details in the two chapters referenced in this paragraph. And with so much scientific research and information supporting the daily need for antioxidants, phytochemicals (plant chemicals), bioflavonoids, and enzymes, I always encourage the regular and consistent inclusion of **The Best Nutritional Support System I Know Of** (chapter.)

For supplements, as with diet, quality, not quantity, is the principle!

THE BEST NUTRITIONAL SUPPORT SYSTEM I KNOW OF!

You know how we always hear and read about how we all need to eat a lot more fruits and vegetables everyday, especially a wide variety of different colored fruits and vegetables?
Well, if I could show you a way to get a lot more fruits and veggies into your diet everyday, in just 2 easy one-minute steps per day, would that be of interest to you?

If your answer is yes, and I expect it is, read on.

Whole Food Nutritional Support System Versus Fractionated, Isolated Nutrients

Let's start with vitamin and mineral isolates. What are they? Well, if we take an orange and examine what's in it, we know that it is a great source of Vitamin C, as well as about 10,000 other nutrients, that work together with each other synergistically to make each of them more available to, and usable by, your body. In Nature, you will never find fractionated (a tiny fraction of the whole), isolated (separating out from, and keeping apart from, the whole) Vitamin C, or any other nutrient for that matter, out there on its own, in high concentrations. Everything in Nature seeks balance, not potency — never too much of any one thing! And on a cellular level, the body does not recognize Vitamin C on its own. It recognizes real food with all of the thousands of nutrients working together in synergy.

Now, let's look at a Vitamin C tablet with just Vitamin C in it. Is this tablet a whole food? Obviously not! The active ingredient, Vitamin C in this case, had to be removed from the orange synthetically, in a laboratory, and then formulated into a tablet or capsule. And then fillers and other ingredients are added that are *not* essential, and may be harmful over time, for your body. All of the 10,000 or so essential nutrients, such as bioflavonoids, enzymes, fiber, and other vitamins, minerals, antioxidants, and phytochemicals, are missing. So, in fact, what you are taking is just one ingredient from the orange. And that one ingredient has been synthetically processed and placed in an unnatural environment. Let' see — 10,000 nutrients in a natural environment versus one nutrient in an unnatural environment — this, to me, is a no brainer! How could one lonely, synthetically processed nutrient ever accomplish what 10,000 natural nutrients, working synergistically together, can do!

Merck Index Discusses Absorption of Vitamin Pills!

According to the Merck Index, the go-to reference guide for generations of health professionals looking for precise, comprehensive information on chemicals, drugs, and biologicals, less than 10% of the vitamins and minerals in supplement form are absorbable by our bodies. Whole foods, by comparison, are generally about 60 to 70 percent absorbable, and assimilable. So, just because you may have a lot of a particular nutrient circulating in your bloodstream, at any given moment, does not mean these fractionated nutrients are reaching the cellular level for absorption and assimilation. More and more research today is determining that disease states are positively impacted to a much greater degree, by eating whole foods, than by the ingestion of isolated nutrients. In fact, there appears to be an increased risk of certain illnesses from taking mega-doses of specific nutrients. Too much of any one thing, whatever it is, will eventually, over time, throw our bodies out of balance. Again, it is all about *Balance*! Everything in the universe — *and your body is its own universe* — strives for homeostasis, or balance.

3 Important Questions That Need to be Addressed

The challenges for most of us today are many, when it comes to eating an abundance of healthy, natural whole foods, including predominantly vegetables, fruits, whole grains, and legumes. We have all heard continually, in the news, that a plant-based diet is by far the most beneficial for optimal, vibrant health and longevity.

> ➢ Yet, can we be assured that the foods we are eating are of high quality are and grown in nutrient-dense soil? The answer to that question is emphatically NO! According to USDA data collected on the nutrient content of 43 fruit and vegetable crops, over the 50-year period between 1950 and 1999, six out of 13 nutrients examined, had declined significantly in value. Donald R. Davis, a research associate with the Biochemical Institute at the University of Texas, in Austin, also found that three minerals, phosphorous, iron and calcium, declined between 9 percent and 16 percent, protein declined 6 percent, riboflavin declined 38 percent, and ascorbic acid, the precursor of vitamin C, declined 15 percent. In Britain, a study of the mineral content of fruits and vegetables grown between 1930 and 1980, showed a similar decrease in nutrient density. Significantly lower levels of calcium, magnesium, copper and sodium were found in vegetables, and significantly lower levels of magnesium, iron, copper and potassium were found in fruit.

> And then the next question we need to ask is whether the produce is picked at the peak of ripeness or not. The answer to that is also NO! Produce is generally picked green and shipped over days and weeks to its destination, where it looks pretty on the shelf, but has very little of the nutritional density it was meant to develop at the peak of ripeness on the vine, tree or in the ground. Produce picked green never fully ripens; it simply softens over time. And of course, if it is not organic, you have to be very careful to wash it thoroughly to remove the many pesticides and herbicides. Be aware, that those chemicals get into the seeds during the growth and development phases of the produce, so you must avoid eating the seeds at any cost. That's a tragedy, since the seeds are so packed full of nutrition in their own right!

> Finally, are you attempting to prepare healthy, wholesome meals everyday? Or are you so spent, fatigued, and completely pooped at the end of the day, that it's way too much effort even just to think about creating a healthy meal? Have you simply given in to the fast food / drive through / frozen meal / canned and packaged foods, way of life, believing that you have no other option?

Well, the fact is, that without your health you have nothing! Health is a "pay me now" or "pay me later" proposition. I know this all too well! The devastating personal journey I experienced with cancer clearly taught me that the more we invest in our health today, the better our payoff will be as we age! We not only feel better physically. But we also experience a better quality of life, and will likely live longer to boot.

Challenge: A Living Body Needs Living Foods to be Fully Alive . . .

Unfortunately, the foods we grab on the run, overall, are the very foods that drain our body's energy resources. They have no life force of their own. In other words, most of those packaged, processed foods are seriously nutrition deficient! And in many cases, almost completely devoid of any nutrients necessary for normal healthy growth! And folks, in case you have forgotten, or are not aware, this body you live in is very much a "living" organism. And it needs living foods to support its existence! Furthermore, the research is globally conclusive. What foods do we need in order to protect our health, and prevent disease, so that we can fully and vibrantly enjoy our lives and our careers? We read about them constantly. We hear about them in the news almost daily! Even the World Health Organization is standing behind the need for more of these foods — not supplements — in our diet.

What are these foods? Well, let me repeat what I wrote a few paragraphs ago: vegetables, fruits, grains and legumes (beans, peas, lentils)! Why these foods? For the thousands of antioxidants, phytochemicals, bioflavonoids, enzymes and fiber, that neutralize the free radicals that contribute to the rampant illnesses and diseases so prevalent today, such as cancer, heart disease, MS, fibromyalgia, lupus, diabetes, Parkinson's, arthritis, kidney disease, chronic fatigue syndrome; and the list goes on . . .

Very healthy cultures, such as the Okinawans in Japan, and the Hunzas in the Himalayas, eat 10 to 14 servings of fruits and vegetables every day. Despite the well documented "5 a day campaign", which had been around for more than a decade in North America, we are not even close to getting the minimum recommendations! And now the recommendation has been increased to 9-13 servings of fresh, raw vegetables and fruits every day! Eating fresh fruits and vegetables daily is always the best way to go. The reality is that no one is doing this! And, as I discussed above, the research proves that vitamin pills, overall, don't work. So what can we do instead?

Though I am a diehard advocate for eating vital living foods that provide the wide range of essential nutrients, I have personally incorporated an outstanding nutritional support system into my daily regime for more than eight years now. That nutritional support system is called Juice Plus+®, the number one, best selling, encapsulated nutritional system in the world. I originally added Juice Plus+® to my personal nutritional program simply for a little extra health insurance. However, I am healthier today, despite being on the road continually, than I have ever been before!

I Was a Hard Sell — It Took Me 3 Years To Look At This Nutritional Support System!

For years, since Juice Plus+® first entered the market in 1993, people would constantly approach me at many of my seminars around the country, telling me how this "amazing" product was *the* perfect match for me with what I was teaching — eat whole foods, with an emphasis on raw produce, and avoid commercial packaged, canned, and bottled foods. As a health professional with a heavy emphasis on biochemistry, I was not interested in, what I thought was, yet another testimonial based product. Without fail, when I asked for research, on those testimonial based products, I would receive a big packet of testimonial letters. And if there was any so-called research, it was generally all done by one doctor or researcher. I was not about to throw away my hard earned credentials for any flash-in-the-pan, miracle cure for everything, from arthritis to cancer to . . .

Well, that changed in July of 1999, the day I finally opened the packet that I had received 3 years earlier — that's right 3 years! I had filed it away for 2 years in a file cabinet — I'm still not certain why I initially kept the packet, unopened as it was. And then, having developed a friendship over those 2 years, with the compassionate and truly caring woman who had sent this information to me, I put that packet in the next best place for filing things — under my bed! (I had been cleaning out my file cabinets, and found this packet still unopened!) Now, well hidden under my bed — the packet stayed there for yet another year.

If my cleaning lady, at the time, had not insisted that I get rid of the many mounds of paper everywhere, I am not certain when I may have opened that packet. But I can assure you, I am so happy that I did. And I wish I had done it years earlier. Oh well, as the saying goes, it's all about timing. Yes, Juice Plus+® made sense to me. However, I personally had to see valid, independent, third party, peer-reviewed, scientific research, which was documented in major scientific publications. You cannot buy your way into such publications! And it had to be done by respected scientists, at respected institutions, and preferably globally represented.

To my surprise, Juice Plus+® had all of that, even then; though nothing compared to what it has today. It has been researched by some of the most respected scientists in the world, at many of the most respected institutions in the world. The research is indisputable and expansive. For more information, on the science of Juice Plus+®, and to make a more informed decision about whether or not Juice Plus+® is for you, contact the person who gave you this book or: visit: www.DrJoyce4Nutrition.com and review the science for yourself. Read the research. Watch the videos. Don't take my word for it! I honestly believe that every single person on the planet would significantly benefit from embracing a healthy, whole food based, nutrition program, lots of purified water, a simple exercise regime, scheduled relaxation and meditation — and Juice Plus+®.

What's The Secret to the Effectiveness of Juice Plus+®?

The secret behind the scientifically proven effectiveness of Juice Plus+® is that it is NOT made up of a large amount of a few separate, isolated nutrients, but contains a little of everything from the 7 fruits, 8 vegetables, and 2 grains, that comprise Juice Plus+®. In other words, it contains a *balance* of all of the thousands of inherent nutritional essences available in these 17 foods. And of course, a substantial amount of the fiber has been removed. (Can you imagine what would happen if you were getting all of that fiber from 17 different fruits and vegetables? I see a long line-up at the rest room!!) Bioavailability, or the synergistic effect found in fruits and vegetables, is missing in vitamin capsules and tablets. We do not compare Juice Plus+® to fragmented vitamin tablets, since such a comparison would be meaningless. It would be like comparing apples and the fruit crates they come in!

I'm On It For Life!

Okay, so why, after all these years, do I continue to take Juice Plus+®, and recommend it to all of my clients and patients, and basically everyone I know? Easy answer! In this day and age, I know of no one who is eating 9-13 servings of fresh, raw fruits and vegetables every single day. Nor are they eating the variety of different fresh fruits and vegetables available in Juice Plus+®, on a daily basis! I eat better than most people I know, or work with, in my busy client/patient practice, and there's no way I can achieve this everyday, especially with respect to variety. Juice Plus+® is simply a very convenient and very inexpensive way to bridge the whole food nutritional gap between what we *are* eating and what we *should be* eating on a daily basis!

So that's where — and why — Juice Plus+® fits in.

So, What's In It & How is it Made?

Juice Plus+® is made from the juices of fresh, high quality, picked at the peak of ripeness, fruits and vegetables, and contains many thousands of vitamins, minerals, antioxidants, phytochemcals, bioflavonoids, enzymes, and some of the fiber present in the original produce. This is in contrast to vitamin pills and tablets that contain only a few vitamins, etc. in fragmented (a few tiny parts separated out from the whole) and unnatural ratios. Nowhere in nature will you find a food that has the vitamin content of a vitamin pill. To protect the purity of Juice Plus+®, it is tested very carefully, throughout every step of production to insure the integrity and value of the product. Using a proprietary water removal system, low temperatures, and an oxygen-free environment, the fruits and vegetables are juiced to extract their nutritional essences, and then reduced to a powder. The ingredients in Juice Plus+® are never exposed to high heat during the manufacturing process, which would destroy the enzymes and other heat-soluble nutrients, such as the B-vitamins and Vitamin C, and who knows what else we will discover in the next 10-20 years!

So, Let's Get Real . . .

Now, let me add a very important disclaimer here. In no way am I saying Juice Plus+® is a cure-all, a magic bullet, or a solution to an illness. I learned, during my journey back to wellness from cancer, that no such things are available. Getting healthy, or getting well from an illness, depends on you making changes in everything in your life — food, exercise, breathing, sleeping enough, effectively handling stress, taking time out to be with your family and friends, relaxation, quiet time with yourself, and an adjustment in attitude, towards yourself and others. In other words — *Balance!* That's right: *Life Balance!*

Simply put, based on the depth and breadth of research, Juice Plus+® is the next best thing to fresh fruits and vegetables, in a convenient, easy to use, form (capsules, chewables, and gummies), that provides some health insurance against the ravages of our hectic stress-filled lifestyles and food grabbed on the run. You can rest knowing that you have taken at least one solid step toward positively caring for your body, and protecting your health against disease.

So, Now Here's The Easy Part We Talked About at the Start of This Chapter! (This is exactly what I *personally* do every day!)

On a count of three, are you ready for one of those 2 one-minute steps per day?

Ready, set, go . . .
Start your stopwatch . . .

Fill a glass with 8 oz of water. Take 2 red capsules out of the red bottle (Orchard Blend) in the morning, and swallow the capsules with the water — a few minutes before breakfast. Stop the stopwatch! How long did it take? Told you — less than a minute, right?

The second step is the same as the first, except that you will take 2 green capsules out of the green bottle (Garden Blend) and swallow them with 8 oz of water a few minutes before dinner.

That's it! How quick — and easy — can it get?

But, of course, just for the record, you can take Juice Plus+® anywhere, anytime. You can mix them up or take the greens in the morning and the reds at night, instead of the reds in the morning and the greens at night. Though I believe it is best to take Juice Plus+® just before eating with water, you can basically take it with or without the addition of food. Everybody is different — and as the saying goes, *"different strokes for different folks!"*

Like we said: quick and easy healthy strategies that can be done by anyone, anywhere, anytime! *Wow, what a concept!*

DR JOYCE RECOMMENDS . . .

I primarily focus on, and work with, whole food-based nutritional support systems and supplementation, versus vitamin, mineral, antioxidant and/or phytochemical formulations, which generally contain mega-doses of only a few nutrients. Also by using this form of supplementation, there is much less likelihood of throwing the body's delicate homeostasis out of balance. In the long run, this will protect the body against the ravages of oxidative stress. In other words, the over-production of free radicals, the underlying cause of all degenerative illnesses!

A growing body of independent, peer-reviewed, clinical, scientific research indicates that the nutrients in whole foods are apparently much more bioavailable to the body than fractionated, isolated, individual nutrients. And hence, they are more readily usable by your body for the thousands of metabolic functions carried out by the body everyday. Refer to the chapter: *The Best Nutritional Support System I Know Of!*

So, with that in mind, following are a few of the nutritional products that I incorporate into the various protocols I have developed for myself and my clients. I will emphasize that in no way do I consider any of the following a replacement for making wise food choices on a daily basis. These are simply added insurance to cover for those days when we inevitably, can't, won't, or don't get all the nutrition we need from the food we eat.

For a complete summary of the basic nutritional support system protocol that I generally recommend go to the end of this chapter.

Juice Plus+® — The Next Best Thing To Fresh Fruits and Vegetables!

As I explained in the previous chapter, Juice Plus+® is not a supplement, as traditionally defined. It is a nutritional support system, basically powdered produce, with most of the sugar, salt and calories eliminated. In other words, you are getting most of the good stuff while eliminating most of the bad stuff. Juice Plus+® maintains, in its production, the wide variety of naturally occurring vitamins, minerals, phytochemicals and antioxidants, as well as active enzymes, some fiber, and chlorophyll*, the substance that makes green plants, green. (For more on this, and other important aspects of Juice Plus+®, visit the website of the creator of these remarkable fruit and vegetable powders at www.smokeysantillo.com.) And Juice Plus+® is labeled as food, not as a supplement. It is, most often referred to, by researchers and health practitioners, as fruit and vegetable concentrates, concentrated fruit and vegetable powders, or whole food-based concentrates.

At this point you must be curious about what makes up Juice Plus+®. Well, it is essentially 7 fruits, 8 vegetables and 2 grains, divided into two types of capsules. One type is called the Orchard Blend (red capsules), and contains the nutritional essences of the following fruits: apple, orange, pineapple, cranberry, peach, papaya and acerola cherry. The other type is called the Garden Blend (green capsules), and is made from the following vegetables: carrots, beets, broccoli, cabbage, kale (When did you last eat raw kale, the number one cancer fighter?), parsley, spinach, tomato, oat bran and brown rice bran. Juice Plus+® is available in Gummies for very young children (And even *big kids* of all ages!), Chewables for older children and adults, and capsules for teenagers and adults (and any child who prefers capsules to chewables).

Juice Plus+® is not a replacement for eating fresh raw fruits and vegetables every day. It is simply a convenient and inexpensive way to add more of the essential nutrients from a wide variety of some of the most nutritionally dense fresh produce and grains available, on a daily basis. And the best news for all of us striving to maintain a plant-based diet is that Juice Plus+® bridges the gap between what we do eat and what we should be eating.

For more information on the science behind Juice Plus+®, and to make a more informed decision about whether or not Juice Plus+® is for you, contact the person who gave you this book, or who invited you to the presentation where you purchased this book, or visit: www.DrJoyce4Nutrition.com; read about the extensive research done with Juice Plus+® and listen to what a variety of leading experts in various fields of health have to say about these fruit and vegetable concentrates.

Juice Plus+® Vineyard Blend

With all of the growing research today focused on the multitude of health benefits derived from berries and grapes, it made sense for NSA to create a berry-based concentrate, in alignment with the original fruit and vegetable concentrate. Also labeled as food, versus a supplement, it was specifically formulated with cardiovascular health in mind. And processed in the same manner as Juice Plus+®, it maintains the maximum nutritional value possible.

The Juice Plus+® Vineyard Blend provides the nutritional essences of 9 varieties of the freshest, highest quality berries and grapes available, including blueberries, blackberries, bilberries, raspberries, cranberries, elderberries, black currents, red currents, and Concord grapes. It also contains a proprietary blend of natural powders and extracts derived from artichoke, green tea, grape seed, grape skin, and gingerroot.

Research to date has indicated that the blood vessels of subjects on a protocol incorporating both Juice Plus+® and the Juice Plus+® Vineyard Blend, compared to subjects receiving placebo capsules, were much better able to respond to blood flow changes following a high fat meal. Instead of the 4-hour impaired response to blood flow after a high fat meal, previously reported by Maryland Researchers, the Juice Plus+® group demonstrated significantly improved circulation. Who do you know who may truly benefit from improved circulation? Look around you — with rampant obesity, a concentration of high fat and high sugar meals, paired with lack of activity, poor circulation is generally the sad result! And it can be fatal!

For clarification here, Juice Plus+® and Juice Plus+® Vineyard Blend always provide the foundation for every program I develop, since together, they include a wonderful variety of fruits and vegetables, providing the complete rainbow of colors necessary for optimum health. And they have sound science to support their inclusion in the diet of everyone I know and work with!

Juice Plus+® Complete

Juice Plus+® Complete is a revolutionary all-natural, identity preserved soy-based, non-dairy, whole food blend of fruit and vegetable powders, natural carbohydrates, vegetable proteins, dietary fiber, extra vitamins and minerals and plant food enzymes. At a base caloric rate of only 110 calories per serving, plus whatever you mix with it (fruit, soymilk, nut-butters, seeds, etc.), it will not likely take a caloric toll with your nutritional regime. It contains no caffeine, sucrose, saturated fat, cholesterol, artificial sweeteners, flavors or preservatives. It is free of corn, wheat, yeast, egg and milk products. And with its proprietary blend of active plant enzymes it is uniquely bioavailable; therefore, easily digested and assimilated by the body.

As part of a healthy weight management program, a complete meal replacement strategy for weight loss, a breakfast on the go, a busy executive's nutritional jumpstart or pickup for the day, a pre-exercise energy boost or a post-workout recovery program, this versatile nutritional powder is an economical foundation for a balanced, healthy and sensible nutritional program for life.

And with 24 grams of isoflavones per serving from soy protein, it may protect against heart disease, as well as protect the health of women of all ages, particularly the baby boomer generation. One serving, not including whatever you may add to it, such as soymilk or organic milk, contains 50% of the RDI for calcium, in a very bioavailable form. Add some *rebounding* on a daily basis, plus some work with the *resistance bands* (see Chapter on **Fit In Fitness** for more details on these amazing exercise systems) and you have the foundation for a healthy bone-building protocol!

So what are you waiting for? Get a JUMP on your day — and get a JUMP in your step, with this great tasting, nutritionally loaded liquid meal! For lots of great recipes using Juice Plus+® Complete, visit <u>www.icantbelieveitstofu.com</u> and get a copy of "I Can't Believe It's Tofu!" in a downloadable PDF format right away. Sign up for the **Tofu Wizard 4 Fun & Health** *Special Report* and receive new ideas and recipes.

Juice Plus+® Thins

I have a personal story to share regarding this Juice Plus+® product. Years ago, when I finally incorporated Juice Plus+® into my own daily protocol, I really did not see the value of the Juice Plus+® Thins for me personally. I had assumed, from the little I had read about this product, that they were basically for people who wanted to lose weight. A few months later I was traveling by plane, with an associate, to another state to facilitate a series of presentations. It was an early AM flight, and I had not taken time to eat anything before racing to the airport. So, I found myself on the plane, famished. You know that feeling I'm talking about? Way beyond hunger!

The flight attendant delivered a small packet of peanuts to each of us — first thing in the morning!! I looked with disdain at this tiny bag of salty, hydrogenated fatty offerings. My associate saw my look of disapproval and offered me some of her Juice Plus+® Thins. I said, *"No thank you!"* I was not trying to lose weight. She assured me that this was not her intent either, and that she ate them when flying in order to appease her hunger with some nutrition, while avoiding the over-processed offerings on most planes. For a short while I resisted. But eventually, the power of my hunger took over. Three Juice Plus+® Thins and a glass of water, and I felt like a new woman. And I got my chocolate fix at the same time, without all of the fat and cholesterol usually found in the chocolate!

Note: For all of you out there, who don't like chocolate, have no fear. The Juice Plus+® Thins come in an apple cinnamon flavor as well.

Now, and for years since that experience, I have carried Juice Plus+® Thins with me on almost every flight. And in fact, everywhere I go! The combination of the soluble and insoluble fibers, along with the chromium and other nutrients included, help to regulate the insulin function, which in turn regulates our blood sugar levels and fat storage. The result: reduced hunger and reduced food cravings. The Juice Plus+® Thins are a wonderful way to add more fiber to a generally fiber-deficient diet. I recommend that you enjoy 2 to 4 Juice Plus+® Thins, with 8 ounces of water, anytime you are hungry between meals. They will stave off hunger, maintain or raise your energy level, and keep your blood sugar levels balanced. It is critical to drink water with the Thins, since fiber requires water in order to do its work. Fiber, without adequate water, can lead to constipation and other digestive distress.

For more information on each of the Juice Plus+® products discussed above, contact the person who gave you this book, or who invited you to the presentation where you purchased this book, or visit: www. DrJoyce4Nutrition.com. You can also email us at: marilyn@marilynjoyce. com. Or call us at 800-352-3443, if you do not have email.

Probiotics — So, How's Your Gut Feeling Today?

When we think of bacteria, we generally associate them with infections, and consider bacteria to be "bad" for us. However, more than 100 different species of microbes naturally inhabit our digestive and intestinal mucosa (the entire lining of the digestive and intestinal walls, from the mouth to the anus). The mucosal microflora (microscopic bacteria) includes beneficial, harmful, and neutral, bacteria. These bacteria are in constant conflict, which we refer to as being dynamic, or continually active. This activity maintains balance, or homeostasis. However, if just one harmful bacteria, such as E.Coli, or H.Pylori, dominates, we can become very ill. And the fact is, that the number and delicate balance of, for example the intestinal microflora, can be disturbed by any number of circumstances, including the use of antibiotics or other prescribed drugs, substance abuse, such as alcohol, tobacco, and recreational drugs, inadequate nutrition, chronic stress, illness and disease, age, and exposure to toxic environmental substances.

And, for many of us born into the baby boomer era, antibiotics became a way of life. From early childhood on, any illness we contracted was treated with ever-stronger forms of antibiotic drugs. The sad part of this scenario was the fact that the more antibiotics we took, the more resistant our bodies became to the particular drugs available. So, stronger and stronger antibiotics had to be created for each new, and even more virulent, strain of an illness such as the flu.

Worse yet, the use of broad-spectrum antibiotics (those that kill many species of bacteria), became the standard and have often been misused, and definitely over-used, by the medical community as a cure-all for everything. And, at the same time, antibiotics, by their very nature, destroy the beneficial or healthy bacteria, in the digestive and intestinal mucosa. So, this resulting imbalance in the mucosal microflora, with a predominance of harmful bacteria, resulted in an increased susceptibility to whatever illness was "going around" at the time. A vicious cycle!

And that is not the end of the story! We do not get antibiotics simply from prescribed medications. A less obvious introduction of antibiotics into our bodies is that from the animal products we ingest. You read that right! Most of our meat, poultry and dairy products come from animals raised in huge commercial operations where they are pumped full of hormones and antibiotics. Every time you eat or drink an animal-based product, unless you have purchased it from a store that carries antibiotic and hormone-free products, you are risking the intake of even more of these harmful substances that destroy your normal digestive and intestinal flora.

The symptoms generally associated with the resulting imbalance of the digestive (including intestinal) microflora include the following:

> - Intermittent or recurrent diarrhea
> - Chronic indigestion and heartburn
> - Acid reflux
> - Bloating
> - Flatulence (gas)
> - Intermittent or chronic constipation
> - Yeast infections
> - Vaginitis and candidiasis
> - Bladder infections
> - Jock-itch and other skin rashes
> - Halitosis (bad breath)
> - Gingivitis (gum disease)
> - A sore throat
> - IBS (irritable bowel syndrome)
> - Inflammatory bowel diseases
> - Autoimmune arthritis
> - Immune function problems
> - Cancer, especially of the breast and colon

Unfortunately, the tendency in the medical establishment is to treat these symptoms with drugs, which generally only serve to prolong or worsen the particular condition. Depending on the severity of the condition, a digestive (including intestinal) mucosal system out of balance, often simply needs to be put back into balance with the addition of beneficial bacteria, and a nutritional program of whole foods, eliminating packaged, processed foods and beverages entirely.

We need beneficial intestinal microbes for various functions throughout the body:

> Efficient vitamin and mineral synthesis
> Prevention of infection
> Stimulation of the immune function
> Prevention of food allergies
> Repair of the digestive and intestinal mucosal (gut) lining
> Prevention of illness, due to an excessive accumulation of toxic pathogens and microbial toxins in the intestine.

Over our life span, the composition of the intestinal flora changes significantly. At birth, our intestine is free of microbes. However, research indicates that within 7 days after birth, the microflora is dominated by the bifidobacteria, simply referred to as Bifidus. Breastfeeding establishes a stable Bifidus-dominated intestinal environment. As we move through childhood, and into adulthood, the bifidobacteria gradually decreases as outside aerobic bacteria, such as E. Coli, and other killer germs, are introduced. And, as we get older, and move into late adulthood, the bifidobacteria decrease significantly in our intestinal mucosa, while harmful bacteria significantly increase.

So, what is the solution? I believe that we most definitely need to include probiotics in our daily nutritional arsenal if we want to maintain optimum health throughout our lifetime, especially as we age. Probiotics are a type of dietary supplement that contain potentially beneficial bacteria. They appear to assist the body's natural microflora in reestablishing and balancing themselves. Also foods such as yogurt, kefir, and milk, often contain probiotics. Just not enough to meet our growing needs, resulting from a lifetime of denatured foods and beverages, and a toxic environment! And if you choose a more plant-based diet, as I personally do — *and that is a healthy thing to do* — you may not be including dairy foods that have added probiotics.

I was very fortunate to have aligned myself many years ago, during my cancer journey, with a wonderful company that has consistently practiced the highest of integrity in the development of pure, excellent quality, non-genetically modified (non-GMO) products. Apart from the production of non-GMO tofu in the US by Morinaga Nutritionals Inc., the parent company in Japan has been the leader in the production of the one of the most scientifically researched probiotic strains in the world — Bifidobacteria longum BB536. Furthermore, for maximum absorption and utilization, this highly concentrated and stable Bifidus powder is housed in a specially formulated capsule that resists disruption in the acidic conditions of the stomach, and then easily dissolves in the non-acidic environment of the intestine. In other words, it gets where it has to go before the capsule breaks down. That's very important!

Though there are many probiotics in the world, our personal choice should take into account several factors. For maximum benefits, it must be confirmed stable and safe, non-GMO, and confirmed effective. Bifidus BB536 is well documented for each of these factors. And the published scientific research to date — from the 1970's to the present — has indicated the following outcomes for BB536:

➢ Improves the intestinal environment
➢ Improves regularity
➢ Helps support a healthy immune system
➢ Helps suppress infection
➢ Helps support healthy cell growth
➢ Helps to enhance bone strength
➢ May prevent diarrhea

As I stated in the previous chapter: **The Best Nutritional Support System I Know Of**, *there are no magic bullets in the nutrition and health arenas. Only sound whole food-based nutrition and healthy lifestyle practices! So, BB536 is not a cure-all; nor is it a magic bullet. It is simply the most scientifically researched probiotic I am aware of, and one that I include in my own daily program.*

For more detailed information you can go to www.morinu.com or call 800-NOW-TOFU, or click on the *"Links"* page at either www.5minutestohealth.com or www.icantbelieveitstofu.com and click on the appropriate button. You can also call us at 800-352-3443.

Udo's Choice® Oil Blend

It is very important to understand that not all fats are *bad*! In fact, good fats, known as essential fatty acids (EFAs) provide many benefits, such as increasing energy and vitality, and helping you to lose fat and build muscle. Therefore, I believe that Udo's Choice® Oil Blend is an essential daily addition to any serious nutritional program. We simply do not, on a daily basis, eat enough healthy fats in a balance that will create and maintain optimum health and vitality. And there are two EFAs that we must get from our foods—omega 3's and omega 6's. You can read all about fats and oils, and EFAs, in the Chapter: **Get the Skinny on Fats!**

Formulated by Udo Erasmus, PhD, renowned author and nutritionist, and world-renowned expert on dietary fats, this well-researched and thoroughly tested oil blend contains a balanced combination of cold-pressed, certified organic, all-natural, unrefined oils and nutritional co-factors. These include the oils of flax, sunflower, and sesame seeds, as well as evening primrose oil, coconut oil and the oils of the bran of rice and oats. This cold pressed oil blend is produced in an oxygen-free environment, with low heat and light, to maximize the nutritional value, stability and freshness of the product.

This oil should never be heated or cooked. And once opened, it should be used within 60 days, or 2 months. The oil is best purchased from a refrigerated case in a store. It is packaged in amber bottles and then boxed to protect the oil from heat, light and oxygen. Once home, it must be refrigerated at all times. To preserve its freshness for longer periods of time, you can freeze the oil. Since oil contracts (shrinks), versus expands, when it freezes, it is safe to freeze it in the glass bottle that it comes in. One to two tablespoons of Udo's oil per day will provide you with all of the EFAs you need. I use 1 tablespoon in my morning smoothie and 1 tablespoon on my evening salad. And the best part is the **WOW** factor. *People will constantly tell you how beautiful your skin looks!*

Perfect Food® — The Next Best Thing to Eating Grass

And who wants to eat grass? After years of growing, and juicing, wheatgrass and barley grass, I was so thoroughly done with all of that work. My lifestyle, like that of many of my clients and patients, is not conducive to this type of activity. Yet, we know from research that all of that "green stuff" is probably an excellent addition to our nutritional program. In my search for something of this nature, in a convenient form, for my clients and myself, this particular product found me. As you will read below, there are certain features in a green product that are essential. So far, this is the only super green food that has fully met with my personal standard and approval.

I often recommend Perfect Food®, produced by Garden of Life, to my clients and patients. It is what we generally refer to as a "super green food". I work with a wide variety of degenerative illnesses and many of them, such as cancer, do not thrive in an aerobic environment. So I feel that it is my responsibility, as an informed health practitioner, to provide as many tools as necessary to assist my client's/patient's body in producing a much more aerobic — oxygenated — environment.

Perfect Food®, is basically a whole food-based, primarily green plant-based, concentrate. Therefore, it is likely that it provides the thousands of nutrients inherent in the included foods, in a balance comparable to the way Mother Nature intended. It is a combination of organic greens, grains and seeds, including green grasses (e.g. wheat, oats, barley and alfalfa), spirulina, chlorella, kelp, and other sea vegetables, as well as enzymes. An important aspect of Perfect Food®, as a super green food, is its high chlorophyll* content (see the box*, below, discussing chlorophyll), which is what makes it so green. And this chlorophyll, in turn, enhances the body's uptake of oxygen, for more efficient and greater production of energy by the body, which then supports all of the many biochemical functions of the body!

It is important to understand that the Juice Plus® Garden Blend (green) is also a valuable source of chlorophyll. However, it also contains the thousands of other nutrients that are normally found in a wide variety of the vegetables we should be eating daily, but are not. For example, when was the last time you had kale on your plate, other than as a garnish? **So, Perfect Food® simply compliments Juice Plus+® — it does not replace it!**

One of the main reasons I include this specific green product with my clients, versus many of the other green products available, is because Perfect Food® does not contain any herbs. Herbs, in general, were not designed, by nature, to be included on a daily basis in your diet. They are similar to though weaker than pharmaceutical drugs. And, if used daily, your body will eventually build up a tolerance to the specific herb, such as Echinacea, Goldenseal, Ginko Biloba, etc. Therefore, when you really need their therapeutic effect, you simply won't get it. If you insist on including herbs in your daily regime, you need to work out a program for rotating your time on, and your time off of taking the herb. Seek the assistance of a qualified health professional in setting up this schedule.

Perfect Food® comes in two forms — caplets and loose green powder. Both are equally bioavailable. The powder is great for adding to a smoothie or a shake, sprinkling on a salad or soup, or for just adding to water. For some extra insurance, when I am under more stress than usual, I will often add it to my delicious daily smoothie (***You can enjoy my special immune-balancing, vitality building, delicious recipe included at the end of this chapter. And then subscribe to my INSTANT E.N.E.R.G.Y.™ site, packed full of lots of great recipes and healthy ideas, by going to:*** www.marilynjoyce.com. The caplets are great to carry with you if you are traveling or on the road a lot with your job, as I am. And they are best taken about 10-15 minutes before you eat with water. The water will activate the enzymes in Perfect Food®, which will then assist with the assimilation and absorption of the nutrients from the food you are about to eat. And you will also plump up the fiber, so that it can function fully to do its clean-up work throughout your entire digestive tract (from your mouth to your anus!).

The number to call, to find out who, in your area, carries this product, is (800) 622-8986. Or you can go to their website at www.gardenoflife.com. Like many other companies, they may recommend that you buy everything, or at least several of the products, that they have to offer. Again, please refer to a qualified health practitioner before you buy the store!

An Important Consideration: *A few carefully selected nutritional support products are generally all that one needs, along with a balanced intake of fresh vegetables, fruits, whole grains, legumes, raw nuts and seeds (and their fresh ground butters), unprocessed oils, and perhaps some cold-water/deep-water wild fish. Though, personally, I am not an advocate of animal food consumption, if you choose to include these foods, consider only grass-fed beef, free-range chicken and eggs, and wild game meat. Avoid all animal products, including fish, eggs and chicken, which have been antibiotic, and hormonally, injected or fed.*

---

*A word on chlorophyll:

Chlorophyll is essential for the body's optimal uptake of oxygen. It is the pigment in green plants that absorbs solar energy. It is to plants what blood is to humans! In fact, the chlorophyll molecule is chemically similar to the human red blood cell (hemoglobin), except that its central atom is magnesium, whereas iron is the central atom of the human blood cell. Chlorophyll is the first product of light, absorbing the sun's nutrients, and therefore, contains more light energy than any other element. It powers the plant. Chlorophyll is high in oxygen, is antibacterial, and research indicates that it may act as a body cleanser, rebuilder and neutralizer of toxins. With its apparent ability to break down poisonous carbon dioxide, it allows more absorption of oxygen into the bloodstream. So, when humans ingest chlorophyll, it appears to enrich and oxygenate the blood. Chlorophyll has also been shown to heighten the efficiency of all the organs and tissues of the body, resulting in more efficient and greater production of ATP (Adenosine Triphosphate), the energy-carrying molecules found in the cells of all living things. This energy, in turn, supports the optimal functioning of the thousands of biochemical systems continually operating throughout the body!

Co-Enzyme Q10 (Co-Q10)

As you have likely gathered from the nutritional items already discussed, I am not a huge proponent of including a lot of fractionated, isolated nutrients in mega-doses, in my client's and my patient's nutritional protocol. If you visit my website at www.marilynjoyce.com and read about my own journey back to health from cancer, you will have a better understanding of why I believe it is so important to derive as much nutrition from natural sources as possible. And that includes the additional nutritional support products we incorporate for extra insurance and peace of mind.

However, in working with many major degenerative illnesses over the years, I have found that Co-enzyme Q10 (Co-Q10) is often a valuable addition to my client's protocol. Co-Q10 is a naturally occurring substance present within every cell in the body of every living plant and animal, including humans. Research indicates that it is a powerful anti-oxidant that plays a vital role in the production of Adenosine Triphosphate (ATP), the most basic unit of energy used by every cell to perform its everyday functions. Remember those energy carrying molecules we talked about that are in Juice Plus+® and in Perfect Food®? Co-Q10 is responsible for the production of about 95% of the life-giving energy in the cells of the body.

Research indicates that many illnesses, as well as aging, or extended periods of physical activity, result in a lower production of Co-Q10 in the mitochondria, the tiny factory within every cell, which is responsible for metabolism and energy production. Co-Q10 is essential for the production of energy in our bodies from the foods we eat. And, remember: those foods must be natural, whole, preferably living foods versus processed, packaged, nutrient-deficient fast foods!

The Key Functions of Co-Enzyme Q10 include:

- ➢ Powerful antioxidant
- ➢ Free radical scavenger in cells; anti-aging factor
- ➢ Protect cell membranes from damage
- ➢ Increase oxygen uptake; enhance aerobic performance
- ➢ Support efficient post-exercise recovery
- ➢ Essential for cellular energy production (ATP)
- ➢ Increase vitality, zest for life, and general well-being
- ➢ Reduce risk of impaired immune function; balance the immune system
- ➢ Reduce risk of weight gain; efficient metabolism has potential to burn fat

> ➢ Benefits shown in treatment of heart disease and high blood pressure
> ➢ Benefits demonstrated in treatment of gum disease, Alzheimer's and obesity

Though there are several good Co-Enzyme Q10 products out there, one of my personal favorites (due to the tremendous amount of research to support its use) is *Super BioActive CoQ10 Ubiquinol*, available through the Life Extension Foundation at www.lef.org/ or call 800-544-4440. For more than 27 years, the Life Extension Foundation (LEF, for short), has been funding scientific research and introducing new and innovative, potentially life saving, medical discoveries. And this foundation has amassed a huge compendium of information in their comprehensive integrative medical book entitled, "Disease Prevention and Treatment". This concise resource and reference manual contains over 1500 pages of the most up-to-date therapies, clinics, doctors, and "inside" information available.

Another personal favorite (again, due to the research behind it) is John O'Neill's Co-Enzyme Q10 from Advanced Life-Products in Australia. For more information go to: www.thexton.com.au/brand/Advanced__Life-Products. You can do a Google search to find a local distributor in your area.

It is recommended that you keep Co-Q10 refrigerated to avoid oxidation. If Co-Q10 becomes oxidized, the protective effects no longer exist. Instead, it becomes a free radical itself. In fact, with all nutritional products and supplements, it is probably best to keep them refrigerated in order to prevent, or at least diminish, the potential for oxidation. And remember that nutrients work best in combination and synergy with each other. No one nutrient works as well in your body, if at all, by itself. For a deeper understanding of this, refer to the chapter: *The Best Nutritional Support System I Know Of!*

Kyolic® Aged Garlic Extract

The benefits of garlic have been touted for thousands of years! And, in cultures that include garlic in their diet on a daily basis, we find some of the healthiest people in the world. Literally hundreds of scientific studies have been, and are being, conducted at major universities and cancer centers worldwide. The results are showing that Aged Garlic Extract (AGE) protects and enhances the health of the cells in the brain, breast, lungs, heart, liver, lungs, stomach, colon, prostate, bladder and the skin. AGE, according to this extensive body of research, can also stimulate circulation, inhibit oxidative damage to the body, lower elevated cholesterol and homocysteine levels, and reduce the progression of plaque in coronary arteries.

And the best part: the research indicates that the form of garlic, whether raw, cooked, as garlic oil, or as aged garlic extract, is not the determining factor as to its value to our health. All of the forms available can work for the protection and treatment of an amazing number of conditions and illnesses.

Now, as delicious as fresh garlic is, there is no question that it can pose a challenge at social functions, especially if there are many folks present who have not partaken of this "stinking rose" (as it has been referred to since Greek and Roman times). So what's the answer to getting the tremendous benefits inherent in garlic without losing all your friends and business contacts? Garlic supplements! However, not all garlic supplements are created equal! And to prevent embarrassment, the supplement must be odorless. For more than 20 years, I have incorporated into my own dietary program, what I believe to be the best garlic supplement on the market, second to none.

Kyolic® (odorless) aged garlic, produced by Wakunaga since 1972, is the result of a manufacturing process that ages organic garlic for up to 20 months. It is available in a liquid extract, capsules, and tablet form at your local health food store. And, without a doubt, Kyolic® garlic is the most researched garlic supplement available. For scientific literature or information on the different Kyolic® formulas, or for a free sample, go to: www.kyolic.com. I'd also like to suggest a book called **"The Garlic Cure,"** which is written in layman's terms, so it's an easy read. The book is co-authored by James F. Scheer, Lynn Allison and Charlie Fox, and the last section is full of enticingly delicious recipes. By the way, if you have never met Charlie Fox, I have to tell you – I have never met a more energetic, physically fit, and enthusiastic human being in my life. And the man is over 80 years *young*!

Caveat: Although I have provided references for you so that you can easily find what I believe to be some of the finest products available, that does not mean that I endorse the multitude of products found on any of the respective websites mentioned; (except Juice Plus+®, which has a very limited number of products, generally based on the same principle of powdered fruits and vegetables in a few different forms, e.g. capsules, chewables, and gummies). In future editions of my *Special Reports*, I will cover this topic much more thoroughly. You can sign up to receive these free Myth Busting Reports at www.marilynjoyce.com.

Important Notice: *Do not stop any treatment or medication you currently use. Consult with your doctor before starting the use of any supplements. The products outlined above are not intended to diagnose, treat, cure, or prevent any disease. And always read the label. Do not use if seal is broken or missing. Use only as directed. If any unusual symptoms occur and persist, see your doctor/healthcare professional. These symptoms may simply* be signs of detoxification occurring in your body, and **that's a good thing** (see the chapter on **Detoxification**). However, don't hesitate to contact us at 800-352-3443 or info@marilynjoyce.com for answers to any questions you may have on supplements, detoxification, or any other concern that arises as you read this book. And allow at least 7 to 14 days for a response, as we receive hundreds of emails each day.

Well, the final segment included in this chapter is my basic nutritional support protocol. Continuously, as I travel around our beautiful planet, addressing the issue of how to develop and implement quick and easy, yet effective, nutrition and lifestyle strategies, on a daily basis, people ask me what I recommend beyond striving to include the most vital and alive foods available. So, I felt that it would be of great value to you to answer this question by including the following easy-to-incorporate, step-by-step, nutritional support system guide, developed specifically for my clients and patients.

And, as you have probably gathered by now, my focus is always on whole food-based nutritional support systems. This type of protocol has been very widely documented throughout the growing body of clinical, scientific research, as being much more bioavailable in the body than fractionated, isolated, individual nutrients. Refer again to the chapter: *The Best Nutritional Support System I Know Of!*

So Here's My Dr Joyce Recommends Basic Nutritional Support Protocol:

Upon arising: Add the **juice of one small lemon** to 8 oz of hot (not boiling) water. Then add 1-2 tsp of pure maple syrup and as much cayenne pepper as you can handle (about 1/10 tsp). The cayenne pepper revs up your peristaltic system, which aids in elimination.

Wait 15-30 min: Perfect Food®: Take 3 caplets with 8 oz of water. (For the greatest benefit and maximum detoxification of the body, it is best to take the *Perfect Food* on an empty stomach, first thing in the AM, and again mid-afternoon, on an empty stomach.)

NOTE: *Start with one caplet in the AM and 1 caplet mid-afternoon for the first month. This is a very potent supplement. Then take 3 caplets (AM) and 2 caplets (mid-afternoon) the following month.*

Breakfast: 2 Juice Plus+®: Orchard blend (red capsules) and 1 **Juice Plus+ Vineyard Blend®** (purple capsules) with 8-10 oz water, 10 minutes before a meal or a shake/smoothie. The water activates the enzymes and plumps up the fiber for maximum utilization of the nutrients available in the meal you are about to consume, which should preferably be no less than 10 minutes and no more than 15 minutes following your intake of *Juice Plus+®.* *

> **Co-Enzyme Q10:** (50 mg) with breakfast. A very large body frame, over 200 pounds would probably do better taking 75-100 mg.

> **Juice Plus+ Complete®:** 1 scoop in a shake/smoothie **

> **Udo's Choice® Oil Blend:** 1 tbsp in shake/smoothie **

NOTE: *Generally the average person, especially if they are taking Juice Plus+® and the Juice Plus+ Vineyard Blend® on a consistent basis (that means everyday!), does not likely require CoQ10. However, from my clinical experience with my clients, I do believe that during, and for at least 1 year following, a major illness, or a prolonged, very stressful event, or for an athlete training for a major sports event, such as a triathlon, or the Olympics, CoQ10 is a very important addition to their program. When we are ill and/or aging, and/or participating in very demanding athletic endeavors, our body's production declines and/or is quickly depleted by the medications or activities. CoQ10 is essential for energy production, and therefore essential for the efficient functioning of all of our metabolic systems throughout the body. As your immune system becomes stronger, more balanced, and more efficient at producing its own CoQ10, via the whole food nutritional support systems outlined here, you will be able to stop taking the CoQ10.*

Lunch: **Bifidus BB536:** (1) capsule with 4-8 oz water, organic milk, or organic soymilk, 5-10 minutes before eating.

Kyolic® Aged Garlic: 1 capsule (600 mg) with meal

Mid-afternoon: **Perfect Food®:** (2) caplets with 8 oz of water on an empty stomach. If choosing to eat a snack, wait at least 15 minutes.

Dinner: **Bifidus BB536:** (1) capsule with 4-8 oz water, organic milk, or organic soymilk, 5-10 minutes before taking Juice Plus.

Juice Plus+®: (2) **Garden blend** (green capsules) and (1) **Juice Plus Vineyard Blend®** with 8-10 oz water 10 minutes before eating. *

* NOTE: *For the first week, start with (1) Juice Plus+® Orchard Blend (red) capsule in the AM, 10 minutes before breakfast, and (1) Juice Plus+® Garden Blend (green) capsule 10 minutes before dinner, with 8 oz of water each time. Then, in the second week, up the intake to the amount outlined above. Add the Juice Plus+ Vineyard Blend® in the AM before breakfast, and in the PM before dinner, in the third or fourth week.*

Some individuals find that they do better taking the Garden Blend (green capsules) in the morning, and the Orchard Blend (red capsules) in the evening. Speak to your Juice Plus+® representative regarding this. There are no hard and fast rules about the best times to take Juice Plus+®. The most important thing is that you take it, and that you take it consistently, everyday!

** NOTE: *See the smoothie recipe that follows. It incorporates all of the life-giving components for optimum health development and maintenance. Enjoy! Enjoy!! We would love to hear from you via email, about anything you have experienced as a result of adding this nutritional support protocol, and/or the smoothie recipe, to your nutritional program.* Contact us anytime at: info@marilynjoyce.com.

SUMPTUOUS IMMUNE BALANCING SMOOTHIE RECIPE
(makes 1 serving)

BASIC SMOOTHIE:
4 oz (½ cup) Mori-Nu tofu   1 tbsp (Flora) golden flaxseeds,
4 oz (½ cup) vanilla soy milk   freshly ground **
½ large banana   1 scoop Juice Plus+ Complete®
½ cup of fresh or frozen berries   1 tbsp Udo's Choice® Oils

ADD THE FOLLOWING:
For a jumpstart to your day or workout, or just to get over an afternoon slump!

1 tsp Perfect Food® (work up to 1 tbsp over 1 month) * — don't use if taking
    caplets
1 tsp Nutritional yeast (work up to 1 tbsp over 1 month) ***
1 tsp Wheat germ (work up to 1 tbsp over 1 month) ****
Add: 3-4 ice cubes, or as desired

You can use any other fresh fruits in season, e.g. peaches, pineapple, nectarines, mangos, papaya, kiwi, pears, cantaloupe, etc. Be adventurous!

* Start with 1 tsp each for the first 2 weeks; then up the amount to 2 tsp each for the next 2 weeks; and finally up the amount to 1 tbsp each from that point on.

** Preferably add 1 tbsp golden flaxseeds, freshly ground just prior to use, instead of the oil. These wholesome seeds are loaded with those essential omega-3 fatty acids we constantly read about in the news!

Add calories with almond butter or sesame tahini.

*** **NOTE:** _Nutritional yeast_ is generally better absorbed, and more easily digested, than Brewer's yeast. It is a primary grown yeast, from pure strains of Saccharomyces cerevisiae, grown on a special growth medium of mixtures of cane and beet molasses. It is therefore NOT a brewery by-product as is brewer's yeast; so it is free of Candida albicans yeast. Nutritional yeast is an excellent source of protein, dietary fiber, vitamins (especially the B-vitamin complex, including B-12) and minerals. It is grown specifically for its nutritive value. Best when stored in a cool, dry place. Very versatile, nutritional yeast can also be used as a seasoning for salads, gravies, soups, and casseroles or in a sandwich spread.

**** **NOTE:** _Wheat germ_, the heart of the wheat berry, is the reproductive area or (living) embryo from which the seed germinates to form the sprout that becomes the green wheat grass. It is the most nutritious portion of the wheat kernel and makes up only about 2 ½% of its weight. Wheat germ is packed with protein, fiber, polyunsaturated fat, vitamins, especially folic acid, and minerals. Its nutty flavor is, in part, due to its high oil content, which in turn, causes it to become rancid quickly. Wheat germ is usually separated from the bran and starch during the milling of flour because the germ's perishable oil content limits the shelf life of the flour. Since wheat germ contains very little of the sticky gluten protein responsible for a wheat allergy reaction in so many people these days, wheat germ is a great way to get the high level of nutrition in wheat without the negative impact of the gluten. Wheat germ oil, an extraction of the germ, is strongly flavored and expensive, and very volatile (unstable shelf life). That is why I always recommend the flaked, dry germ form, versus the oil.

LET'S WAKE UP TO THE HEALTH OF OUR CHILDREN OR RATHER, LACK OF HEALTH!

Wake up folks! It is more important than ever before to take steps to protect our families. Statistically children born since the year 2000 will not only live shorter lives than their parents, they will be facing epidemic rates of diabetes, obesity, heart disease, cancer, ADHD, Autism, and the multitude of other degenerative diseases.

The SAD (Standard American Diet) State of Affairs!

We often hear the statement that our children are our future. At least we hope they are! Can we really be sure at this time in history that this will be the case? Today we see younger and younger children being diagnosed with diseases that were once generally only seen in adults, such as Type 2 Diabetes, which used to be called Adult Onset Diabetes, for that very reason—it was a disease that developed in adults who had poor diet and lifestyle habits! Asthma has increased in incidence at an alarming rate. Leukemia and lymphoma are much more prevalent among unborn and newly born babies than ever before. And obesity among our young people, according to the National Center for Health Statistics, has tripled since 1980. That equates to almost ten million children between the ages of 6 and 19, or one in five American children. And that is only taking into account the US. The statistics, percentage wise, are similar in Canada, and fast increasing in most of the other developed nations on the planet.

Being overweight and obese sets the stage for early development of life threatening illnesses. Obesity has been linked in the research to such illnesses as high blood pressure, hypertension, insulin resistance, type 2 diabetes, heart disease, dyslipidemia, stroke, gall bladder disease, osteoarthritis, osteoporosis, respiratory disorders, sleep apnea, breathlessness, asthma, steatohepatitis, hyperuricaemia, various cancers, reproductive hormone abnormalities, polycystic ovarian syndrome, infertility, lower back pain, and other chronic conditions and illnesses. Apart from developing serious illnesses earlier in life, overweight and obese children have a substantially reduced quality of life and a shorter life expectancy. Dr. David Ludwig, the director of the obesity program at Children's Hospital Boston, states that, "Obesity is such that this generation of children could be the first, basically in the history of the United States, to live less healthful and shorter lives than their parents."

What is causing this sad state of affairs for our youth? Well, when you consider that the average young person eats the equivalent of five pounds of sugar per week — that is ¾ pound of sugar a day — the amount that was the entire ration per person per year during both, World War 1 and World War 2 — it is easier to understand the situation! Many children that I have worked with didn't even know what a fresh fruit or vegetable tasted like prior to our work together.

Sodas, chips, french fries, lunchables, candy, and the plethora of processed, packaged, and canned foods, that fill up our grocery store shelves, where once there used to be primarily whole foods, is the root cause of this critical situation. These foods have little or no life enhancement value, and are generally devoid of any wholesome nutrients compared to whole foods. They are filled with artificial substances and flavors, trans fats, simple white sugar, over-processed white flour, fillers, emulsifiers, additives, food dyes, preservatives, and often pesticide, herbicide, antibiotic and hormone residues. What chance do our children have for optimum health? In a nutshell, our kids are overfed and severely undernourished!

A *"must see"* for the entire family, is a movie that clearly covers the issues that we are facing today with our own health and that of our children. Many of you have probably heard of it, and even watched it — *"Super Size Me"* — produced by Morgan Spurlock. You can read more about it at www. supersizeme.com. The website outlines some surprising statistics that in no way would make us proud! And there is also an educationally enhanced version of the movie now available, which is very appropriate for younger audiences and has great value for classroom viewing. Spurlock has also authored an eye opening book, *"Don't Eat This Book"*, which thoroughly compliments what he has covered in the film.

According to the Surgeon General, David Satcher:
"Fast food is a major contributor to the obesity epidemic."

Let Me Again Emphasize A Very Important Note:

"The average school age child eats a 5lb bag of sugar per week!"

So, what does that mean when it comes to your child's health? Keep reading . . .

Sugar depresses immunity. Research has shown that the amount of sugar in two average 12-ounce sodas can suppress the body's immune responses very noticeably two hours after ingestion, yet still evident five hours after ingestion.

Sugar negatively impacts behavior, attention, and learning. Study after study has shown a significant relationship between the effects of sugar consumption and ADD and ADHD (Attention Deficit Disorder and Attention Deficit Hyperactivity Disorder) in both children and adults. There is a growing consensus that many children and adults are sugar sensitive, reflected by inappropriate behavior, poor attention span and concentration, and compromised learning ability which deteriorates in proportion to the amount of sugar they consume. According to the renowned pediatrician, Dr William Sears, MD many of the children diagnosed with ADD actually have NDD (Nutritional Deficit Disorder).

Sugar highs impact children and adults alike. They are followed by serious lows, often referred to as "sugar blues". Studies done globally have shown that some children with Attention Deficit Hyperactivity Disorder (ADHD) react to glucose-tolerance tests with a dip to low blood-sugar levels resulting in abnormal or inappropriate behavior. High adrenaline levels or low blood-sugar levels produce this abnormal behavior. And the tragedy of constant sugar highs and lows may be fatal—as in suicide!

This does not apply to complex carbohydrates, which are high in fiber, and found in fresh vegetables, whole natural grains, and fresh fruits. These foods are good for you. It's the simple sugars found in sodas, candies, frostings, and packaged foods and treats that can seriously harm. *It's as "simple" as that.* Avoid "simple"—reach for "complex"!

Sugar increases insulin levels. This can lead to high blood pressure, high cholesterol, heart disease, diabetes, weight gain, premature aging and many more negative side effects. One of the most important things you can do to optimize your health is control your insulin levels. I don't think there is a health professional alive who would dispute the fact that avoiding simple sugar in any form is essential to achieving this.

Sugar promotes cravings and fat storage. The more sugar you eat, the more sugar you want! A high-sugar meal raises your blood-glucose level. This triggers an outpouring of insulin that has no place to go. This excess insulin then triggers a craving for more sugar. Your blood sugar is continually out of balance, sending your body into a perpetual biochemical roller-coaster ride.

Eventually, as you eat excess carbohydrates in an attempt to stave off the cravings, your body turns these sugars into fat—the body's safeguard against starvation. This generally results in higher blood triglycerides, a major risk factor in cardiovascular disease, which is becoming a common occurrence in younger and younger children every year.

Get Rid of These NOW:

Soft Drinks. There are absolutely no redeeming qualities inherent in soft drinks—just a whole lot of sugar and caffeine! The sugars in soft drinks destroy many of the healthy nutrients that make it into our bodies from the foods we eat before the body has an chance to absorb, assimilate and use them. High doses of sugar, as well as the various artificial sweeteners used in the soft drink industry, increase urinary excretion of calcium, which leads to osteoporosis (thinning of bone density), and to deposits of calcium in the kidneys (i.e., kidney stones.). The phosphoric acid present in most soft drinks adds insult to injury by depleting the body of calcium, by significantly increasing the loss of magnesium and calcium in your urine.

Packaged, processed, commercial bakery goods. The combination of white over-processed flour, completely refined brilliant white sugar, and hydrogenated and partially hydrogenated fats (trans-fats), makes these commercial packaged baked goods less nutritious than the boxes and cartons they are packaged in! Avoid them like the plague that they are!! Look for whole grains, with nothing added, and create your own healthy combinations from scratch. There are many great ideas throughout this book. What are you waiting for? Go to the recipe index at the back of the book and "pin the tail on the donkey"—in other words, any recipe here will help to make a healthy body!

Did you know that a 12 oz can of soda can contain as much a 13 teaspoons of sugar? And it is in one of the most deadly forms of sugar ever invented—high fructose corn syrup!! Kids consume and average of 2 sodas per day!

By The Way:

You can figure out how many teaspoons of sugar your child is eating by dividing the number of grams listed on the label of the package, bottle, or can by 4. And remember to take into account the number of servings contained in the package, as this can be very misleading. For example, a 15-ounce bottle of a name brand beverage lists the amount of sugar as 14 grams. One assumes that the bottle is a serving. So that would be 3.5 teaspoons of sugar. Right? Wrong! The label states there are 2.5 servings. So, if you were to drink the whole bottle—and most of us would—there are 2.5 servings, times 3.5

teaspoons per serving. So you would be consuming almost 9 teaspoons of sugar! *READ THE LABEL!!*

Stevia, Sucanat, raw honey & pure maple syrup are better choices.

READ YOUR LABELS . . .

Many packaged foods contain <u>harmful</u> ingredients.
Dr Joyce's top dozen — that's 12! — WORST ingredients:

1. Sugar — 4 Grams = 1 Teaspoon
   (sucrose, corn syrup, high fructose corn syrup, brown sugar, Turbinado sugar, raw sugar, honey, molasses, fructose, dextrose)
2. Caffeine (coffee, lattes, sodas, hot chocolate, black tea, chocolate bars)
3. Sugar Substitutes, e.g. Nutrasweet and Equal which are Aspartame, Sweet and Low, Splenda (chlorinated sugar molecules)
4. Monosodium Glutamate — (MSG)
5. Hydrolyzed Vegetable Protein
6. Hydrogenated Fats, Partially Hydrogenated Fats (Trans Fats)
7. Refined, Enriched and Fortified Anything — including White Flour
8. Nitrates and Nitrites (preservatives)
9. Sulfates and Sulfites (preservatives)
10. Food Colorings and Food Dyes
11. Other Preservatives
    (e.g calcium propionate,sodium nitrate, sodium nitrite, sulphites {sulfur dioxide, sodium bisulfite, potassium hydrogen sulfite, etc.} and disodium EDTA, BHA and BHT, formaldehyde, glutaraldehyde, diatomaceous earth kills insects, ethanol, dimethyl dicarbonate and methylchloroisothiazolinone)
12. Pesticides
    (e.g. organochlorides and organophosphates, and a list far too long to include here)

Note: For more information on deciphering food labels, see the chapter, *So What's on a Label.*

Traffic Light Eating

So, my first step in working with a family — and it is critical to work with the entire family, so that everyone is on the same page — is education. It is important for each member of the family to understand that different foods have different values. A system that has been particularly simple to use is based on Red – Amber – Green Light food lists. A wonderful resource for educating our younger population, that incorporates this system, is the book, "Eat Healthy, Feel Great," by Dr. William Sears and Martha Sears, RN. Traffic Light eating is a way to identify foods that are good for you and foods that are not.

"Green-light" foods are "go for it" foods, the healthy choices. They're the unprocessed or minimally processed foods that are full of lots of nutrients, and great for your health – eat all you want of these. The label, if there is one, usually includes a very short list of readable ingredients. These foods and beverages will keep you energized, alert, focused, at a healthy weight, and more able to avoid illness.

"Yellow-light" foods are "think about it" foods. These foods are processed and the drinks may have a small amount of nutritional value. Moderate levels of saturated fats may be present. And the ingredient list tends to be quite long with a lot of words the average person can't pronounce. They are okay in moderation but should be reserved for treats and eaten only occasionally, not as a steady diet. Over time you are more likely to gain weight, feel sluggish, tired, easily hungry, and eventually you may develop an illness.

"Red-light" foods are "stop, say no, bad for you" foods. They are highly processed and full of "empty" calories, with next to no nutritional value. Generally the ingredient list is very long and full of words the average person has never heard of and can't pronounce. My theory is: *If you can't read it, or you can't pronounce it, don't buy it!* These foods and beverages may cause you, and especially your children, to feel continually tired, sleepy, sluggish, nervous, and irritable, as well as unable to concentrate and focus, and more likely to gain weight, eventually leading to obesity, Type 2 Diabetes, and other serious and chronic degenerative illnesses.

Here are Samples of Food Items for Each Category:

GREEN-LIGHT FOODS	YELLOW-LIGHT FOODS	RED-LIGHT FOODS
vegetables, fresh	pies (no trans fats)	hot dogs (most)
legumes (beans, peas, lentils)	cakes (no trans fats)	nitrate-containing meats
fruits, fruit leathers, dried fruit	butter	& cold cuts
fish, deep water, wild salmon	chocolate, natural	packaged foods w/
sprouted grains & breads	crackers	hydrogenated oils
	(no trans fats)	hydrogenated oils
		marshmallows

pasta, whole grain
nuts and seeds, raw
soy foods, tofu (non-GMO)
edamame (non-GMO)
eggs (cage-free/no hormones)
vegetable oils (olive, sesame, flax)
avocados
healthy treats (no trans fats)
homemade soups, stews
natural nut butters (almond,
   peanut, cashew, sesame
   tahini)
steel-cut oatmeal
wild rice, brown rice, quinoa
other whole grains
meat and poultry (hormone-free)

fast foods (not fried)
fruit drinks
white bread
spritzers
frozen yogurt
canned soups
cookies (no trans fats)
pastries (no trans fats)
white flour tortilla, pita
commercial salad
   dressings
organic dairy products

punches and drinks with
   added colorings
candy, candy bars
doughnuts
crushed ice drinks &
   diet sodas (are mostly
   syrups & dyes)
cereals with dyes and
   hydrogenated oils
fast foods fried in
   hydrogenated oils
pre-packaged foods (e.g.
   Lunchables)
crackers & chips w/
   hydrogenated oils
mayonnaise, regular or
   low-fat
margarine
sodas

When it Comes to Fresh Fruits and Vegetables—More is Better!
Here are just a few reasons:

➢ The thousands of nutrients in raw fruits and vegetables are primary building blocks for healthy bodies. You know the expression: "You are what you eat!"

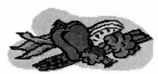

➢ Free radicals (lipid peroxides) are a major by-product of metabolism in every living person, including children. They cause break down and destruction of your body's trillions of cells, leading to eventual aging of your body, often resulting in degenerative illnesses, such as cancer. Exercise is very important. However, the more active a child is, the more free radicals their bodies create! The many thousands of vitamins, minerals, antioxidants, phytochemicals (plant chemicals), and bioflavonoids in raw fruits and vegetables neutralize these free radicals.

➢ There are over 25,000 known phytochemicals in plant foods. These nutrients create the colors in the different fruits and vegetables— greens, whites, yellows, browns, reds, purples, blues, and oranges. And we need to try to eat some of each of these colors every day.

Each, of a single apple or tomato, has at least 10,000 phytochemicals. *(Phytochemicals have been shown in research to prevent disease and reduce the risk of many degenerative illnesses.)*

➢ Fruits and vegetables are loaded with many minerals, including calcium, magnesium, sodium and potassium, which are critical for normal bodily function, efficient metabolism, and the development of strong bones and teeth.

➢ The soluble and insoluble fibers in raw plant foods can lower cholesterol, scrub the intestinal walls, reduce or eliminate constipation (a significant health challenge in our culture for young and old alike), reduce the risk of diabetes by slowing carbohydrate absorption (another health challenge in our culture for all ages!), and reduce the risk of many types of cancer and other degenerative illnesses.

Enticing Ways to Encourage Your Kids to Eat More Fruits and Vegetables:

First let me emphasize: *Eat your produce (fruits and vegetables); don't drink it!* While 100% fruit or vegetable juices are good choices, whole or cut-up fruit or vegetables have the added benefit of fiber.

➢ Have fruit washed and easily available in a bowl on the counter.
➢ Cut up veggies and have them ready in the refrigerator to eat for snacks.
➢ Use fresh fruit and *real* fruit leathers (read the label) for a sweet snack.
➢ At breakfast, add fruit to yogurt, or whole grain pancakes, waffles, or cereal.
➢ Top low fat yogurt with crunchy granola and wheat germ, and lots of fresh berries (blueberries, blackberries, raspberries, strawberries), and/or other fresh fruits in season—for a healthy breakfast or snack
➢ Send fruits and vegetables as a snack in packed lunches.
➢ Serve fruit and vegetables (with healthy dips) as a snack at home.
➢ Freeze grapes, watermelon, and bananas for a refreshing and cool treat.
➢ Whip up a smoothie made with fruit and low fat or nonfat yogurt for a quick, nourishing snack or meal.
➢ Serve salads with homemade dressings first at dinnertime, when kids are hungriest.

- ➤ Serve a salad full of fruits and/or veggies each night with dinner. Just go easy on the dressing and high fat toppings.
- ➤ Grill fruits and vegetables to make them sweeter and more delicious.
- ➤ Chop, dice, or shred vegetables into muffins, stews, lasagna, meatloaf, and casseroles.
- ➤ Use pureed vegetables to thicken soups, stews, gravies, and casseroles.
- ➤ Flavor vegetables with fresh or dried herbs and a splash of lemon juice or balsamic vinegar. Skip the sauces.
- ➤ Vary the texture. Kids tend to like raw, crunchy fruits and veggies with dips, such as hummus, salsa, or low fat yogurt-based dips.
- ➤ Try shredding veggies to top sandwiches or salads.
- ➤ Decorate plates with edible garnishes, like cucumber twists, red pepper strips, or cantaloupe slices.
- ➤ Offer new fruits and vegetables — don't assume your kids won't like them. (Sometimes a child needs to be exposed to a new food 14, or more, times before they'll eat it.)
- ➤ Serve yams and sweet potatoes instead of white potatoes for more potassium and beta-carotene.
- ➤ Have a total vegetarian meal at least once a week. It can be as simple as soup and salad, or a stir-fry meal.
- ➤ Add veggies, such as mushrooms, carrots, onions, green, yellow and red peppers, squash, and fresh tomatoes to spaghetti sauce.
- ➤ Experiment with new ways to serve fruits and veggies — for example, a broccoli slaw salad mix, or pomegranate juice. Just because your children didn't like certain fruits and veggies initially doesn't mean they won't like them as they get older. Our taste buds do change.
- ➤ Give your kids concentrated fruit and vegetable snack foods. (Juice Plus+® Gummies and Chewables. See chapter: **Dr. Joyce Recommends.**)

Add the Power of a Healthy Lifestyle — & You've Got a Healthy Happy Kid!

As we know, there's more to health than food . . .
If we are to overcome this sad state of health that is sweeping the globe, we have to instill healthy lifestyle habits into the lives of our kids! So here are some recommendations to add to the pot.

Drink, drink, drink! Water, that is! Promote hydration with water! Encourage your kids to carry full water bottles with them wherever they go. Make yours and your kids' beverage of choice fresh pure water. Invest in a complete house filter system. Or, at the very least, a kitchen and a shower filter. See the chapter *Water: The Elixir Of Life!*

If anyone is going to be healthy, no matter what age they are, activity must play an important role! Our kids today spend a huge amount of time, sitting on their duff, in front of a screen of one kind or another — whether it be a computer or a TV. This, together with their very SAD diet, has led to major health challenges. It is time to stop, and reverse, this negative direction in its tracks right now! There is a saying that *the family that plays together stays together!* Why not get active together?

Find fun activities to do as a family. Hike, climb, swim, ice or roller-skate, bike, jump rope, disco or rap dance, toss a Frisbee, play some tennis or volleyball, run a marathon, take a yoga class, join a gym class, sign the family up for karate or judo, take walks after dinner, see who can last the longest on the treadmill, take the stairs at the mall, race around your block, see who can shoot the most hoops, play catch at the local baseball field, compete in a triathlon, plan adventure trips — I think you get the picture. The sky is the limit! Get out, and get active!

Eat more meals together. We are always on the run these days, and meals seem to be gobbled down while standing at the kitchen counter on the way out the door to a game or a meeting or some sort of training. Or they are mindlessly consumed in front of the TV or computer. Turn off the computer and the TV and sit down together and eat a wholesome meal with shared love and conversation. The healthiest cultures in the world eat meals together with conscious connection and sharing.

On that note, cut down TV, computer and video game time, other than for educational purposes! One to two hours per day is absolute max! Inactivity = ill health. And could very likely lead to overweight, and worse, obesity.

Let your kids participate in the meal preparation and service of the food. They know how much they need to eat better than we do. That "clean your plate" philosophy is very passé these days and should not be encouraged. Generally speaking, our children certainly do not need more food on their plate. Remember, a child's stomach is about the size of their closed fist. So use this as a measure for their personal food portions. When kids are allowed to serve themselves early in their development, they tend to make better choices and develop more appropriate cues for hunger and satiety — that feeling of fullness or satisfaction.

Be a role model! Set a great example! If you want your children to reach and maintain a healthy weight, do it yourself. You'll be slimmer, healthier, more energetic, and more fun to be around. Your kids will love playing with you, and that activity will keep all of you slimmer and healthier.

No food or drinks for rewards! Praise and non-edible rewards are the best way to teach self-respect and self-esteem. Seek to know your child's deepest dreams and desires, and reward with the training or material items that will support them in their dreams and visions. Consistently give them love and encouraging words. Be there for them during their greatest accomplishments. Let them know that your deepest desire is supporting them in their dreams.

And **always** have healthy snacks and beverages available for your kids — at home, in the car, in their lunch box or bag for school, on a road trip. This will prevent the temptation to stop at the nearest drive-though — just this once! *Which, of course, is never just this once.*

Finally, in this hustle, bustle, world, kids think they have to be busy doing something all the time. Why not teach them (by example), that it is okay to take time out just to sit and be still. Many times our best answers to our most challenging questions arise from those quiet moments of being still. Teach by doing just that — by being still. My daughter, many years ago now, said to me that I was a great and caring mother, but a lousy role model. That was like a dagger in my heart until she explained what she meant. I had taught her that it was not okay to take time out to take care of yourself. I had spent all of my life taking care of others' needs — but never my own. She learned from my example that it was not okay to take care of your own needs, only those needs of others. Wow, what a wake-up call. Of course, that all followed my journey through cancer! Crazy isn't it, that it took such a dramatic journey to wake me up!

Children's Nutrition

Fruit Smoothie Recipe (makes 2 servings)

4 oz Mori-Nu tofu, soft or firm	8 oz Vanilla soy milk	1 large banana
1 scoop vanilla Juice Plus+® Complete	½ cup fresh strawberries	3-4 ice cubes

Blend all ingredients in a blender until smooth and creamy.

You can use other fresh fruits in season, e.g. peaches, pineapple, nectarines, mangos, papaya, kiwi, pears, cantaloupe, etc. You can also vary the berries, or use frozen berries instead of fresh. Be adventurous!

Natural Candy

1 cup natural almond butter	¼ cup raisins	¼ cup mashed banana
¼ cup carob powder	2 tsp pure vanilla	ground cinnamon

Mix together, shape into balls, and roll in ground cinnamon. If desired, press an almond or walnut half on top of each ball. Natural peanut butter can be substituted for the almond butter.

Granola

2 ½ cups raw steel-cut rolled oats	¼ cup raw sesame seeds
1 cup shredded natural coconut	¼ cup raw sunflower seeds
½ cup each chopped almonds,	½ cup raw wheat germ
walnuts, pecans	½ cup honey

¼ cup cold-pressed peanut or sunflower oil
1 cup dried fruit, e.g. raisins, chopped dates, apricots, currants, etc.

Mix dry ingredients together (except dried fruit), and then add honey and oil. Spread on a cookie sheet. Bake in oven at 275 degrees until lightly browned, turning several times. Add dried fruit after baking.

Healthy Snacks

Vegetable sticks and onion dip	Rice cakes with tahini or peanut butter
Fresh fruit dipped in healthy pudding	Brown rice pudding
Hummus and whole grain crackers	Granola with soy milk or 2% organic milk
Low fat plain yogurt with fruits & nuts	Corn on the cob
Wholegrain crackers with fruit preserves	Fruit sticks or fruit kabobs
English muffin vegetarian pizzas	Baked apples
Homemade applesauce with tofu cream	Carrot sticks or baby carrots
Celery with almond or peanut butter	Smoothies (see above recipe)
Low-fat cheese (dairy or soy) & crackers	Soy or tofu dogs in wheat tortillas
Frozen grapes	Celery with cream cheese and raisins

For more great ideas, refer to the chapter on **Snack Attack**. And then sign up for my Special Report at <u>www.icantbelieveitstofu.com</u>.

Suggested Reading for You & Your Kids

Beating Cancer with Nutrition	Patrick Quillin, PhD., R.D., C.N.S./Noreen Quillin
Beating the Food Giants	Paul Stitt
Chew on This	Eric Schlosser
Don't Eat This Book	Morgan Spurlock
Dr. Atwood's Low Fat Prescription for Kids	Charles Atwood, M.D.
Eat Healthy, Feel Great	William Sears, MD & Martha Sears, RN
Enzymes, the Missing Link to Radiant Health	Humbart "Smokey" Santillo, N.D.
Excitotoxins, The Taste that Kills	Russell L. Blaylock, M.D.
Family Nutrition Book	William Sears, M.D.
Fast Food Nation	Eric Schlosser
Fat Land	Greg Critser
Food and Behavior	Barbara Reed Stitt
Food Politics	Marion Nestle
Foods That Heal	Bernard Jensen, D.C.
I Can't Believe It's Tofu!	Dr. Marilyn Joyce, PhD, R.D.
INSTANT *E.N.E.R.G.Y.*™ (Health Guide & Cookbook)	Dr. Marilyn Joyce, PhD, R.D.
Prescription for Nutritional Healing	James F. Balch, M.D. / Phyllis A. Balch, C.N.C.
Spontaneous Healing	Andrew Weil, M.D.
The Food Revolution	John Robbins
Your Body, Your Castle, Your Kingdom, Your Home	Nikki McAdoo
What Your Doctor Didn't Learn in Medical School	Stuart M. Berger, M.D.

For More Info: Dr. Marilyn Joyce, PhD, RD — 800-352-3443 or info@marilynjoyce.com
Websites: www.marilynjoyce.com or www.DrJoyce4Nutrition.com

And some other wonderful resources are:

- ❖ Natural Ovens Bakery — www.naturalovens.com
- ❖ Appleton Alternative High School — http://www.aasd.k12.wi.us/aca/default.htm
- ❖ United States Department of Agriculture (USDA) — www.usda.gov
- ❖ Nutrition.gov — www.nutrition.gov
- ❖ National Center for Health Statistics — www.cdc.gov
- ❖ No Junk Food — http://www.nojunkfood.org/
- ❖ Healthy Kids — Governor Doyle's Healthy Kids Initiative — http://healthykids.wisconsin.gov/index.asp
- ❖ Feingold Association of the United States — www.feingold.org
- ❖ *Christopher Kimball is the founder of* America's Test Kitchen *and* Parents Against Junk Food (www.parentsagainstjunkfood.org).

FIT IN FITNESS

It's been said by many fitness experts that, "the exercise for you is the exercise you'll do!" It doesn't matter what you do, just do something you love, and you are more likely to do it. And we all know that if you keep doing what you've always been doing, you'll keep getting what you've always gotten. And if that is an unhealthy, unfit body — well . . . you get my drift.

Yet in a world where we are always on the go (in the car, on a train, or a plane) on the way to one appointment or the other, or we are tied to a desk at the computer or on the phone, it sometimes seems daunting to attempt to fit exercise into our already packed day. Research has shown, time and again, that those folks who have a high fitness level are much less likely to die prematurely for any reason. So, the *Master of 5-minute health strategies* is here to help you with this matter as well. Along with a healthy diet, not instead of a healthy diet, research proves that we must have a healthy fitness routine.

I realized years ago that it was more important to fit in short workouts, as possible throughout the day, than not to exercise at all. It may not make you an Olympic champion, a marathon runner, a basketball superstar, or a body building king or queen, but there's a lot more to fitness than being a fitness hero.

What will physical activity do for you?

> Relieve tension, anxiety and stress (the cause of all degenerative illnesses today)
> Help your heart work more efficiently reducing risk of heart disease and stroke
> Improve circulation of your blood
> Reduce brain fog — those moments when the brain seems to freeze and you can't remember names or anything that you've always known!
> Keep your weight at a balanced range
> Lower your risk of developing diabetes
> Create an appealing tone to your muscles (and it seems every baby boomer today wants to look like they did 20 years earlier, so the muscles are not such a bad thing to have!)
> Slow down the loss of bone mass and development of osteoporosis
> Strengthen muscles, bones and joints
> Reduce blood pressure
> Balance and improve immune function

➢ Reduce risk of colon, breast, and prostate cancers (likely most other cancers as well since cancer does not thrive well in an aerobic environment)
➢ Increase self-confidence and self-esteem
➢ Improve your energy level
➢ Provide a vibrant quality of life for a lifetime

But there is so much more to fitness than that. You will have the energy and strength to do everything you want to do or need to do to enjoy your life fully and take care of your daily activities — walk where you need to walk without a walker, carry groceries into the house, pick up and play with your children or grandchildren, keep up with our fast-paced society, care for yourself as you get older, and you may actually significantly slow or even reverse, to an extent, the aging process.

Unfortunately, for the younger folks, that may not mean much. But I can assure you that, as we get older, this becomes a major objective! No one wants to be struggling through each day barely able to walk, with little to no energy, and breathing heavily with every step we take. I watched my mother unable to climb two stairs without physical assistance when she was only 45 years of age — that is significantly younger than I am now. So if you want to be healthy, get that body of yours moving!

So what is this section of the book about?

It's the same as the whole book — a *lifestyle* approach to health and fitness. Simply add short segments of physical activity into your daily life. Increase activity any way you can. Include aerobics, stretching and outdoor activities. Other strategies include:

➢ Walk or run upstairs whenever possible
➢ Take the stairs instead of the elevator or escalator
➢ Stand up and do calf raises while talking on the phone
➢ Walk to the store
➢ Ride a bicycle around the block
➢ Do neck and shoulder stretches when sitting in traffic
➢ Wash the dishes by hand
➢ Plant a garden
➢ Park the car a farther distance from your destination
➢ Put some music on and just move to it
➢ Try a new dance video or DVD — learn some steps while loosening up
➢ Take a walk during lunch break / go for a swim

> ➤ Jump rope — the new rage
> ➤ Use the hoola hoop to music for 5 minutes — a flash from the past
> ➤ Find a buddy to stretch with
> ➤ Do the sun salutation 5 times (a series of yoga movements)
> ➤ Conduct meetings while walking instead of sitting
> ➤ Go for a walk after dinner (take a partner or loved one — seems to lengthen the walk)
> ➤ Use a push mower to cut grass
> ➤ Bounce for 5 minutes on a rebounder (mini-trampoline) — *my absolute favorite*

Simply search every aspect of your life to find opportunities to integrate physical activity into your daily routine. For more details on specific activities, refer to page 88? in *"I Can't Believe Its Tofu!"*

The Rebounder

Now, let me tell you about the rebounder, my absolute favorite exercise. You can easily do this exercise in your living room, bedroom or family room, office, backyard, even a hotel room. Folding rebounders are available. And I personally love my quarter fold rebounder by ReboundAIR™. However, it is not always possible to carry it when I travel — but that does not mean I don't rebound on the road. Beds can be very useful substitutes as long as the ceiling is not too low, and the mattress is fairly firm. I am sure many hotel maids have wondered what the heck went on the night before in the rooms I have stayed in!

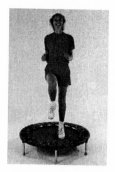

The Rebounder in Motion

Among the many benefits of rebounding are the following:

> ➤ Reduces your body fat and likelihood of obesity
> ➤ Rids your body of toxins
> ➤ Enhances your digestion and elimination processes
> ➤ Minimizes the frequency of colds, allergies, digestive disturbances, and abdominal problems

- ➤ Increases the capacity for respiration
- ➤ Circulates more oxygen to the tissues
- ➤ Aids the lymphatic circulation throughout your body
- ➤ Detoxes the lymphatic system
- ➤ Moves fluids containing waste products of metabolism around and out of the body
- ➤ Aids the flow of blood in the veins of the circulatory system
- ➤ Improves cellular stimulation and function
- ➤ Expands the body's capacity for fuel storage and endurance
- ➤ Strengthens the heart and other muscles in the body so that they work more efficiently
- ➤ Provides an increased G-force (gravitational load), which strengthens the musculoskeletal systems
- ➤ Tones the glandular system, especially the thyroid, increasing its efficiency of output
- ➤ Promotes body growth and repair
- ➤ Provides an aerobic effect for your heart
- ➤ Stimulates your metabolism
- ➤ Firms your legs, thighs, abdomen, arms, and hips
- ➤ Increases your agility and coordination
- ➤ Improves your sense of balance
- ➤ Offers relief from neck and back pains, headaches, and other pain resulting from lack of exercise
- ➤ Releases tension, anxiety and stress
- ➤ Leads to better mental performance and more efficient learning processes
- ➤ Relieves fatigue and menstrual discomfort for women
- ➤ Rejuvenates your body when it's tired
- ➤ Results in better and easier relaxation and sleep
- ➤ Increases oxygen to the cells.
- ➤ Appears to slow down the aging process

And the list goes on . . .

A note on the lymphatic system:

The lymphatic system is the metabolic sewer system of your body. It rids your body of toxins including dead and cancerous cells, heavy metals, nitrogenous wastes, fat, infectious viruses, and other waste byproducts cast off by the cells and metabolic processes. The liquid movement performed in rebounding simulates the flow of fluids throughout your body, and provides the stimulus for a free-flowing system that drains away these potential poisons.

While the cardiovascular system has the heart to move blood through the vessels, the lymphatic system does not have its own pump. The lymphatic flow requires muscular contraction from exercise and movement, as well as gravitational pressure, both of which are provided by rebounding. And then the internal massage to the valves of lymph ducts, caused by the bouncing motion of rebounding, moves and recycles the lymphatic fluids and the blood throughout our circulatory system.

Though you can achieve similar results with a jump rope, the jarring effect from hitting the ground can be very hard on your knees, ankles and lower back. One of my strategies when jumping rope when I am traveling (rope is small and light weight enough to pack in my suitcase), is to go to a climbing gym in the off-peak hours and jump on the cushioned floor. Next best approach is to find a cinder track to jump on.

James White, Ph.D., director of research and rehabilitation in the physical education department at the University of California at San Diego (UCSD), has explained that, "Rebounding allows the muscles to go through the full range of motion at equal force. It helps people learn to shift their weight properly and to be aware of body positions and balance."

Based on research performed by Victor. L. Katch, Ph.D., in the Department of Physical Education at the University of Michigan at Ann Arbor, rebounding offers a less stressful means of reducing body fat while simultaneously firming body tissues. Furthermore, running in place on a rebounder burns calories more effectively than jogging. For example, the total calories spent by a 125 pound individual jogging for 12 minutes at 5 MPH were 59 compared to 70 rebounding.

So, do you see why I am addicted to my rebounder? And now, you may be asking, "Where do I buy one and what do I look for?" There are many brands out there, but I would avoid the department store variety. They are generally poor quality and cheaply made, and will not stand up to regular use, especially if you weigh over 100 pounds. As well, they could be harmful to your joints, muscles and nerves. I would check out what is available at a reliable sporting goods store, or by mail order. Some health food stores also carry them. It's probably best to purchase your rebounder directly from the manufacturer.

My absolute favorites, which are extremely well made, are the ReboundAIR™ (regular and ½ fold), and the Ultimate Rebound™, which is a quarter-fold portable model. For the business, or simply avid, traveler who wants to maintain optimum fitness even on the road, this quarter-fold rebounder with it's own cover and airport dolly is a dream come true. *I love it!* To compare these rebounders and determine the right one for you, visit the American Institute of Reboundology at www.ultimate-rebound.com or 1-888-464-JUMP [5867].

Personally, I believe that you get what you pay for when it comes to rebounders. And even the most expensive rebounder is cheap compared to the myriad of other exercise equipment sold at 5 to 10 times the cost. And they have no scientifically proven benefits other than from what is provided by the manufacturer's sales copy.

If you are concerned about losing your balance or falling, or you are on the other side of 50, and have only minimally exercised of late, it is advised that you purchase a stability bar that you hold onto. It attaches to the rebounder, and is likened to training wheels on a bicycle. Any reputable rebounder company has these bars available for a minimal additional cost.

And one more thing about rebounding—I add weights to my workout by using 1 and 2 pound dumbbells in each hand, or wrist or palm weights, while I'm bouncing. You can also get Velcro glove weights that may be easier for someone just starting a rebounding program (available at www.ultimate-rebound.com). This is a great way to work on the upper body muscles at the same time. There are DVD's available with a wide variety of exercises that you can incorporate into your routine. So, just get on that rebounder NOW and have FUN!

Resistance Bands & Tubes

Another very effective portable exercise system uses rubber bands, referred to as resistance bands or tubing. It is referred to as rubberized resistance, and incorporates different levels of resistance. The variety of exercises that you can do with these bands is limitless. And they are a great replacement for free weights.

However, unlike free weights for strengthening the muscles, resistance bands provide constant tension during each phase of an exercise, and you can create resistance from all directions—from overhead, from below, from the side, etc. And done with proper form and tension, your muscles won't know the difference between a workout with the bands or free weights. And the bands are a whole lot easier to pack into a suitcase when traveling, since they are much more compact, and a fraction of the weight of free weights.

For sleek, toned, strong muscles, fitness band exercises are great. Women love them because they do not have to worry about getting huge muscles. Fitness bands operate according to the principle of resistance, so they gradually strengthen and tone muscles in a natural way. And resistance band exercises can benefit you, regardless of your level of fitness, because you can easily increase or decrease the resistance you experience with the bands, by shortening or lengthening them. If you are relatively weak when you first start your workout plan, you can start with minimum resistance. As you build up strength, you can gradually increase the resistance by shortening the bands. The shorter the band, the more intense the workout!

In addition to building strength, these exercises significantly improve flexibility. One major problem many people have with stretching is that they are unable to adequately reach key parts of their body to apply the pressure needed for a full and complete stretch. Fitness bands solve the problem by giving people an extended focused reach that gradually increases flexibility.

So, I'm sure you are asking where in the heck do I start? Well, one of the best resources I am aware of was produced by my dear friend and associate, Toni Branner, a world renowned exercise physiologist and wellness consultant. Toni was one of my inspirations when I first introduced the bands into my 5-minute workout routines. Her DVD, *The Safe Exercise Workout,* is very user-friendly. And Toni will dispel a lot of those established myths about exercise as well. You can order the DVD at www.tonibranner.com or call 704-551-9051.

Dyna-Flex Exerflex Exercise Balls

Another great and versatile addition to almost any workout, including your resistance band program, are the exercise balls (www.dynaflex-intl.com or call 800-480-8084). They have established a prominent place in every self-respecting health and fitness club across the nation. As far as I know, Dyna-Flex International is the only company to produce an adjustable ball (50-65 cm), and each ball comes with a pump and instructional video. Great for stretching back muscles, strengthening abdominals and obliques, and for developing balance, health practitioners of all types, including chiropractors, dance instructors, and fitness trainers, highly recommend the incorporation of this ball into your daily routine. The price is miniscule compared to the phenomenal results you can achieve in 5-minute bites throughout the day. And they're fun to boot!

Yoga:
Last in this section, but not least!

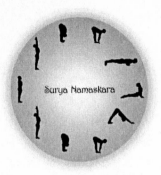

This chapter would never be complete without a word on yoga. After all, I spent most of my late teen years and well into my thirties, studying Ashtanga Yoga (an 8-path system of Yoga), initially focusing on the path of Hatha Yoga — meditation through asanas or movement — and later focusing on the practice of Bhakti yoga (another of the 8 paths), the path of pure spiritual devotion to God. So yoga has been a very significant part of my entire life and, although I am including some information about it in this section, look for more in the section entitled *Master Your Breath-Master Your Life*. My clients continually tell me that the introduction to yoga was one of the best moves (no pun intended) they have included in their daily regime.

So, where does one start with the incorporation of yoga movements into a daily program? The Sun Salutation is a basic set of movements that can be done easily in 5-minute segments, at any time during your day. I recommend starting and finishing your day with this series of stretches. And it is very important to breathe throughout the entire salute to the sun. In step number one, below, breathe out completely, and then follow the pattern outlined in the diagram below. Start with one set of the series of stretches, and gradually build up to 5 rounds done continually without stopping. Remember to keep the movement flowing throughout, from one stretch through to the other.

The Salute to the Sun exercises all major muscles and joints and helps you establish a state of calm as you begin and end your day. Center yourself before you begin. Stretch slowly and be careful not to strain. Repeat the whole exercise several time alternating legs for better results. Enjoy!

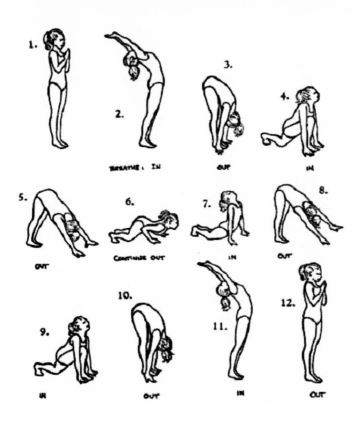

Yoga asanas / movements, done properly, assist anyone who practices it regularly, in developing a much more flexible and stream-lined musculature, at the same time as finding balance, a sense of calm, and inner peace. One of my favorite yoga resources is www.yogaheart.com at 800-558-YOGA (9642), with Susan Winter Ward. Her videos, DVD's and CD's are so easy to follow and completely user-friendly. No matter how little or how much experience you have had with yoga, you will love Susan's calm, compassionate approach to teaching and guiding the listener / watcher. So, what are you waiting for? And then call or email me and let me know how you are doing.

WATCH OUT FOR THE VICTIM TRAP!

The focus of this entire book is to provide easy-to-implement 5-minute health strategies to create and maintain your health and vitality in all aspects of your life. *And this is done by focusing on what you want versus what you don't want, and on becoming a whole and centered person mentally, emotionally, physically and spiritually.* At the same time, there are lifetime patterns that can get in the way if we are not aware of them. It is clear that a person achieves the greatest results in life when they operate from an inner locus of control (look further in this chapter, for an explanation about locus of control) and a deep sense of self-empowerment.

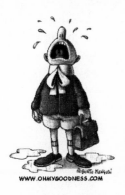

WWW.OHMYGOODNESS.COM

Yet, most of the world's population operates on a vicious triangle—the victim triangle—that forms the foundation of negative co-dependency versus healthy interdependency. This is a style of connectedness, or rather lack of connectedness, and communication that is based on a lack of personal power, and the individual's inability to set boundaries in his/her life. We often refer to this pattern as dysfunctional behavior, affecting approximately 90% of our families overall. However, this whole victim trap is rampant throughout every institution of life—home, work, school, church, the government—it is everywhere! In fact, the victim mentality is the foundation for everything we see that removes the responsibility for our own life. It is based on the blame game! And it is rooted in manipulation of others for a perceived gain. However, no one gains! Everyone loses!

So What Do You Mean — Teach Someone to Fish?

We have all heard the saying that if you give fish to someone, you feed them for a day. If you teach them how to fish, they will have food for a lifetime. But how often do we see organizations, and even parents, give food, shelter, and other basics of life, even lavishing unearned rights and privileges on others, without providing opportunities for learning how to fend for, and be responsible for, one's own life. Having been homeless in my youth, I can honestly say that it becomes a pattern of learned helplessness to receive handouts without some form of accountability — some expectation of me taking some action or actions toward becoming responsible for my own life.

I believe that many of the challenges we are facing with our youth today, such as gangs, violence, drive by shootings, drugs, development of destructive computer viruses, and early promiscuity, are because they have been given too much time and freedom without any accountability. They are not expected to do anything to earn certain rights and privileges, such a driving a car, or having a credit card before learning anything about handling money. And with this we have lost a great deal of respect for the very principle that built all of the strongest nations in history. It is called a work ethic – the knowledge that with effort, education, and applied skills we can build a productive, fulfilling and joyful life.

Today, we are living in a predominantly victim-based, divide and conquer world; where everyone is quick to blame someone else or something else for all that is not working in their lives. If we spent some quality time at home, in the schools and in our religious and spiritual institutions, teaching accountability, self-esteem and self-empowerment to our youth, I am convinced that we would see a healthier, less violent, more self-determinant generation moving into their respective communities. Instead we have created a me-first, instant gratification, what's-in-it-for-me, self-indulgent, blame the world for my problems mentality. Don't get me wrong; I know the world has a lot of problems and challenges. But, as the late President John F. Kennedy said: Ask not what your country can do for you – ask what you can do for your country!" That statement could substitute for "country", any of: family, community, city, state/province, continent, the world. After all, we are all on this planet together! As each of us becomes more self-reliant and self-determinant, we will become the role models that will inspire others to become more of who they truly were meant to be. And that is not a VICTIM!

And any parent, teacher, counselor, or clergy person, who tries to be a friend versus an adult role model and mentor, preparing our children and teens for a future as healthy, self-determinant, contributing members of society, is operating from a victim perspective as well. Doing this is a grave disservice to this future generation! We need to do whatever we have to do to become better parents and mentors, providing our children with the appropriate guidelines and opportunities for inner growth, a more balanced locus of control, and development of fully realized self-esteem.

Who Did You Say Controls Everything At Home? – Your Kid? But, They're Just a Kid!

By the way, when a child controls the home, you will likely see the victim triangle operating full throttle. So, what does this look like? Well, at the foundation of this vicious triangle are 3 characters operating at any given time: the victim, the persecutor, and the rescuer. When I explain this trio to attendees at my seminars and workshops, it is amazing how almost everyone will identify themselves as one of these three characters. The fact is that we are all three at some point in the victim game; though we may gravitate to one style of communication more readily than others.

I'll use my own example – the reason that I was a homeless youth. Yes, I was one of those lost kids on the streets for a while. It was a long time ago, and seems like another lifetime! Anyway, my mother, now deceased, for most of her adult life, suffered with a mental illness that caused her to be very violent towards me. I don't remember a day at home that was not frightening. I truly walked on pins and needles, never knowing what might happen in the next minute to completely turn my world upside down every minute of every day. Chaos was the theme of my childhood home life – and well into my adult life, until I finally gained an understanding of where my need for chaos originated. That's another story, and not important to this section.

On the surface, most people would determine my character as the victim, and my mother the persecutor. So who was the rescuer? Well, when my dad was around, at times he would be that rescuer. Other times it would be the school guidance counselor. Other times it would be the local hospital. However, let's take a closer look at this whole situation. When I could not take anymore abuse quietly, I viciously grabbed the soaked belt from out of my mother's hand, her usual daily punishment on bare skin, and began to whip her repeatedly until my father ran into the room and grabbed the belt from my hand. So now, who was the persecutor? And who was the victim? And when the school guidance counselor pulled me out of my home, who was the persecutor, and to whom? Would it not be the counselor who was the persecutor? And my parents, the victims? Yet was she not also a rescuer of me? And it doesn't stop there! When my parents threatened the counselor for her action, who then was the victim? That's right, the counselor. And around and around the cycle goes.

Now, after being on that triangle for all of my childhood, and a large part of my adult life, what role did I begin to adopt – the rescuer of course! I had developed such a sense of indignation for the suffering victims, I tried to rescue everyone from their tormented life, or from whatever illness they were enduring. However, for many years, I was not very effective, until I began to understand the cycle of the victim trap.

So, let's take a look at what happened in my nutrition and lifestyle counseling practice. My clients would not take responsibility for their own lives because

I was so busy rescuing them. They, in turn, took advantage of my willingness to let them off the hook for things such as showing up for appointments, or payment for my services. Of course, when I did not get paid, what role did I take? The victim, of course! Because, from my victim perspective at the time, they did not appreciate the work I had done for them. The martyr perspective of the rescuer also surfaced — *"Poor me, after all I have done for them, and they can't even pay me what they owe me!"* And then, in anger, I became the persecutor, refusing to see them again, cutting them off. So with just one client — and there were many — what roles did I assume throughout our relationship? That's right — all three! The rescuer first, followed by the victim, and finally the persecutor. Was I conscious of all of this at the time? NO!

Can We Break Free From This Perpetual *Nightmare*?

The only way to stop perpetuating this triangle in your life is to understand that any time you feel like a victim to anyone, or anything, and your response is to blame someone, or something, you are in the midst of that trap. How can you get out of it and stay out of it? First, you must understand how each of the characters behaves as they move around the triangle. And second, you need to understand fully the root cause of this triangle, which is negative co-dependency.

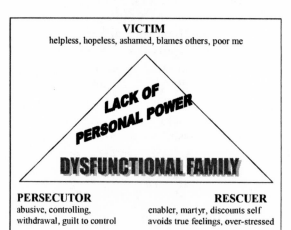

So, as I explained above, the whole victim triangle, often described as the drama triangle, is the result of a lack of a developed internal locus of control, or a lack of a sense of personal power, within the participants on the triangle. The victim is operating from a sense of helplessness, the "poor me" perspective, feeling oppressed, helpless, powerless, ashamed, victimized and hopeless. Their reactions are based on self-pity and the blaming of others for everything. They rarely make good decisions, and experience very little self-understanding and joy for life. Often substance abuse dominates his/her life.

The persecutor, also a victim, abuses others in an attempt to gain control, and uses guilt and withdrawal to control. It is always the other person's fault.

They continually criticize, blame, and oppress the victim. They are rigid and authoritative, setting very strict standards and limits for those around them. Like my mother, they will act out and react as the rigid, critical parent! The persecutor is also often a user of drugs and alcohol.

And the rescuer, also a victim, is the enabler of the victim's behavior—the "let me help you overcome your problems" attitude. As martyrs, they suffer for others, and discount themselves and their own needs. They rescue others even when they don't really want to, and are filled with guilt if they don't rescue the victim. The rescuer also uses guilt to control (i.e., "I've done all of this for you, and this is the thanks I get!"), keeping the victim dependent, and avoids expressing their true feelings. They generally expect to fail in their attempt to rescue the victim, which gives the victim permission to fail. And this person will generally appear, and is, over-stressed. We often refer to the parent who is generally a rescuer, as the "marshmallow" parent!

So what is underlying all of this? Well, as explained, it is a lack of personal power, which results in the unfulfilling games of manipulation, guilt and blame. Let's go deeper though. Most of us have two separate selves—the private self, that is hidden away, and the public self, that is expressed when around others, in our community, at work, at church, etc. Neither of these is our real, or true, self. Our private self is the one that has internalized all of our fears, insecurities, judgments, buried secrets, and feelings of self-doubt. Our public self is the one that puts on the façade, creates the image we think others expect, and covers up our secrets. It is the one that projects fake smiles, and develops roles that he/she perceives is expected or will be respected, admired, or loved. And this same public self is based on pretenses, even about family roles, or community roles (We have seen or heard about the model father or mother on the surface, or the model clergy person on the surface, being revealed as a completely different character in reality).

The Solution is Simple—Not Easy—But Simple!

What is the solution? The only way to end this triangle and create wholeness, both individually and globally, is for each and every individual to realize and accept their true self—the real person underneath the façade, and the fears (False Expectations Appearing Real) and secrets. The real self is anxiously waiting to be expressed. That means we must be willing to be vulnerable and tell the truth about who we really are. Our value does not depend on another's perception of our value. Our value is an individual inside job. Of course, to achieve this, we must be willing to forgive ourselves for our own self-judgments, and the judgments of others. Perfection is not the goal here—it is simply being the best we can be in any given moment. And by being honest about who we are, and by being willing to be vulnerable, we are, in fact, opening the door for everyone we meet, and inviting them, to do the same thing — be real and be vulnerable. This whole way of being is so freeing! I am convinced that this is what every living being truly wants. They just need permission — after years of not having it. Why not give it — permission — by being it — vulnerable? And in this equation: vulnerable = permission!

I once came across an interesting thought — Permission = per our mission! Is not one of our missions to be a whole, fulfilled and joyful person? And can we truly be all of that without assisting others in achieving that also? Not very likely, since whatever each of us does impacts the whole. The world has become too small now to think otherwise.

So Exactly What Is A Locus of Control?

On the next page is an outline of what makes up the internal and external loci of control, or personality constructs, as they are generally termed. The important thing for all of us to understand is that the victim triangle cannot exist if, one or both parties involved, have a highly developed internal locus of control, a balance of both loci, and do not buy into the victim perspective. By seeing someone as whole, and leaving ownership of the challenge or problem to the person projecting a victim perspective — and that person still believes that circumstances outside of him/herself determines the quality, or lack of quality, of his/her life — you are helping this person to grow as well. There is a saying that it takes two hands to clap. That statement saved my life and my sanity. When I made the decision not to participate in any more cycles around that crazy drama machine, the means by which I was able to stop it in its ugly tracks, was simply not to join in. If it takes two hands to clap, this hand would just not clap anymore. It worked!

I know what you're thinking! Do I forget sometimes? Of course — I am human — and I grew up, and lived much of my life, on that endless triangle. However, the more aware we become of our reactions in the moment, and the more developed our inner locus of control becomes, the easier it gets to nip the situation in the bud immediately. I promise you this works! Just remember the following statement — I know — I use a lot of repetition, but repetition is the mother/father of invention! The next time you find yourself in a situation that triggers your old victim behavior, REPEAT OUT LOUD:

"IT TAKES TWO HANDS TO CLAP,
AND MY HAND IS NOT CLAPPING!"

Let me assure you that you can develop a very strong internal locus of control, despite how entangled you may feel right now on that distorted victim triangle! Life is anything but static, so just as life is ever changing, so are you. If you *believe* that you can change, you will *achieve* that desired change. It is all based on your focus — and what is it that you are to focus on? That's right! Focus on what you want — not on what you don't want! And when you watch the movie, The Secret (www.thesecret.tv), you will completely understand why! Have you not bought it yet? What are you waiting for? I assure you, I make no material profit from recommending this to you — I just know the positive changes it has created in everyone I have shared it with!

They Say A Picture Speak Volumes . . .

So, following is a diagram that outlines the general processes involved in the inner and outer loci of control. Where do you fit on the chart? You can go the web, google "*test locus of control*" and test yourself to see where you fit as far as inner versus outer locus of control is concerned. Neither is good or bad. We just know that, overall, the inner locus folks seem to experience more control of their lives, more success, more peace, and a greater sense of achievement. And their lives are not dictated by others!

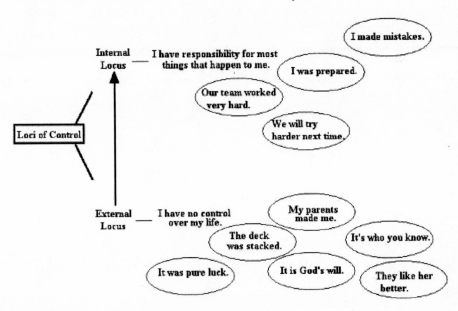

So, here is a linear summary of the characteristics of Outer / Inner Loci of Control:

Outer / External Locus of Control	Inner / Internal Locus of Control
Perception: I generally have no control	Perception: I control my destiny
Things outside of self have control	Inner thoughts and energies = results
Destiny is result of fate, luck, outside circumstances	Actions determine the rewards

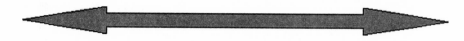

> *"Time is the coin of your life. It is the only coin you have, and only you can determine how it will be spent. Be careful lest you let other people spend it for you."*
> — Carl Sandburg

Rules to Live By — Overcome The Victim Trap
Develop a Strong Locus of Control©

Listen with your heart.

Tell the truth — there is no room for denial!

Love unconditionally — yourself and others.

Remember: Responsible = ability to respond.

Fully participate in life with joyous enthusiasm.

Act — don't react! — Reacting is from a point of weakness.

Believe: "I can. I am able — I can do it." Believe. Commit!

Dare to be different and revel in your unique talents and gifts.

Embody: I am 100% accountable for my life (No Blame Game!)

Maintain personal integrity — If you commit to something — Do it!

Accept yourself fully for who you are — with love and forgiveness.

Have expectations of yourself and others — You get what you expect!

Be a risk-taker — your choices and decisions impact everything positively.

Use words of empowerment, versus words of disempowerment
(see Attitude Chapter).

"I lead my life in a self-determinant way that creates the results I want!!"

Okay, so you are working toward being fully realized, and never the pawn in anyone else's victim-based life. That's great. One word of caution; always maintain your compassion and love for others. Remember, what goes around, comes around! Give out good — receive in good — and always be ready and open to receive. It is always wonderful to give. However, the universe needs a balance in everything, including your receiving as well as your giving. That's called flow! _And Balance!_ So go for the flow in everything, and your life will flow in every way!

CONQUER WORRY!
The Seed of All Discontent & an Attitude Destroyer

The Facts Against Worrying:

Fact: Worry is not logical!

Fact: Worry stifles creative solutions!

Fact: Worry is a wasteful form of procrastination.

Fact: Worry does no one any good whatsoever! It just wastes valuable time and energy!

Fact: Worry is founded on FEAR (False Expectations Appearing Real) of the unknown.

Fact: Worry generally has no basis for the energy wasted on it.

Fact: Worry is not the result of a problem — it is the actual cause!

Fact: Worry takes us away from thinking about the things we want — we are too busy worrying about what we don't want!

Fact: Worry prevents us from thinking about, and working on, things that can create good for others and ourselves.

Fact: Worry about the past is futile — the past is done, gone, caput! You can't change the past!

Fact: Worry about the future is futile — it is not here yet, so it is based on projected thoughts about something that will likely never happen.

Fact: Worry makes you miserable and unhappy, therefore unresourceful and unproductive.

Fact: Worry makes you age faster, and creates deep unhappy lines on your face.

Fact: Worry makes you sick — all of those free radicals that are produced due to the stress caused in your body by your focus on worry.

Fact: Worry creates problems in our minds — versus opportunities for growth.

Fact: Worry alienates others — people want to be around happy vibrant energy.

Fact: Worry never solves a problem — positive action does!

Fact: The longer you worry, the more miserable you become!

The Strategies for Preventing or Overcoming Worry:

> Stop the worry thought in its tracks — see a big red stop sign and shout STOP to yourself!

> Identify the source of what is bothering you — ask yourself why it is bothering you. Keep asking why this is bothering you until you get to the root cause. Think about how you would describe your concern to someone else.
> After you have identified the source of your worry, take out a notepad, write out the problem or concern, and then start writing down every possible solution.
> Determine whether you can solve the problem or problems by yourself — or do you need help from others?
> Determine how much time you need in order to solve the issue — and schedule a realistic time frame.
> Break the solution down into short-term goals, or steps, that will eventually get you to your desired outcome.
> If you need more information in order to understand the problem, do some research.
> If you just can't determine a solution for your concern on your own, confide in someone you trust and respect, and ask for his/her input. By simply sharing and discussing a problem with a friend, it often diminishes the seriousness of the concern.
> If you are worried about your health, plan a strategy to begin to take control of it — maybe it is just adding 5 minutes a day on your Rebounder, see the chapter, *Fit in Fitness,* — the released endorphins, alone, will relax you and ease your worrying.
> If you are worried about finances, consult with a financial advisor, and then take action to learn how to best handle your finances. Knowledge is power — you will have the power of knowing, with the help of an advisor / specialist, exactly what is happening with your finances; and then establish a plan for effectively handling them.
> If you are worried about your significant relationship — maybe they have not been very attentive lately — make a decision to speak your truth to your partner about your concerns, and invite them to do the same. Then work together on strategies to improve, eliminate, or overcome, any issues or obstacles that may presently exist.
> If you are worrying about someone else, remember that you can't help anyone with worry — just as for yourself, only actions can help another. And only if they want your help! Remember, you can't be responsible for another — only yourself!

You know how a stitch in time saves nine? Taking action right away, at the onset of a situation, concern or worry, can save many hours, days, weeks, even years — of wasted time, energy, and stress — and maybe even prevent an illness from developing, due to your chronic worrying.

And just a little more food for thought regarding worry:

When we live each of the aspects of our lives — personal, professional, and spiritual — with full focus and concentration, in the now, the present, without wasted thoughts about the past, the future, or other things that we have no control over, or can't do anything about, we experience a profound sense of satisfaction, fulfillment, peace and joy in the achievement of each of our desired goals and dreams. We feel vibrant, alert, enthusiastic and passionate about our lives when we focus our full attention, right now, in this moment, on the things that will actually move us closer to the achievement of our precious dreams. Any other thoughts that get in the way of this focus, and have no relevance to our desired end result, are simply wasted thoughts. Worry is just that — wasted thoughts!

In Zelinski's book *"The Joy of Not Working: A Book for the Retired, Unemployed, and Overworked,"* we find a table about wasted worries. The table indicates that 96% of our worries are wasted time. Wasted Worries according to E. Zelinski:

40% of our worries have to do with events that will never take place
30% of our worries have to do with events that have already taken place
22% of our worries have to do with unimportant events
4% of our worries have to do with events that we cannot change
4% of our worries have to do with events that we can do something about

Let me repeat — only 4% of our worries have to do with events that we can do something about.

As the saying goes: ***Where your attention goes, your energy flows.*** Why not have your energy flow toward your dream, versus toward the worry, which is most likely unfounded to begin with?

WORRY

<u>W</u>asted time & life!
<u>O</u>verstressed & exhausted!
<u>R</u>elationships broken!
<u>R</u>estlessness & insomnia!
<u>Y</u>oke that will destroy you!

Worry my child, is a silent killer.
When you least expect, it sneaks up on you.
In your quiet time, in the middle of the night,
In your car while driving, yes, even at work.
It does you no good, it fixes nothing.
It simply adds to your misery, and saps your energy.
Before you know it, it's become your best pal,
Going with you, wherever you go.
The good Lord told you, there's no need to worry.
Why not listen and obey, the best teacher there is?
Don't worry, my child!

—Anonymous

SO WHAT'S THE BIG DEAL ABOUT BELIEFTS
Change Your Beliefs — Change Your Life!

"If you think you can or you think you can't, you are right!"
— Henry Ford

How many times have you thought to yourself, or even expressed to others . . .
"Wow, I've done everything I can and still I am not getting the results I expected in my life?"

Or . . .
"I'll believe it when I see it!" And then never see it!

Or . . .
"I can't believe how difficult it is to _____!" (You get to fill in the blanks.)
Well, obviously you do believe how difficult it is, because that is exactly what you're getting — DIFFICULT!

And how many times have you felt like a complete victim of life? The harder you try to make things happen, or to find happiness and satisfaction, the more dissatisfied and unhappy you have become.

It is amazing how many of my patients and clients have called me over the years, trembling with incredible fear in their voices — fear that they will not be able to overcome a particular health challenge, or that they do not have the capacity to take charge of a specific life situation. Well-meaning friends, family members, and various health professionals have inflicted their own fear-based doubts and beliefs upon this already, physically or emotionally, compromised individual.

And then this challenged individual buys into, and internalizes, the fear-based beliefs of those people they trust, who have been so convincing; hence, feeling completely defeated before they have even begun to personally address the situation at hand. I have gone there myself many times over my own lifetime! So what belief are we all coming from? It is certainly not a belief that we will, or do, have the resources to find a solution to a particular situation, or to overcome a particular health challenge!

We are coming from the belief that:

I will believe it when I see it. Or: I have to see it to believe it!

104

Well, let's stop and think about this for a minute. Take some time right now, and *think of a time when you achieved a major desired outcome?* How did you do it? You might say by taking action—or you might say it was from your behavior, or your sense of expectation, both of which, by the way, determine your action. Okay, but from what place inside you did that behavior, expectation, or action blossom? FROM BELIEF! FROM THE BELIEF THAT YOU COULD DO IT—AND THAT YOU WOULD DO IT! Where there is belief, there is no doubt! Only faith, that it is so!

Of course, if your belief is that the cup is ½ empty, you have no doubt that it is just that. So you create, by your expectations, behaviors, and actions, more of that ½ empty outcome! For great "cup ½ full", versus the "cup ½ empty", results, we have to internalize and embody healthy, happy, optimistic, fulfilling, positive, and rewarding beliefs into our very own biology.

And remember: Behavior is simply your belief expressing itself, and cannot be changed simply by changing your mind. What drives your behavior is not what you *think*, but what you actually *believe*. And as far as your expectations are concerned, they are also very firmly rooted in your beliefs. So, expectations alone simply won't drive you home to your desired results. People say you get what you expect. *No, you get what you believe you expect!*

Everything—and I mean *everything*—starts with BELIEF!

You see: BELIEF DRIVES EVERYTHING!

You don't believe what you see. You see what you believe.
You don't believe what you think. You think what you believe.

So, how can we adjust our thoughts, in order to then experience our desired outcomes? By adjusting our beliefs! And you ask: How do I adjust my beliefs—I've had them all of my life!

Well, like everything in life, we have to stop what we are doing—get off the roller coaster of life—and take the time to ask ourselves, and sincerely answer, some deeply introspective questions. This is the only way to truly uncover our hidden beliefs about ourselves, about life, in particular our own life, and about the world around us, as well as how we individually perceive that world around us impacts our personal and private world. We are all the centers of our own universes. And what we believe about ourselves, and our relationship to our surrounding universe is what we experience in our daily lives. If our experience is unsatisfactory, we need to get to the root of the internal beliefs that are responsible for this external expression, and change them at a cellular level.

Choice, in every aspect of our life, is a human privilege. However, having the right and ability to choose what we want in our lives, is a double-edged sword; it can work for us, or against us. Regarding belief, each of us has a choice. We can believe one of four things:

1. What everyone else believes.
2. What we would rather believe.
3. What other people, and/or industries, and/or the government, want us to believe.
4. What is actual reality, or the truth.

Which one do you think is in your best interest? Which one is in another's best interest? Which one would most other people like you to embrace? Generally speaking, everyone has his or her own specific agenda, which just may not be in your best interest. By knowing yourself and your own deep-seated beliefs, you can make much wiser and more informed choices. Of course, if a belief you hold is not serving you in a healthy and fulfilling manner, change it! Now!

Since awareness is the key to changing your beliefs, you have to ask yourself the right questions in order to get to that place of awareness. And then appropriate actions, coupled with this new awareness, result in acts of power, mastery, and co-creation. So let's start by changing the quality of the questions you ask yourself, in order to really get to the depth of the beliefs that may be holding you back in your life.

To determine the power of what you believe, a very insightful process is to write down 5 things you believe about yourself and the world around you. If you are stumped by this, ask others in your life what they believe about you. Remember, what they believe about you is something that you have reflected to them about you, so it is reflective of your beliefs about yourself. You may be very surprised by what others share with you about yourself.

Each of us creates the specific life we experience every single day. Whether we are held back by an invisible or insignificant restraint (or limiting belief), or motivated by investing all of our faith into empowering beliefs, such as "I can do, I can be, I can have, etc.", we are each the creator of our specific life, and the one with all the power. Only you have the power to agree on what to believe in your life!

And it is critical for you to really see, and acknowledge, the beliefs that you hold about your life, about others, about abundance (or lack of it), about health, about the world, etc. Understand that YOU *created* these beliefs; therefore, you *can create* different beliefs. It is important to ask yourself what agreements you have made with yourself about what you will believe, or not believe, about yourself, your life, the things that happen to you, the things that happen to others, and your attachment to each of these beliefs. Sounds too ethereal and too out there for you? Trust me, if you will take the time to work through my 8-Step Process, your life may just never be the same again! And I mean that in the most positive way!

Creating New Beliefs

Okay, so let's get started. Remember: If you want quality change in your beliefs, and hence, in your life, you have to schedule quality time without interruption to go through this process. Answer the questions honestly, and then write about what you notice arising within you (emotionally — hate, anger, frustration, love joy, etc; physically — wrenching gut, neck pain, tense muscles, tight throat, perspiration, relaxed, etc; mentally — anxiety, denial, blame, guilt, self-determined, relaxed, etc; spiritually — emptiness, peace, fulfillment, etc) after each answer. In other words, ask yourself not only the question, but also _why_ you answered the way you did:

Here's my 8-Step Process to get you there:

I. Become aware, and conscious, of your present beliefs. You created these beliefs — you can create different beliefs. Ask yourself some or all of these questions in order to uncover your personal beliefs. Really contemplate your answers. Do not rush through this process if you are serious about creating lasting change. Write your answers down with clarity and simplicity.

1. Am I realizing my deepest desires and achieving my soul's purpose? *What are they? List them — write them down.*
2. How does my outlook or perspective hinder me realizing my desired outcomes?
3. Do I have a habit of assuming things without knowing all of the facts? *Observe how often you make assumptions over the course of one full day.*
4. What do I constantly tell myself is impossible, can't be done?
5. What do I tell others about myself? How do I introduce myself? What stories do I share with others, about me, and about my life?
6. What is one thing that is working in my life? What belief do I have about that?

7. What is one thing that is not working in my life? What belief do I have about that?

8. What is my unique perspective or belief that drives everything in my life—my opinions, attitudes, decisions, intentions, actions, and reactions?

9. Who are the people that are closest to me in my life—personally, professionally? *List them.*

10. How does each one of them reflect my beliefs—about my life, about my relationship to the world around me, about my relationship to others?

11. What are 5 emotional attachments that are hot buttons in my life? *For example: I am still angry that my parents ripped my brother and I away from our extended family in our homeland of Scotland—not once, but 3 times! So I have never had a sense of true family connection. Actually, to a large extent, I have overcome this emotional charge. However, since it was a very high-temperature hot button for much of my life, I used this as an example to assist you, the reader, in understanding what is being asked for in this question. And then ask yourself* "How does my response make me feel?"

12. What is one thing I most want to accomplish in my life before I die? Why?

13. What TV show or movie best reflects and represents my life? Why?

14. What are 10 things that make you me happy or bring the most joy in my life?

15. What award would hold the most value for me? *Employee of the month, Parent of the year, Professional of the Year, Humanitarian of the Year, Nobel prize, Pulitzer, Emmy, Oscar etc?*

II. Look for the limiting beliefs that surfaced as you answered the questions. Some examples of limiting beliefs are:

I'm just not enough as I am.
Money never comes easily to me.
I don't belong here.
I wasn't wanted.
I am not good enough.
I feel ashamed and guilty.
I will never be any good.
I always lose some of myself in relationships.
I feel a deep sense of sadness inside.
I can't feel joy.
I don't feel safe.
People can't be trusted.

I am safer on my own.
Men / women can't be trusted.
I don't feel safe in relationships.
I would like a relationship but I would only get hurt.
I'm too sensitive.
I am to blame for everything.
I am not lovable.
I don't measure up.
I am no good.
I don't deserve anything.
I am afraid of success.
Bad things happen to me all the time.
I am not safe.
I am still angry with my mother/father.
I find it hard to forgive and let go.
I can't let go of the past.
Life is difficult.
There is no peace in this world.
Why can't I be happy like others?
I don't like myself, and all of my weaknesses.
I can't take a compliment.
Why can't I see what other people see in me?
I'm always trying to sabotage myself, and all of my efforts.
What's wrong with me that I always attract narcissistic men/women?
I'm too vulnerable.
I am too exposed.
I am angry with God.
I punish myself.
I can't let go of the sadness and pain.
I'm just going to die anyway.

III. Determine the consequences of not changing your beliefs that are limiting you. There are four key questions that form the basis of what is referred to as NLP (Neuro-Linguistic Programming) based explorations. NLP is one of the most powerful processes you can go through on your journey of self discovery. Before you answer these questions:

- Pick any belief you've determined for yourself that you want to change.
- Run through each of the following four questions, one by one, and take the time to sincerely answer each one.
- Notice how differently you feel with each question.

So, here are the 4 key questions — and don't skip any of them:

1. **What would happen if you eliminated this belief?**
2. **What would happen if you did not eliminate this belief?**
3. **What would not happen if you eliminated this belief?**
4. **What would not happen if you did not eliminate this belief?**

Question #4 is perhaps one of the most mind-provoking, and mind-expanding, questions you can address with yourself. Or, for that matter, with a loved one, or a team member, or business partner! This last question will truly have you thinking outside of the box of conditioned mass consciousness thinking and belief patterning. You'll get new answers, an important step in changing your mind, and hence your belief.

IV. Assume responsibility for the beliefs you have created in your life. Realize you have a choice about what you believe, and DECIDE to change any of your limiting beliefs that you discovered during steps 1 and 2.

V. Interrupt your old belief pattern by replacing that belief with a new one that makes you feel great. An example may be, "I am absolutely enough in everything I do. I achieve everything in my life easily, and effortlessly, with grace and ease." Or, "I am the kind of person who attracts money easily and effortlessly every day in every way. I live a fully abundant life, simply because I AM the kind of person to whom financial well-being flows."

VI. Install the new belief by repeating and reinforcing it daily, as often as possible throughout the day. Preferably, stand in your power, and express this belief affirmatively, with passion, enthusiasm and gratitude — gratitude for this belief, as if you have already firmly embodied it. Place a copy of your new belief everywhere you are most likely to see it — on your office wall, on your refrigerator, in the bathroom, on your Palm, on your computer monitor, etc. (I personally love the **Dream Wizard** software that you can program all of your dreams and visions into, and hear about them at scheduled intervals throughout the day, when you are working on your computer.)

VII. Most importantly, come from a place of Love — eliminate Fear (False Expectations Appearing Real). These are the only 2 emotions attached to any belief you have, or agreement you have made with yourself — you make the choice.

Fear begets Loss; Love begets Abundance.

VIII. Always express an Attitude of Gratitude for this expansive belief, or beliefs, in your life. Reward yourself for making this shift in consciousness. Make it a positive reward, perhaps a spa day, a new outfit, a special dinner with close friends, a movie night, a weekend cruise with that special person in your life—you name it . . .

If you believe it, you will achieve it!
So go get it—whatever it is you want, with the belief that anything is possible. And it is, if you believe it is!

You have the power to change the very foundation of your life—
YOUR BELIEFS!

I PROMISE, YOUR LIFE WILL NEVER BE THE SAME AGAIN!

THE AGING MOUNTAIN THEORY & PROCESS:
A Guide to Overcoming Any Obstacles
And Challenges in Your Life!

About one year after my initial diagnosis with cancer, I attended a 5-day intensive retreat program on a beautiful mountainous island off the coast of Washington State, in the US. We experienced five of the most extraordinarily beautiful sunny and warm days imaginable in an area that rarely experiences a day without rain. The bulk of our time, outside of workshops, was spent in complete silence, with every activity being some form of meditation.

On the third afternoon of the retreat I experienced an event so significant that it has left a permanent imprint on my life that impacts everything I do to this day! It was our lunch break, and we were surrounded by magical and wondrous beauty! I found myself sitting on the edge of a majestic cliff by the water's edge, gazing at some of the most breathtaking, rolling mountains I had ever seen. Though not very rugged in nature, they were truly majestic in their own right.

The Aging of a Mountain

I found my mind wandering to all of the places in the world that I had had the good fortune of traveling to. Wherever I have gone, mountains have always held me in awe! Some of my most spiritually progressive experiences were in mountainous regions including Nepal, the Hunza Valley, India, parts of Japan, Mexico, South America, New Mexico and Arizona, the state of Georgia in Russia, and the Great Wall of China, just to mention a few.

It was fascinating to think about the many heights, shapes and sizes, from high, jagged peaks to low, rolling hills, and everything in between. Now, what is the determining factor in all of this? The age of the mountain! It determines the height, and the jagged and rough edges versus the soft, smooth and gently rolling nature of the hills. Is this not much like the aging of humans? That is exactly what I asked myself on that peaceful reflective afternoon. Reviewing my own life, I could definitely relate my own transformations throughout my life, to the transformations the mountain goes through with each passing year.

A young mountain reaches for the heavens, statuesquely and uniquely cut, awesome to view, boasting its power with jagged, rough, and barren peaks, and often razor sharp edges; dangerous at the best of times, with extreme behaviors in temperature and climate, generally fairly arid, and difficult to climb, often claiming the lives of even the most athletic individuals. The aging mountain, on the other hand, softens, as its edges are smoothed out due to weathering and breakdown over time. Easier to climb and more lush, due to the much lower elevation and more temperate climate, these low lying mountains invite us to enjoy comfortable walks, hikes, and picnics with our family and friends.

We Age Gracefully Like The Mountain

Both the young and the old mountains are beautiful in their own right! Think of a young person and their characteristics, and an older person and their characteristics. We are so much like those mountains I viewed on that heavenly day. Like the mountain, we define ourselves in our youth by our individuality, competitiveness, extremes, our need to be right — sometimes at any cost! We express our sharp, rough edges for all to see — and experience. Our tempers may be hot, our dispositions cold, and our patience minimal, with war and violence often our solution to everything.

As we age, we tone down. Like the mountain edges, we become smoother, less defined, more flowing and more refined. We blend into the community, while still maintaining our individuality. It is more important to live by example with integrity, and to assist others in creating the same for themselves. We want to work and play within a cooperative team-based structure, and understand and perpetuate the value of each person's unique gift to the whole. We blend into the culture without becoming it.

Just as not every mountain ages with incredible beauty and elegance, neither does every human. For example, a mountain may face a major earthquake, or spit forth, from its deep interior, hot volcanic juices. Obviously the outcome may resemble a very disrupted figure with little obvious beauty — remember perception is everything and always very individual in nature — and only hot cinders. Perhaps this could be compared to an individual who is experiencing his/her own personal earthquake in life, such as dying of cancer in a hospital bed. There are simply some energies that may not be within our control at our present level of consciousness!

However, what we may not understand on a purely physical dimension, we can grasp on a more universal level, if we are willing to do the work, to go back to our center. The human trait is to go into fear and worry, doubt and frustration, and then to act out of these conditions of consciousness, as soon as something does not fit the picture we have brought into the particular scenario. If, like the mountain, we could simply remain in our center of consciousness, our center of knowledge of our oneness with all things, we would tap into the universal unconscious and understand that something greater than us, yet which encompasses and embodies us, is at work. When we realize that we are not our bodies, or our minds, or our emotions, but that we are spirit experiencing itself in a physical form, we can live more fully the moments we do have in this present form, with the understanding that it is but a temporary stop-over in the universal journey that each of us in on.

Energy can neither be created nor destroyed! It simply changes form. The life force within our bodies is that energy. To be at peace with the chaos that presents itself throughout human existence, the key is to get to that place within each of us, which is unaffected and immovable — our essence!

The Aging Mountain Theory Emerges & Unfolds:
On Becoming Centered

So, that day sitting on that cliff, watching the stillness of the mountains, and realizing that, as the years and the elements wore them down, they stood strongly and boldly, ever-changing, yet centered, seeming to know, and joyfully accept, their place in the universe, without question or doubt. That was where I wanted to be! The journey began. And with it is my theory — The Aging Mountain Theory. In the following learning sheets, all of the processes and qualities are fully covered, and they will fully move you out of a victim consciousness, into taking responsibility for your own outcomes in life.

Our inner locus of control (not affected by what is happening outside of ourselves and around us, but by our inner core values and sense of self-worth), which forms the basis of this centering exercise, is comparable in my Aging Mountain Theory to the immovability of the mountain from its position despite the elements and circumstances it faces daily. The mountain is unaffected by what is done to it, apart from becoming more approachable, softer and gentler to all who experience it. However, just as the mountain is very unique in its own right, expressing its character with its own unique curves and twists and definite slopes, so too is each of us with our own unique and individual talents and gifts. As we each become more centered in our individual wholeness, we can then become centered in our unique positioning in the universe, just as the mountain becomes centered in its unique positioning within its universe.

Finally, passion for life and for the expression of one's unique gift, is the motivation and the fire that keeps us going when things seem off balance, or when things seem not to be running according to our design. Passion is the driving spirit that galvanizes our purpose, and propels it unceasingly forward, so that it continually unfolds for the benefit of both ourselves, and all those we share it with. And our passion is what inspires others to grab onto whatever it is that we have that they want, as well as inspiring them to develop their own unique gifts in order to share them with the world.

The Oneness of All Incorporates the Uniqueness of One

From my experience and perspective, a healthy individual is one who has a highly developed understanding of the oneness of all things in the universe, yet a realization of his/her unique contribution to the whole, and the importance of that contribution to the existence of the whole. This individual is living every moment fully, operating in the passion of their unique talent/gift. This evolved being radiates love, peace, harmony, joy, bliss, compassion, generosity, integrity, enthusiasm, gratitude and appreciation for everything.

To discover your own unique gift, the following worksheet moves you from the base of the mountain in your life, which is survival, though to the summit or the peak, which represents self-realization or a completely committed relationship with God. In some philosophies this would be called Oneness with God. Please understand that this is not a religious perspective, but rather a philosophical perspective. It is not contrary to any religious beliefs one may carry. I have worked with people from every faith on this planet, using this process. It is simply a joining of hearts!

What the Heck are Tolerations?

Let's talk about "tolerations" in the second step of the process, or worksheet. What are you tolerating in your life right now? What are you putting up with that you truly don't want in your life. I know that our focus has to be on what we do want in order to get our desired outcomes in life. However, if you aren't clear about what you have in your life right now that you simply want to end or get rid of, your lack of awareness about these things allows them to remain in your life and fester, like a wound that never heals and becomes infected. With awareness, you can work toward eliminating them once and for all. And usually that is by being pro-active and taking action steps to change them. And, of course, at the same time, by changing your thoughts and words from a focus on what you don't want, to a focus on what you do want, you will eventually stop creating, in your life, those "tolerations" those things you don't want.

So, what are some examples of things you may be tolerating? Perhaps you are in a job you hate, or working with a boss or manager that you can't stand. Maybe you are enmeshed in a toxic relationship with a significant other, or another family member, and spend most of your time with them racing around the Victim Triangle (see the chapter: **The Victim Trap**). Do you have a health challenge that you have been putting off doing something about? Or a bill that is so large you never get around to paying it? Maybe you have a lot of debts and have not yet figured out how to handle them. Perhaps your house needs a lot of repairs that you just don't ever seem to get around to doing. Or maybe it is simply a few plants that desperately need repotting, and you simply keep forgetting—except when you walk past them every other day. Get them all out on paper and then you can start to deal with what needs to be dealt with in a much more effective manner.

How to Get the Most Out of the Following Worksheets:

With increased self-awareness we are generally much better equipped to create a more balanced and harmonious approach to life, with realistic goals for each area of our life. This, in turn, leads to greater self-confidence in our own ability to make daily choices that are most beneficial for our overall health, and therefore assist us in maintaining lower stress levels.

Though I have created worksheets that follow for you to use, I suggest that for the first time doing this process, you take out a legal size notepad, and on the top of each of 3 separate pages you put the headings from the first page:

> WHAT YOU LIKE ABOUT YOUR LIFE RIGHT NOW
> WHAT YOU ARE TOLERATING IN YOUR LIFE RIGHT NOW
> WHAT YOU WOULD LIKE YOUR IDEAL LIFE TO LOOK LIKE

Your Life Right Now

We begin with what you like about your life right now. It is very powerful to start with the positive things in your life—the things that you are most appreciative of, and that move you in the direction of realizing your own personal values, such as peace, joy, happiness, fulfillment, and balance. To assist you in determining your own specific values, see the **Values** list at the end of this chapter. You can start by making a list of 3-5 values that are absolutely essential in your life. Or you can write your list of what is great in your life right now, and then determine your values from that list. You may think of more things in your life that you are grateful for, or that you truly do enjoy, as you move through the rest of the exercise. That's why having this extra space to write a longer list is invaluable. Use more than one page for each of the first 3 steps if you need to. There is no limit to how much you can write. Just write until you can't think of anything else.

Those Darned Tolerations

Do the same thing with the tolerations list, which was discussed previously in this chapter. And in this section you can also list your fears that may be getting in the way of achieving all of your dreams. Perhaps you are afraid of dying in a plane crash, or worried that your business won't bring in enough money to pay bills, or that you will lose your house due to financial challenges or foreclosure. Maybe you are afraid that you will get stuck in a relationship that takes away your freedom. Perhaps you are already in such a relationship right now. Again there is no limit to what you can write. Just write until there is nothing more coming from your brain to write on that page.

And What's Your Ideal Life?

And then do the same process with what you desire in your ideal life. These could include material things such as the house of your dreams, a specific car you desire, your ideal job, artwork or furniture you desire, a home theatre, gym or sauna, a face lift, a new wardrobe, or a boat to sail around the world in. In this segment, you may also design your career, develop a TV or radio show, create a massive publishing company, or launch a huge charitable organization that ends hunger/poverty/homelessness. Perhaps you would like to adopt a child from a less fortunate population. It's your life. Be creative and allow your deepest desires and dreams to make it onto that page. If you could snap your fingers and have anything in life, what would that be? Or what would your life look like?

Once you realize where you are right now — the positive, the negative, and the dreams and desires you have — then the next step is to determine, from everything that you have written in the three lists, **the 5 most important things** to you right now. Write them down in the space provided on the worksheets. You may want to make several copies of each of the pages of the worksheets for future use. Think about what would most effectively alleviate at least a couple of the tolerations you have been putting up with. Tolerations drain us of our precious energy. Remember, where our focus goes energy flows. And though we may not be aware on a conscious level that this is occurring, these tolerations are wreaking havoc with our immune system on a cellular level, as a result of an underlying current of unresolved chronic stress.

You may decide that you need to increase your income in order to pay off large credit card debts. You may need to get counseling on your relationship situation, or even get out of a toxic relationship. Perhaps you are dealing with a major weight issue, or life challenging illness, and the time has come to hire a life coach or health practitioner to assist you in creating an effective detox, and/or wellness, program. If overwhelming worry or fear, (False Expectations Appearing Real) are controlling your life, it may be a good time to seek out a ropes course or some other form of personal growth program. Once you have addressed the most pressing items you place in this short list today, you can come back to this list and select 5 more items to address.

Heart—Centered Intention

Okay, the moment of truth arrives. What, in this short list of 5 items, are you truly ready to commit to changing right now? It is a fact that we cannot achieve great results in many things at the same time. So, we have to be gut-wrenchingly honest with ourselves about what we are truly ready, at this moment in time, to address head-on, with heart-centered intention and conviction for change.

The Power of Affirmations with "Feeling" . . .

Affirmations are a powerful step in this process. But only if there is a tremendous amount of feeling attached to the affirmation. Well, by this point, after working through all of the previous steps in this process, you should have come to a place of deep emotional connection to those things you want to change right now. So let's look at an example of how to create the most appropriate affirmation based on what you may have written and worked through so far.

Perhaps one of your tolerations is that you have been diagnosed with cancer. And your fear is that you will die. A concern you have is that you have no idea where to start with the journey back to excellent health. And in the life you desire, what you most want right now is to be completely healthy, and living a vibrant, full life everyday. So an affirmation for you may be, **"I am healthy, vital, balanced, and brimming with boundless energy, because I make excellent nutrition, lifestyle, and attitude choices every day in every way!"** When you state this intention, stand up straight, center yourself in your power, and repeat it clearly and loudly while allowing yourself, with your mind's help, to deeply feel these expressions of health vibrating throughout your entire body. Feel your complete health and vitality as if it is a reality right now. Again: *everything that exists began with a thought and a conviction or intention (affirmation) that it could actually exist.* Any great athlete will tell you that first they affirmed they were going to win. And then they took that thought and used it to visualize the moment of winning, which they pictured in their mind, and at the same time, *felt in their body, as though it had already happened!*

If you Fail to Plan, You Plan to Fail!

Congratulations! You have now come to the point of scheduling what you are willing to do each day of the week in order to achieve your desired results. You know the expression: *If you fail to plan, you plan to fail*. So getting a system established on a daily basis sets you up for success. Your consistency of efforts is the only proven strategy for maximum results/success. You can't get fit from one long workout each week—but you can from one relatively short workout 5-6 times each week. It's the action that becomes a habit that leads to your destiny! I love the following quote, which I think says it all:

> Watch your *thoughts*; they become *words*.
> Watch your *words*; they become *actions*.
> Watch your *actions*; they become *habits*.
> Watch your *habits*; they become *character*.
> Watch your *character*; it becomes your *destiny*.
> —Frank Outlaw

So determine what you will do each day and for how long. For example, you may (and I recommend this) choose to repeat your affirmation three times each day, morning, noon and evening. Plus each day you may also choose to take some action step that will move you towards clearing one of the tolerations off your list.

Inner Reflection = Inner Balance

I have found, that without adequate quiet time for inner reflection, which encompasses relaxation, prayer, and meditation, the hustle and bustle of our everyday lives eventually stretches us to a point of no return on every level of our existence: physically, mentally, emotionally and spiritually. Without regularly scheduled time for relaxation, reflection and renewal, our outlook on life becomes strained, unfocused, cluttered, anxious, and fragmented. In other words, we can't see the forest for the trees! Efficiency of thought, word, and action is hampered and everything seems like a huge effort, with significantly diminishing returns. Our nerves eventually feel like elastic bands ready to snap! Relaxation is as important to regaining and maintaining our health, preventing an illness, and creating overall well being, as is exercise and the food we eat.

This time out does not have to be an hour—or even a half hour. In fact, a dedicated 5-10 minutes daily of quiet time can make a powerful impact on your outward expression to the world. Just *letting a situation be* for a few minutes while you breath deeply, slowly and rhythmically, allows you to become calm and balanced in the face of a problem, and in turn, to experience a healthier relationship with what is disturbing you. I recommend a minimum of 5 minutes twice a day, in the morning, and again in the late afternoon or evening. However, if taking time out works best for you once a day for 10-15 minutes, at a particular time of the day that fits better into your schedule, just schedule it for that time. Again, remember, that consistency – doing it everyday, or almost everyday – will reap maximum benefits for you. For more detailed information on relaxation, prayer and meditation, see the chapter: **Balance From the Inside Out: The Power of Time Out.**

Two of my favorite CD's, for taking my patients and me quickly and easily to that place of inner peace and harmony, during those precious stolen moments throughout our hectic days are, **The 5 Minute Hour** and **The 5 Minute Hour 2.** Each of these unique CD's include five, 5-minute, healing flute melodies. Created by the incredibly gifted and world-renowned flutist, Maria Kostelas, these musical masterpieces are highly effective in releasing tension and restoring vitality and wellbeing. You will literally experience 60 minutes of relaxation in just a short five minutes. The CD's are available in the products section of my website: www.marilynjoyce.com.

Of course, breathing is a critical part of the relaxation and renewal process. There is no life without breath! And remember that to fill your body with this precious life force enhancer you have to breathe deeply, extending your abdomen fully with each breath in, and contracting it completely with each breath out. See the chapter: **Balance From the Inside Out: The Power of Time Out** for more information on this subject, plus a simple 5-minute breathing technique I teach my patients and clients that can be done anywhere, anytime.

Journaling: The Road to Self-Awareness

And now we arrive at the final step of the Aging Mountain Process, other than the Commitment Contract. I personally believe that *journaling* is an essential step in any health and wellness program. It is one of the keys to self-discovery and self-awareness. By journaling, you reach inside yourself to places you may otherwise never explore. And at the same time, you connect, far beyond yourself, with the universal rhythms and forces of nature, and of God. Journaling helps you to gain clarity, solve problems, and discover valuable insights. You are, in essence, inviting answers and insights, both from within yourself, and from God and the universe, for whatever you are dealing with in your life right now. For more details on how to most effectively journal, see the chapter: **Balance From the Inside Out: The Power of Time Out.**

"The reason most people never reach their goals is that they
don't define them,
or ever seriously consider them as believable or achievable.
Winners can tell you where they are going, what they plan to do
along the way,
and who will be sharing the adventure with them."

Denis Waitley

NOW—Get Committed!

Are you asking why I have included a Commitment Contract? Let's face it. Humans are a strange breed! Without some form of accountability we just don't seem to get much done. We need a simple system for tracking what we say we are going to do, with a specific timeline attached, in order to prevent our commitments from somehow falling through the cracks. Otherwise, we come up with more excuses for why we were not able to accomplish our tasks, goals, dreams, visions—well, let's just say, our life, in general!

Yet, I have never found any value in having some kind of punishment attached to not achieving something we say we are going to do. Punishment has a negative connotation, and sets a person up for failure overall, due to the guilt and shame one may feel, based on a false perception that they are not doing or being enough. If we are always focused on the resulting pain (punishment) associated with not doing what we say we are going to do, in a time frame we have established, this negative energy expands, and ripples into everything else in our lives. We feel that we are not enough, or we are not good enough. Or we don't deserve success! Or we are just one big failure! So we continue to fail at everything we do—or at least, a lot of what we attempt to do.

However, it creates a completely different outcome when, instead of punishment for not achieving what we say we are going to do, we receive rewards for what we, in fact, do accomplish. The good feelings—good vibrational frequencies—generated by the rewards then set us up to succeed in future endeavors. Remember: Focus on what you want, not on what you don't want! You want good energy and positive outcomes. So by rewarding yourself for what you do accomplish, you set yourself up to accomplish more of what you commit to.

And, what the heck . . .

So what if you don't get everything done that you say you are going to do in the time frame that you set up to achieve those objectives and commitments! It is not the end of the world. Just recommit to the incomplete objective, and then reward yourself when you achieve it. There is simply no reward, in this process, when you do not achieve something you have committed to. That's it in a nutshell. No hard or bad feelings are necessary. Just let it be—and get back to work.

> "Finish every day and be done with it . . . You have done what you could; some blunders and absurdities no doubt crept in; forget them as soon as you can. Tomorrow is a new day; you shall begin it well and serenely and with too high a spirit to be cumbered with your old nonsense. This day is all that is good and fair. It is too dear, with its hopes and invitations, to waste a moment on the rotten yesterdays."
>
> —Ralph Waldo Emerson

Finally, when you write an explanation (as required on the contract) for why you did not achieve your goal or objective, this allows you to better understand what may be standing in your way. And this awareness can assist you in removing the block or blocks so that achievement is possible at a later date. Journaling can also help you with this process by taking you to a deeper level of understanding regarding anything that may be standing in the way of your success.

How Often Can I Do the Process?

This Aging Mountain process can be done as often as needed to get, and keep, your life on track. Many of my patients and clients do this process on a monthly basis. I personally do it every 2 - 3 months. Your *initial* time investment may range from one hour to as many as 3 hours. However, it is well worth the time and effort for the long-term benefits you will derive. Subsequent visits to this process may take as little as 10 - 30 minutes. It all depends on what you want to get out of doing the process, and what you desire in, and for, your life. I would love to hear about your experiences as a result of working through these worksheets, and any of the outcomes you have realized as a result—positive, negative or neutral. Just email me at: info@marilynjoyce.com.

So go ahead . . .

Fly like an Eagle
&
Realize your Dreams!

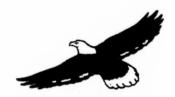

AGING MOUNTAIN WORKSHEETS
& COMMITMENT FORM

WHAT DO YOU LIKE ABOUT YOUR LIFE RIGHT NOW?

1)
2)
3)
4)
5)
6)
7)
8)
9)
10)

WHAT ARE YOU TOLERATING (PUTTING UP WITH) IN YOUR LIFE RIGHT NOW?

1)
2)
3)
4)
5)
6)
7)
8)
9)
10)

WHAT WOULD YOU LIKE YOUR IDEAL LIFE TO LOOK LIKE?

1)
2)
3)
4)
5)
6)

7)
8)
9)
10)

WHAT OUT OF THE ABOVE IS MOST IMPORTANT TO YOU AT THIS TIME?

1)
2)
3)
4)
5)

WHAT ARE YOU WILLING TO COMMIT TO CHANGE RIGHT NOW?

1)
2)
3)

WHAT QUALITY DO YOU WANT TO DEVELOP WITHIN YOURSELF?
(Examples: love, forgiveness, compassion, health, self-nurturing, joyfulness, confidence, happiness, fearlessness, self-empowerment, non-judgment, kindness (even to yourself), balance, harmony, vitality, etc)

CREATE AN AFFIRMATION THAT INCORPORATES YOUR QUALITY(S).
(Must be affirmative, present-tense, I am statement, i.e. "I am completely healthy, fulfilled, and radiating God's gifts of vitality and Love, with grace and ease.")

WHAT STEPS ARE YOU WILLING TO TAKE EACH DAY THIS WEEK?

1)
2)
3)
4)
5)
6)
7)

RELAXATION & PRAYER / MEDITATION: MINIMUM OF 10 MINUTES A DAY

Mon.
Tues.
Wed.
Thurs.
Fri.
Sat.
Sun.

JOURNALING: MINIMUM OF 10 MINUTES A DAY IN AM &/OR PM

Mon.
Tues.
Wed.
Thurs.
Fri.
Sat.
Sun.

COMMITMENT CONTRACT

I, _____, on this day, (Month) _____, (Day)_____,
(Year)_____, commit to the completion of all of the above activities over a
_____ period of time, ending on (M/D/Y) _____.

My reward for achieving said goals & objectives is: _____
....
....
....

If, in the event that I do not achieve one or more of the above goals & objectives,
I agree that I will not receive my reward. **Note**: There is no punishment or
judgment in this process; simply no reward!
Signed: _____   Dated: _____

I achieved my goals and objectives for this contract: _____ YES _____ NO

Explain: _____
....
....
....

VALUES AND QUALITIES

VALUES

Accomplishment
Achievement
Adventure
Authenticity
Balance
Beauty
Collaboration
Comfort
Community
Connectedness
Creativity
Ecology
Excellence
Family
Free Time
Freedom
Happiness
Harmony
Health
Humor
Independence
Inner Peace
Integrity
Learning
Loyalty
Nature
Non-Judgment
Orderliness
Optimism
Participation
Passion
Power

Productivity
Recognition
Relationships
Resourcefulness
Security
Self-discipline
Self-expression
Service
Simplicity
Spirituality
Success
Trust
Unconditional Love
Vitality
Wisdom

QUALITIES

Adventurous
Ambitious
Articulate
Artistic
Authentic
Balanced
Caring
Committed
Compassionate
Confident
Conscientious
Considerate
Courageous
Creative
Curious
Dedicated

Disciplined
Elegant
Energetic
Enthusiastic
Fair-minded
Fearless
Fun-Loving
Generous
Gentle
Giving
Happy
Health Conscious
Heart-centered
Honest
Humorous
Independent
Innovative
Intelligent
Intuitive
Joyful
Kind
Light-Hearted
Loving
Loyal
Organized
Passionate
Positive
Resourceful
Respectful
Self-empowered
Tolerant
Trustworthy

BALANCE FROM THE INSIDE OUT
THE POWER OF TIME OUT

"It has often occurred to me that a seeker after truth has to be silent."
—Gandhi

"When you change the way you look at things,
the things you look at change."
—Wayne Dyer

I can just hear some of you as you read the title to this chapter. "Time out! You must be kidding me, right? Who has time to stop and just be still? With a never-ending list of responsibilities at work, at home, in the community, with the family, and with my partner, there is never enough time to get all of that done, far less take time out for me." Well, let's face it, no matter how many hours you put into your day, you will never get everything done. Your to-do list is, and will always be, a never-ending, continually growing list of tasks, opportunities, events, and activities demanding attention. As fast as you clear some items, there are 10 more items added to the list! Think of it like washing dishes, or doing laundry. As quickly as you get one load done, there is another load waiting to be done!

According to Topher Morrison, in his tremendously insightful and easy to read book, *Settle for Excellence*, "When you are too busy to spend time with yourself during the day, you are saying that you are the least important aspect of existence." Repeat that statement to yourself, out loud as follows: "When I am too busy to spend time with myself during the day, I am saying that I am the least important aspect of existence." How does that make you feel? Invest in yourself now, or . . .

So, our lives are generally about running continuously on empty, never stopping to gas up our engine. And the truth is that if we don't *choose* to schedule time out for a few minutes each day to unwind, reflect, rejuvenate, and refuel our engine, eventually we'll stall and we won't have a choice about stopping to gas up our tank. It will be forced upon us! Or worse, there will be no tank to gas up! Our body, mind and spirit demand balance in all areas of our life. All work and no play, or relaxation, does not only make you a dull person, but also a hyper, agitated, stressed-out, burned-out, completely fatigued, and chronically ill person. As I have said at many of my events: *Ignore your health, and it will go away!*

For practical purposes, let's look at a tangible example of the necessity for balance. Imagine a 3-legged stool. In order for that stool to stand firmly without wobbling or falling over, all three legs must be equally strong, balanced and the same length. Well, the same is true in our lives. For total wellbeing, all 3 areas or aspects of our life — body, mind and spirit — must be equally attended to and nourished on a daily basis. Balance and harmony are the result of integrating all 3 parts of our whole being throughout each and every day.

Forget Multi-Tasking

That always brings me back to the statement made by T. Harv Eker, who wrote the very thought-provoking book, *Secrets of the Millionaire Mind* (for information on this book and his programs go to: www. secretsofthemillionairemind.com/a/?wid=137674&page=/preview/tele). Harv states that, "How you do anything is how you do everything." For example, if you decide to multi-task in order to get more things done in a shorter amount of time, and you try to answer emails while you are listening to a meditation CD, which aspect of yourself is being best served, your mind or your spirit? Obviously — neither. Where your attention goes, energy flows. Where is the energy flowing? Basically nowhere! Or worse, all over the place! Neither aspect can be served when you try to do both at the same time! Forget multi-tasking. Focus on one aspect of your whole being fully at one time, and watch your entire disposition shift — positively. Something to think about . . .

Many chapters in this book more than adequately address how to care for and nourish your body. Other chapters explore how to change your mind to change your life addressing attitudes, beliefs, behaviors, and thought processes. The following chapters, and to a large extent the previous chapter, *The Aging Mountain Theory*, address much more fully the spiritual "leg" of our life's 3-legged "stool". To more passionately live our lives to the fullest, we need the various gifts contributed by our spirit or soul aspect — emotion, intuition, faith, trust, love, compassion, connection, and gratitude.

NOTE: *As you read through the following chapters, you may see a fair amount of overlap. That is intentional. Because many of the processes both, stand alone, and work together, I have written these chapters so that you can go to any one of the processes or exercises and perform it individually, without having to do another, or several processes, prior to the one you select to explore or implement. As always, we are sincerely interested in your thoughts and experiences regarding anything you read, and try throughout the following chapters. Just drop us an email at* info@marilynjoyce.com. *And let us know if we can share any of your insights, experiences, or challenges with our Ezine readership (To sign up to receive your own copy of our free **Special Report**, don't forget to go to* www.marilynjoyce.com*)*.

The next two chapters will explore two potentially life altering *"quiet time"* practices, often mistaken as the same process. Yet each is very unique in its approach. And when both are practiced consistently on a daily basis, they can have a profound impact on the outcomes we experience in our lives on all levels of consciousness, physically, mentally, emotionally and spiritually. You are about to explore . . .

Prayer & Meditation: What's the Difference? **Well, simply put, prayer is asking the question — meditation is listening, in silence, for the answer.**

However, before we fully delve into each of these two practices, let's first address a major concern that continually arises in the coaching I do with my patients and clients around the issue of *focus* during their quiet times, especially the meditative and breathing processes.

How Can I Get and Stay Positively Centered During My Quiet Times?

I remember, years ago, being asked by many of my patients what they should focus on during their prayer and meditation. First of all, there is nothing one "should" specifically focus on, simply some things that seem to result in a more rewarding experience. At the time, I made a few suggestions and all seemed well. Yet, though many incorporated regular prayer into their lives, very few of my patients, ever fully embraced meditation in a meaningful way. As I began to facilitate seminars and workshops, more and more people asked for lists of ideas to help them stay focused during their quiet times. You see, the main challenge for many people is that they are programmed to think of what they don't want versus what they do want. So, instead of creating positive changes in their lives, they continued to create the same old things in their lives that they had always been creating.

In other words, the quality of their thoughts, intentions and objectives, was not stated in a *positive*, present tense format. For example, if you want to create positive emotions in your life, stating that, *"Negative thoughts destroy only me,"* will only bring more of that kind of energy frequency, instead of the frequency required to produce your true desired results. The Universe picks up on your words, *negative* and *destroy*, and their frequencies, and gives you more of what you have stated energetically. So, you'll get *negative thoughts that destroy only you*, and no one else around you. The Universe does not get that this is something you don't want. The frequency of the words you use is what vibrates through you, and around you, attracting more of that same vibrational frequency.

A better way to reframe the above statement to reflect a more positive, expansive energetic frequency might be: *"Positive thoughts and feelings expand and empower me."* Repeat each of the 2 statements out loud: *"Negative thoughts destroy only me,"* and *"Positive thoughts and feelings expand and empower me."* Which one feels better, more expansive, more empowering? Of course, the second one does. It all goes back to focusing on what you do want—not on what you don't want! So, below is a list of suggested *focus statements* to assist you on your journey. By all means, feel free to develop your own as well. And if you are uncertain about whether your statement is expressed in the most optimal way to enhance the outcome of your meditation, just send us an email with your statement to: marilyn@marilynjoyce.com, and we'll evaluate it for you, and coach you on more expansive, or more empowering, ways to express it.

POINTS TO PRAY OR MEDITATE ON

Positive emotions expand and empower me.
Happiness is an emotion I am internalizing and expressing to
the world.
Challenges stretch me and make me stronger and more resilient.
I am given only challenges that I am ready for.
I am what I think & *feel*.
I am the only person I can change.
I consciously and joyfully accept responsibility and
accountability for everything in my life.
My life is extraordinary everyday in every way.
I dare to be different, and to march to my own drummer.
I am worthy of all the good that comes into my life.
The fundamental objective of my life is to experience joy in my
emotional and spiritual growth.
The past is gone forever, and only the choices I make today
determine my future.
The future is only a dream, so I choose to live my life fully
today, in every way.
Today is the first day of the rest of my life.
This moment is the only moment in my life that exists.
Enthusiasm is my daily exercise.
I am a competent person and have much to give to others.
I am blessed with the knowledge of my purpose for being, and
with the ability to fulfill this purpose fully and easily.
Abundance is mine in every aspect of my life.
All my love given freely, and without condition, returns to me
many fold.
My open expression, and extension, of love to all can change the
course of my world and theirs.
I am a messenger of God's Love and Joy.
I am here now to fulfill my mission in a way that is for the
highest good for all.
I am 100% accountable for everything I attract into my life.
I lead my life in all the ways that create all the results I desire.
I am a magnetic for good!
I can, I am able—I can do it!

SO, WHAT EXACTLY IS PRAYER?

IT IS ASKING THE QUESTION. In order to get the most out of your quiet time, I believe that you do, in fact, need both *Prayer & Meditation*. Since, as stated previously, most people mistake these as the same process, I felt that it would be useful to provide an overall definition of each for clarification. So, let's start with prayer. Regardless of your religious affiliation, *prayer is spiritual communication between God (whatever you perceive God to be) and you. It is a two-way relationship in which you not only talk to God, but also listen to God.* Prayer is how we begin a conversation with God—how we say hello. Its purpose is to assist us in building our relationship with God. Praying to God is our opportunity to offer gratitude, praise, to make a request, or to express our own thoughts and emotions about whatever is on our mind, at the time of prayer.

One of the Scriptures that has remained very deeply embedded in my memory from my childhood religious studies emphasizes God's intention for us through prayer. "Ask and it will be given to you; seek and you will find; knock and the door will be opened unto you" (Matthew 7:7). And another affirmation emphasizing our relationship to God and the Universe is the Law of Pure Potentiality from the book, *The Seven Spiritual Laws of Success*, by Deepak Chopra: "The source of all creation is pure consciousness . . . pure potentiality seeking expression from the un-manifest to the manifest. When we realize that our true self is one of pure potentiality, we align with the power that manifests everything in the universe." I call that power God.

Whatever your spiritual beliefs and practices are, it has been well documented globally that prayer heals. Studies have linked prayer to positive outcomes with such ailments as headaches, anxiety, asthma, high blood pressure, heart attacks and cancer. Because of Western medicine's focus on science and quantifiable results, prayer as a potential healing agent has generally been swept under the carpet, so to speak. Yet, this form of therapy has been practiced universally since ancient times. And even if it is simply an induced sense of wellbeing that results within us from prayer, that knowing in our heart and soul that we are loved by an unconditionally loving God connects us to the eternal significance of life—our reason for being. Through prayer, we infuse within us a deep sense of peace, which carries us more effectively through the most difficult and challenging experiences we may encounter as we move through this thing called *life*!

Personally, I know the positive impact of prayer in my own life. During some of my darkest hours and worst hardships, communication with God moved me to a place of knowing that I could not only *survive*, but *thrive*, beyond the seemingly insurmountable situations I found myself confronted with. Over the years, I have moved from a place of fearing a punishing God, to honoring, embracing and embodying a loving God. I have learned to express gratitude in prayer for all that I have in my life right now, as well as for all those things I desire, both tangible and intangible, as if they are already present in my life right now.

When I express doubt in my prayer to God, such as pleading for something over and over again, I am expressing a lack of trust in God's love for me, in God's willingness to hear me, and in God's ability to assist me. I am forgetting my oneness and unity with the Universe and God's infinite love. This doubt feels a lot like that *Victim Trap* we talked about earlier in this book. And since we are created in the image and likeness of God, we are not created as victims, unless we choose, through our free will, to ignore God's sacred gift of our creation. My personal belief is that God is Love, unconditional and eternal — and God exists within all that exists, and all that exists, exists within God. This creates such a wonderful feeling of relief, knowing that I am simply a vessel that receives God's messages regarding what I must do, and a vehicle for carrying out my specific aspect of God's work. In other words, I am not the message; I am simply the messenger. Whew! What a weight off my mind and shoulders!

Personally, prayer is much more fulfilling and rewarding, and I experience a much deeper sense of connection with God and the Universe, when I follow these simple steps:

1. Recognize God's eternal and infinite capacity for unconditional love and understanding, for me, for others, and for all that is. There is One Life and that Life is God, and God is the Love of all that is.
2. Continue the prayer with my affirmation that God is all that there is therefore there is nothing outside of God, nothing separate from God. So all that is, all that will be, is One with God. I am One with God.
3. Realize the attributes or qualities of God that I want to embody and express, qualities that I want to be more conscious of in my daily life, such as integrity, peace, unconditional love, charity, compassion and prosperousness. I know that these Divine qualities are within me, and I choose to fully live and express these qualities at any given moment and at all times; and become the very best vessel for God's purpose in my life, and the most committed vehicle for expressing God through me at all times.

4. Express gratitude and acceptance for the guidance and transformation of my consciousness so that I may always live my life for the highest good of myself, and others; express gratitude for the answers and understanding that are mine. It is so.

5. And finally, I release control of the outcome, letting go and letting God, knowing in my heart that, at the perfect time, in the perfect way, the perfect answer will come that is for the highest good of all concerned. I allow God to do the work. It is done. And so it is. Amen.

Though these are the general steps I use in my own prayer, I do not limit myself to a certain time of the day to pray. We can be in prayer frequently or continuously throughout the day, expressing and demonstrating our gratitude to God, and the Universe, as we go about our daily tasks, and experience breakthroughs and insights regarding challenges we are facing, as well as when unexpected good things occur. In other words there is no set time or protocol for prayer. Communication with God, I believe, should be an ongoing conversation throughout the day.

Some examples of things that you could immediately express gratitude for might be the car accident that almost happened but did not;, the fire that came close but did not do any significant damage to your property;, the check that should have bounced but somehow the money was there in time to cover it; the person who shows up in your life with a service you desperately need at just the moment you were thinking about how much you need that service;, the phone call from a loved one that you had just been thinking about; the unexpected thank you card that arrives in the mail on a day when you were feeling completely unappreciated in life; and the list goes on.

OKAY, SO LET'S TAKE A LOOK AT MEDITATION. WHAT EXACTLY IS MEDITATION?

IT IS LISTENING, IN SILENCE, FOR THE ANSWER. Basically, it means awareness, and whatever you do with awareness is meditation. It is a state of consciousness, whereby the mind is free of scattered thoughts, and other distractions. Meditation can simply be watching your breath, or walking through the woods and listening to the sounds of nature (No cell phones or headphones allowed!), or listening to the chirping of birds, or the melodious sounds of wind chimes outside your window. It can be painting a wall using the same stroke throughout (remember the movie, *The Karate Kid*) or listening to the waves as you sit by the ocean. Even gardening can be a form of meditation; or sitting in that very expensive massage chair you bought on a whim, and just focusing your awareness on the movement of the massage from your head down to your feet, and back up your body again—and remember to breathe through the entire process. One of my most absolutely favorite forms of meditation is walking a labyrinth. It is always out in nature, and usually in some of the most awe-inspiring places on the planet! The most important thing to remember is that you become the *observer* of this sound, thought, movement, breath, or beautiful environment, realizing that all the activity of your mind is reduced to this one observation.

The word meditation is derived from two Latin words. The first word, *meditari* means to think, or to dwell upon, to exercise the mind. The second word, *mederi* means to heal. And the Sanskrit derivation is *medha*, which means wisdom. Imagine all of that embodied in one little word. Not bad, is it?

So Just Where Does Yoga Fit into This Picture of Meditation?

Rather than go into a lengthy explanation about meditation here, I will cover some of the steps I personally use, and share, with my patients and clients. First, however, let me explain how I came upon the concept of meditation, and how it became an important part of my life. In my quest for inner peace when I was barely 16 years of age, a troubled suicidal run-away kid, escaping a violently abusive home environment, and just off the streets of Toronto, I stumbled upon a yoga class being taught at the local YMCA. That was in the 60's—that's right, the 1960's! It was the beginning of the mind-blowing "Beatles" era—the era of the hippies, flower power, "if it feels good, do it" generation. Except that I did not feel good at all!

John, the instructor, was probably one of the most balanced, loving human beings I had ever met at that point in my life — or possibly ever! Somehow he saw some redeeming qualities in me that I did not see in myself at the time. So he decided to take me under his wings, and teach me the fundamentals for creating inner peace through the control of my thoughts, using slow bodily movements and focused breathing techniques. That was my introduction to Hatha yoga. And for the first time in my life, I experienced some sense of calm and inner peace — fleeting though those moments may have been. All the same, those experiences opened me to the possibility that inner peace, versus inner turmoil, could exist in my life.

John further inspired in me, a craving for exploration and travel — both internal and external. He shared fascinating stories, and often showed sensory stimulating slides, of the incredible journeys that he and his wife had experienced, around the world, and particularly in India, the original home of yoga. I continued to study with John for several years. And then the day of reckoning arrived — John did not show up for class! I lived for that class. I was devastated! And then the office manager for the YMCA approached me and informed me that John had instructed him that I was to teach the class. Oh my goodness — *how could he do this to me?* I was a student, not a teacher.

But an astounding thing happened! The entire class of more than 100 students stood up and applauded as I squirmed with embarrassment. So, that day is a day I shall never forget! Never, in my life, up to that point in time, had I ever felt more validated and supported. Not to mention more frightened initially — followed by complete calm as I moved into the zone, that place of knowing that you are doing exactly what you are meant to be doing in that moment! The entire classroom of students stood up at the end of class and again loudly applauded with sincere appreciation. So, began my yoga teaching career. In fact, I was one of the original members of the Federation of Ontario Yoga Teachers. So, also, began my speaking career!

You see, I had been assisting John for some time, correcting people's postures and insuring that the students were relaxed during the meditation at the end of each class. However, I had not been aware of the fact that he was priming me to become a yoga teacher. He had set me up that day for an amazing unfolding of life experiences that I could never have foreseen in my childhood years. The study and dedicated practice of yoga became major priorities in my youth. So began my own global journeys, in my quest to become the best and most advanced yoga teacher possible. As a result of my travels, and my yoga studies, in both North America, and in India, I developed a fairly extensive background in Ashtanga Yoga, the 8-limb path of Yoga. Hence, I tend to incorporate the philosophy and systems that have been taught for many thousands of years, versus some of the newer inventions. Hatha Yoga, the most familiar term in the Western world, focuses mainly on the 3rd and 4th limbs of Ashtanga Yoga—the 3rd being asanas or postures, basically meditation in motion, and the 4th being pranayama or breath control.

Many of the newer versions of yoga are merely jazzed up forms of cardiovascular exercise. If you attend a yoga class and the movement is fast, and then they add insult to injury by adding extremely high heat, that is not true yoga! That is simply another form of cardio. And these forms of exercise defeat the whole purpose of yoga, which—let me repeat—is meditation in motion! True Hatha yoga definitely *does* exercise your body, but it is achieved using extremely slow movements, focused breath control, and complete attention/focus on the entire stretch, or contraction, of each and every muscle throughout the posture.

Yogic asanas (postures) are called meditation in motion for a reason! Your focus is entirely on the movement, or posture, as you move into it, hold it, and gradually release it. Many yogis have been known to hold a posture for up to 2 or more hours. A personal example of what I mean by this depth of practice, was during the 1976 Montreal Olympics. Several of us, who were certified and practicing yoga teachers, at the time, were selected to do headstands on top of a 6-foot high, 2-foot wide, wall. Our mission was to stay completely poised and still, in a headstand, for a minimum of 1½ hours. There is only one way that a human being can achieve such a stance for that long, and it is by meditating in the position. I guarantee you that, if most of us were to try to do this by sheer strength alone, very few of us, especially women, could do it. Well the fact is, that I remained in that position, on that wall, for almost 2 hours, and only stopped because we were politely asked to finish our demonstration.

Believe me, with yoga as a definite passion of mine, this could easily have become a much longer chapter on the subject. The abomination of yoga that I see in the Western world, with its focus teetering so intently towards the physical, versus the spiritual, aspects, has ignited in me the need to re-establish, in the hearts, minds and souls of those people who come into my life, the deeper purpose for the practice of yoga.

Based on more than 40 years of personal experience, it is apparent to me that the regular practice of a balanced series of yogic techniques has a tremendous potential for assisting anyone, anywhere, in increasing their energy and vitality, while liberating their mind, expanding their quality of consciousness, and eventually attaining deep relaxation, inner peace, and a much deeper level of awareness of God through meditation. Yoga is neither eastern, nor western — it is universal in its approach and application. Because I so frequently receive emails and calls about this subject, I have decided to address the various yoga systems and practices, in much more detail; and you will find this information at my **INSTANT *E.N.E.R.G.Y.*™** site at **www. InstantEnergyToday.com**.

> *"When you're in tune with life you will find yourself doing everything at the right time. All you have to do to get into tune, is take time to go into the silence, to find your direct contact with Me. This is why those times of peace and stillness are so vitally important for you, far more important than you realize. A musical instrument, when it is out of tune, creates discord; you, when you are out of tune, do the same. A musical instrument has to be kept in tune; you, too, have to keep yourself in tune, and you cannot do it unless you take time to be still. It cannot be done when you are rushing around, anymore than a musical instrument can be tuned while it is being played. It is in the silence that the notes can be heard and be readjusted. It is in the silence that you can hear My voice, and I can tell you what to do."*
>
> —Eileen Caddy
> Co-Founder of Findhorn, Northern Scotland
> expressing the still small voice of the God within each of us.

So, Where Do We Begin with Meditation?

Over the years, I have constantly been asked by my students, patients, clients and seminar attendees, "Okay, I get the importance of incorporating meditation into my daily life, but where do I begin? How do I get started? I don't have time for — or I don't want to go away to — a yoga school to learn how to do it! Please give me some guidelines to get started. What are the most effective steps for beginning the process?"

Well, since you asked, here's my:

12 Most Effective Steps for Getting Started with Meditation:

1. Set an intention for your meditation. It may be contemplation on a goal, or a challenging question or situation that you are facing. Know your purpose for doing it. Since 90% of accomplishing anything is intention, have a plan or idea for what you want to meditate on.

2. Select a quiet area that is familiar to you and comfortable. Make sure that you won't be disturbed for the period of time you schedule to meditate. I have personally established a specific area in my home that is only for this practice, and in it I have surrounded and filled the space with only that which is pertinent to my quiet time.

3. Sit in a comfortable position, either cross-legged on the floor, or sitting in a straight-backed chair, with your back straight, feet together, and hands at your sides or on your knees. I choose to close my aura—a subject for another book—by joining the thumb and forefinger of both of my hands, and resting my hands on my knees, as I sit cross-legged on the floor. I prop a cushion behind my lower back to assist me in keeping my back straight throughout the meditation.

4. Get comfortable. Make sure you are wearing loose, non-restrictive clothing devoid of any accessories, such as belts and tight fitting undergarments.

5. First, exhale completely. Then take 3 deep breaths, exhaling forcibly after each. Breathe very deeply, down into the solar plexus and stomach area. This deep breath draws in a greater amount of oxygen, and relaxes the body and emotions more fully.

6. Close your eyes, gently. Your face, especially your jaw area, should feel relaxed.

7. Become aware of your consciousness centered in the pituitary gland, which is above and between your eyes. This is often referred to as the *conscious Self-center or 3rd eye*. Believe it or not, you are there anyway—just focus on becoming aware of it. *Always start here and finish here.* And always know where you are.

8. Now just relax—sense and feel what it is like to be centered, and aware, with no outside influences. Your body may become restless, and want to twitch, itch or move. Just ignore these impulses. They are simply your mind's way of attempting to distract you. When your mind starts to wander, just notice the extraneous thoughts, release them, and see them floating away.

9. The goal of meditation is to learn to guide and control our will, which is the spiritual power we have available to us, to use any time we choose to use it. Will is the energy behind all of our actions. Desire moves Will, and Intention sets the direction of the movement. The glue that holds it all together is, what else, but LOVE! So, with all of this in mind, when you are ready, begin to move your consciousness to your left foot. Use your Will to relax your left foot—each muscle and each nerve. Do not try to force it!

10. After you have willed each part of your left foot to relax, move to your right foot. Then move up to the ankles on each foot, and then the

calves of each leg, one part at a time, focusing on each part becoming completely relaxed. The goal is to move slowly through each part of your body until your entire body is totally at ease and completely relaxed.

11. You are now back in your pituitary gland, centered, relaxed, and aware, and ready to meditate on whatever topic, concern, question, or purpose you have selected during the Intention stage (step 1).

12. To assist you in determining some areas that may have relevance for meditation, I am listing a few questions my patients, clients, and I have often used. These are simply examples that may prompt your own brain to formulate your own areas of intention. With any question you ask, or intention you set, allow yourself to be aware of both, the hard facts of the situation or intention, as well as any feelings you may experience, in relationship to the questions and answers you receive.

❖ What are my core values, beliefs and ideals?

❖ What qualities are important to me: in my business, my relationships, and within myself?

❖ Are my actions in alignment with my core values and beliefs?

❖ How do I envision my life?

❖ How do I feel about my life as a whole?

❖ What are the things I like most, even love, about my life?

❖ What am I tolerating in my life, and how can I change or eliminate these tolerations?

❖ How can I create a synergy between my body, mind and spirit in everything I do?

❖ How can I become more in touch with what my mind, body, and spirit are telling or teaching me?

❖ How can I be more continuously in touch with my intuition and follow its guidance without question or doubt?

❖ In what ways can I change my inner daily thoughts so that they can express themselves as a more abundant outer world?

❖ In what ways does my external life express my higher self?

❖ What choices can I make that will better honor my inner needs as well as my external needs?

❖ How can I experience an on-going Oneness with God everyday of my life?

And remember to check the list of suggested focus points included in the chapter: *Balance from the Inside Out: The Power of Time Out.*

A Simple Meditation

(I recommend you record your own voice on a tape or mp3 player, slowly taking yourself through this meditation. Then you can play it, preferably with some relaxing meditative music in the background, while you actually do the meditation.)

Okay, you are now relaxed and centered again in your pituitary area (above and between your eyes). Imagine yourself beside a deep pool of water, in the middle of a forest. You are surrounded by huge, beautiful trees, which are majestically standing over the pond, as if protecting it from the elements. The sun is shining softly through the trees, reflecting off the pool, and providing just enough warmth for comfort. The pond is deep and still – very still – like a glass surface, not a ripple in sight. Lilly pads and flowers adorn the pond's surface, floating aimlessly and peacefully, with no apparent direction in mind. You decide to wade, or jump, into the pool – it really doesn't matter what you do. But you feel the water as you go into it. It feels refreshing and warm. Just keep going out into the pool, until you sink deeper and deeper into the pool. Now you are sitting on the bottom; and you become aware of the sun's rays shining on the surface of the pool. You notice bubbles of air all around you rising and floating to the surface of the pool. Just be still and observe the bubbles floating to the surface. These bubbles are your thoughts – but they have nothing to do with you. Reach out and touch one – hold it – examine it – and then let it go. When you examine it, feel it – its texture – its weight – its substance – its size – what does it really feel like? Then let the bubble go, and watch it just float up to the surface of the pool and burst into the sunlight. Enjoy the peace and tranquility of this beautiful setting. And when you eventually come to a place of complete peace within yourself, allow yourself to float to the surface of the pool and move gently to the shore. Come back to your body – and when you are ready, open your eyes.

> *"Who looks outside, dreams;*
> *who looks inside, awakes."*
>
> Carl Gustav Jung,
> Psychologist

VISUALIZATION & "FEELIZATION"
THE REAL SECRETS TO SUCCESS ON EVERY LEVEL!

I will never forget the day, many years ago, when I read the book, *Creative Visualization*, by Shakti Gawain. What a revelation! It made complete sense to me, that if we could create a picture in our mind's eye of what we wanted, and then visualize it, it could become a reality. Well, at least on paper it made sense! Somehow — for me — it did not seem to work in my real life circumstances. There was a piece of the puzzle that seemed to be missing.

Are You Getting What You Want? — Or What You Don't Want?

Well, in fact, there was. The aspect of *deeply feeling* the outcome we have visualized, as though we had already achieved it, was the missing component. Now, what I mean here, is not simply having a mild experience of what we think it may feel like. It was years after reading Ms Gawain's book, that I learned the power of *feeling the experience* right to the very marrow of my bones. Many top athletes have used this technique to win in competition. *Feelization* is really the heart and soul of visualization. Visualization is basically inert without the added experience of *deeply feeling and internalizing* the outcome, as if it had actually occurred in this present moment.

So, lets get down to how to make this whole process work for you. As with everything else outlined in this chapter, it is critical to determine what you want to focus on for the process, your intention. To imprint this even more deeply into your mind and heart, find a picture or photo that represents your intention. As the saying goes — A picture is worth a thousand words. I am not sure where that cliché came from, but it has always proven true in my life! This is like a new seed being planted deep within the garden of your consciousness. Of course, we have to nurture that seed in order for it to germinate and grow into a healthy plant.

I realize that what I am about to write, has been written in many ways, many times, throughout this book, yet it is key to everything that we experience in our lives. Energy flows where intention goes. Let me expand on that thought — *Energy flows where emotional intention goes*. I think most of us can relate to the negative side of this coin. For example, someone borrows a healthy sum of money from you, with the promise that they will pay it back within, say, one month. And it was, in fact, a hardship for you to part with that money at that time. However, for one month, it seemed the right thing to do, to help out a friend in need. Well, one month passes, and nothing. Two months, three months, a year, two years . . . And nothing! So, what goes on within you, frustration perhaps, then anger, even anxiety, especially as you are unable to pay some of your own bills as a result of this loan? You swear you will never be duped by anyone ever again. You decide never to lend money to another living soul. You carry resentment and anger — and voila — what keeps showing up in your life? Sick plants! Dead plants! Do you see what has happened in this picture? Your energy flowed in the direction of your disturbed emotions.

Okay, so are we clear that this is not the direction we want our emotions to go? Can you see how your feelings, in this situation, magnetically attracted what you don't want? This is the direction of pain and disharmony. Our objective, here, is to take that emotion, that is actually energy in motion, and attach it to a clearly defined and desired intention — something that is for the good of all concerned, including yourself. And then to, magnetically, attract what *you do want* into your life, using *feelization* positively (versus negatively)! Because emotions are the fuel that ignites our intentions, we have to get to that place within, where the power of our thought and imagination meet with and marry our feelings, so that our mental creation of the physical expression of these emotions is so real, that it is as if we have actually achieved our intent, goal, or objective. Now, what kind of plants do you see growing from the seeds of your consciousness? Probably very vibrant and vigorous plants!

Are you ready to try this out? *"What are we waiting for?"* you ask. Okay then, hold on for the ride of your life! *Because what you see, and feel, is what you get!*

How to Effectively Visualize & *"Feelize"* Your Intentions!

Just follow the steps below to most effectively visualize & feelize your intentions:

> ➢ Determine the intention you want to focus on.
> ➢ Close your eyes, and vibrantly visualize, in your mind's eye, every detail of what that intention looks like, and the exact outcome you desire.
> ➢ Now, use all of your inner senses to *feel* your intention as if it was actually manifesting right now, in this present moment.
> ➢ Feel the joy of your accomplishment, the thrill of your achievement, the ecstasy of your fulfillment. — *feel* all of these feelings surge through every cell of your body.
> ➢ *Feel* the emotional magnetic field that you have created around you, that begins to attract everything you need to fulfill your intention easily and effortlessly.

➤ Acknowledge yourself for a job well done. "We have to celebrate to accelerate." (a quote by dear friend, Tim Meyers). The increased sense of self, along with the positive energy and attitude you have created by this step, expands all of your future possibilities.

➤ Express and *deeply feel* gratitude for the achievement of your intention as if it is present right now. This creates within you a sense of having, and opens you up to receive more.

➤ Return to this feeling of manifestation any time that you feel yourself out of alignment with your intentions, and the vision you have for your life.

This simple *visualization and feelization* process functions, almost miraculously, in getting you fully in touch and engaged with your true inner Self, and your realization of a deep sense of fulfillment of your bigger vision for your life. It achieves this outcome by re-focusing your intent on *that which you want in your life versus that which you do not want*. And then ignites it with your deepest of feelings, married to your detailed vision of what you desire. See *Points to Pray or Meditate On* in the *Balance From the Inside Out* chapter. And then, by the Law of Attraction, you draw to you more of the same on an ongoing basis, due to the positive magnetic energy field you have created around you.

Remember that everything that exists began with a thought and a conviction or intention (affirmation) that it could actually exist. Any great athlete will tell you that first they affirmed, confidently and competently, that they were going to win. And then they took that thought and used it to visualize every detail of the moment of winning, which they pictured in their mind, and at the same time, *felt in every cell of their body, as though it had already happened!* What you experience in your life, generally, perhaps always, reflects that which you have specifically rehearsed in your mind (*visualized*) and your body (*feelized*), with the full anticipation and expectation of achieving the extraordinary outcome you desire.

So, what are you waiting for? Go get 'em tiger!

JOURNALING –
THE INNER DIALOGUE THAT MAKES IT TO PRINT!

I am a complete advocate for the process of journaling. This is the act of writing down your thoughts, actions, concerns, and feelings, preferably by hand in a notebook, so that you incorporate the-mind-to-hand-to-page connection. This process has resulted in significant healing, for me personally, as well as for my clients and patients. The mind is like a parachute – it's no good unless it is open! And journaling seems to open our minds up to realizations, insights, understandings, knowledge and wisdom that are, otherwise, unavailable to us on a conscious level.

Though journaling can be done very effectively on its own, and provide amazing answers and insights to the most challenging of questions or concerns, the value is potentially tenfold, when it follows either, the breathing technique outlined previously in this chapter, or the meditation, also included in this section. You can actually use the questions listed in #12 of my *12 Most Effective Steps for Getting Started with Meditation*. Or just write about whatever comes up for you; that you are experiencing, sensing or feeling, about a particular situation in your life. It may be a past, unresolved situation, a present circumstance, or a future uncertainty – anything. There are no hard and fast rules for what you can journal about.

For example, I personally love to write about my goals, ideas, learning experiences, and my vision for the future – both personally and globally. However, my most joyful subject to journal about involves my "Aha" moments, those moments that sweep my body, mind and spirit off their respective seats – their physical, emotional and celestial seats! You know the moments I am talking about – when goose bumps invade every inch of your skin! Perhaps it's that great feeling I get while I am writing about the "Aha" experience that fills me up with optimism, joy and certainty, so that by the Law of Attraction, I continue to attract more of the same kinds of experiences. And based on the many books I have read by some of the most accomplished masters on the planet, it is apparent that they focus their thoughts, attention and activities on the things that make them feel great. I am not talking about self-centered narcissism here. True masters, generally, spend their lives joyfully in service to others, as they realize, live, and fulfill, their unique destiny or purpose for being here now. (See the *References and Resources* chapter for lists of recommended books by some incredible masters.)

Journaling is also a wonderful tool for personal inner reflection, with no particular issue or concern to explore, solve or evaluate. If you simply find yourself in a contemplative mode of thought—maybe it's time to go deeper into the *soul* of who you are, or it's time to *release* some past mistakes or thought patterns that no longer serve you, or you have an overwhelming desire to offer praise to God for some of your amazing accomplishments, victories and blessings—you may choose to ask yourself some of the following questions:

❖ Who am I?
❖ What is my background—physically, mentally, emotionally and spiritually?
❖ What experiences brought me to this time and place in my life?
❖ What life changing mistakes have I made that it is time to release?
❖ Are there any buried mistakes in my life that still hold me back?
❖ Have I released my mistakes to God, and/or the Universe, so I can experience God's and the Universe's true blessings for my life?
❖ What event or series of events in my life brought me to my knees in surrender?
❖ Where did I focus my thoughts and efforts during crisis?
❖ When did I turn it all over to God, the Creator, the Universe?
❖ What victories have I experienced in my life?
❖ What blessings has God brought my way?
❖ Think about God's role in my life, my connection to the Universe, and give thanks to God and the Universe for all I have?

Nip a Crisis in the Bud!

Of course, journaling is an invaluable tool for dealing with life's many frustrating moments, even apparent crises. And often this is an individual's first introduction to the process of journaling, as many therapists, today, have incorporated it into their counseling strategies for this very purpose. Getting challenging, frustrating, painful, or anxiety-ridden experiences out of your head and onto paper, is tremendously freeing. Perhaps the tremendous sense of relief that follows, allows your mind to become a clear and open vessel for the receiving of insights, ideas, solutions, even game plans, for handling a particular situation that may never have, otherwise, surfaced from the your prior cluttered, fragmented, scattered consciousness. In other words, *clarity and empowerment* now reign where, once, confusion, uncertainty, and anxiety ruled.

Some examples of situations that can be alleviated, or even eliminated, by journaling include, overwhelming fatigue, challenges with your argumentative, self-perpetuated teenager, disharmony with your partner or other loved ones, a disagreement with your doctor, boss, or a friend, always too much month at the end of your money, your journey past any present health challenges, your fear about a potential disastrous outcome resulting from a diagnosis of illness, and any negative thoughts about it, too many deadlines in every area of your life, loss of a significant other, loss of your home due to a fire, flood, or other natural disaster, or any other event that brings up uncomfortable thoughts, feelings, or frustration.

Once you have determined the root of your discomfort or frustration, just go ahead and cry, scream, punch a punching bag, hit a pillow—do whatever it takes to release all of that tension within you. Of course, the overall criteria here, is that, whatever you do does not harm you or anyone else!

Now, at the same time, or just following this physical action of the release of pent-up emotion and tension, write in a journal about the experience, asking yourself the following questions:

1) What about this situation or concern is bothering you?
2) How does it make you feel? (Very important!)
3) What outcome would you like to see happen?
4) How would that outcome make you feel? (Very important) *Feel that feeling* as if the desired outcome had already been realized.

Just let whatever comes up, come out of you, and end up, in writing, on the page. Do not think before you write. The whole purpose of this process is to release everything—every thought and every feeling you experience about an issue or an event—onto that page. Then bask in the feeling you have as you *visualize and feelize* (see the previous section of this chapter) the experience of your desired outcome as if it had already actually occurred. Acknowledge yourself for a job well done. And express gratitude to God, and the Universe, for assisting you in gaining the clarity and understanding you required to positively impact your situation. My journal actually has this type of journaling in the front, and I track my gratitudes in the back (see the next section on Gratitudes). It is small enough to fit into my purse, so I can therefore carry it with me wherever I go. And what a blessing it has been.

A BRIEF WORD ON
MIND – BODY – SPIRIT EXERCISES

Have you ever watched as someone moves fluidly through a series of yoga postures, or artfully glides through their Qigong practice, or gracefully dances through a series of Tai Chi poses? There is a degree of grace, ease, focus, and fluidity, expressed throughout each movement, which can only be accomplished by the harmonious union of the mind, body and spirit of the practitioner. The amazing power and agility demonstrated by those who have mastered one or more of the various forms of martial arts are simply breath-taking to watch. These forms of exercise are actually meditation in motion. Every millimeter of the move is performed with laser focus, and experienced fully, from the start to the finish, as I explained earlier in this chapter during the discussion on yoga.

In 1995, I had the opportunity to facilitate a group tour to China. Definitely a different world compared to the West! I remember, one morning, looking down from the top floor of the very tall hotel I was staying in, and seeing an awe-inspiring sight. There were probably about 100 Chinese men and women, of all ages, moving through a series of Qigong postures, with such incredible grace and fluidity; I was literally overwhelmed by the uniformity and synchronicity of the dance taking place far below me. It appeared to be perfectly choreographed, like something you might spend more than $100.00 a ticket to see on stage in America. More amazing was that it was not yet 6:00 AM! And this happened every morning at the same time – with the same number of people participating! And, it happened in every city we visited – as well as in every countryside location we had the occasion to explore.

What I have come to understand is, that to achieve success in these art forms of exercise, we must incorporate all parts of our whole being. These truly are meditations in motion, as they intertwine our bodily movements with a centering deep within ourselves. By practicing one of these forms of meditation in motion, we can develop a deeper sense of purpose, clarity, self-determination, resilience, endurance, precision, confidence, and balance – balance in every aspect of our lives: mentally, physically, emotionally and spiritually. And then we can take those experiences, and inject them into every other part of our lives. Imagine the results you would get with a balanced, focused calm approach to everything you do!

Instead we go to the gym, and rush through a series of exercises, while having a conversation with the person next to us, and while also watching, and thinking envious thoughts about, a *beautiful body* working out, *with focus*, on a machine in front of us. What kind of results do we expect to get? Can you imagine a serious athlete working out in that manner in preparation for a competition? Not a chance! The professional athlete has learned how to embody the mind-body-spirit component, just as the martial artist has. Scattered, ineffective thoughts lead to scattered, ineffective actions that result in scattered, ineffective outcomes.

For anyone with an interest in exploring *Tai Chi*, I recommend anything by *David Dorian-Ross*, a US and world Tai Chi medalist and Master of his art. He truly makes it look like a dance as he assists even the novice student in feeling as though they will one day be able to master the practice of Tai Chi. And for more information on yoga, Susan Winter Ward's compassionate and calm teaching style puts even the least experienced yoga student at ease in her *Yoga for the Young* at Heart DVD and book. To find out more about Susan's materials go to the products page at www.marilynjoyce.com, or email us at: info@marilynjoyce.com.

And One Final Thought:

Affirm continuously to yourself:

"I am in the right place, at the right time, for the right purpose."
—Ursula Roberts

SO WHAT THE HECK ARE GRATITUDES?

Well years ago, before writing lists of things that we are grateful for in a journal, became popularized by the media, and TV shows such as Oprah Winfrey, I was introduced to this gratitude journaling concept, while traversing my journey with cancer. Dr Bernie Siegel, an amazing oncologist who, in my estimation, was way ahead of his time, facilitated a seminar in Toronto, Canada, that I had the good fortune to attend—in a wheelchair, and a mere 88 pounds, soaking wet. I would never have expressed it as good fortune at the time—but you know what they say about hindsight...

My personal journey was, at that point in time—just before being introduced to this gratitude concept by Dr Siegel—a tortured, emotionally painful, experience. Forget the *"chip on the shoulder"* perspective. *I had blocks the size of tree stumps on each shoulder!* I was so weighted down with indignation, shame, frustration, anger and self-pity—definitely a master victim—that almost no one cared to spend time with me. Following a short, however inspirational and memorable, conversation with this compassionate, loving doctor, I was opened up to the possibility that a gratitude journal may have some value. I want to be clear here, though, that I was not 100% convinced; simply willing to give it a shot! After all, what did I have to lose? Nothing else seemed to be working! Well, the first time I attempted to write even one single thing in this gratitude journal, I was completely stumped (no pun intended)—nothing—nada—came to my mind! It was a dismal failure. I was told that "5" was the magic number, and not even "one" gratitude came to mind!

I remember crying out to God, "Give me just one good reason to continue with this ridiculous exercise!" That particular day was a very gray, overcast winter day—anyone who has spent a mid-winter day in Toronto, Canada, knows the kind of depressing day I am talking about—and then the most amazing thing happened! For just a brief moment—I mean a fraction of a minute—the sun shone brightly through the dark, heavy clouds. I was awestruck! In my heart, it was the answer to my prayer. It was validation that this *gratitude thing* was a process I had to continue with, and somehow embrace, on a daily basis. And I did! That day I thanked God 5 times for the sun shining upon me. It was less than a month later that I entered over 100 different gratitudes in my journal for just one single day! And my life has never been the same since!

Since that time, we have come to understand, through the science of psychoneuroimmunology, that maintaining a great attitude is essential to optimum health and prevention of illness, as well as for overcoming a life challenging illness. *I hear you: easier said than done!* Yes, on the surface, maintaining a great attitude in the face of endless problems that arise daily—both personally and globally—seems like an absolute impossibility. However, we have already discussed the fact that what we focus on expands. That's the *Law of Attraction*. Remember?

So, by writing our long—or maybe it's short to begin with—list of things we are truly thankful for, we create an energetic frequency that attracts more of the same—more things to be grateful for. When we focus on what we are grateful for, we attract so much more to be grateful for. It just keeps expanding and filling our lives with people, places, events, and things to be thankful for. *That attitude of gratitude thing—with all of its good emotional feelings—really works!*

The Magic is in the Number 5!

I recommend writing a minimum of 5 gratitudes each day, the same number that the heart-centered, compassionate doctor recommended I write. And, it can look like this: Dear God: Thank you for the sun, Thank you for my excellent health (also serves as a positive affirmation), Thank you for my wonderful friends, Thank you for my amazing career, Thank you for assisting me in discovering my purpose, Thank you for protecting my house from the wild fire, Thank you for my wonderful neighbors who truly care about each other, Thank you for my amazing Dream Team, Thank you for my tremendously improving family relationships, etc. etc.

Some of my patients and clients choose to give thanks by simply expressing as: I am grateful for . . . (each item that they are grateful for). Or I am filled with appreciation and gratitude for . . . (again, stating each item that they are thankful for). Some choose to thank God, others the Universe, others the Creator, and others give no specific name or title in their address. I use the word "God," as it is a universally accepted term, and what feels closet to my heart when I am addressing that which is Omni-present in my life. I choose not to get wrapped up in semantics or religious discussions about what is the correct, or not correct, regarding this matter. Words, after all, are extremely limiting as a form of expression, in comparison to the limitless capacity of an open and unconditionally loving heart.

For gratitudes to be effective they need to be written as positive, present tense statements, in the same way that affirmations need to be stated. As I stated previously, I personally carry a little journal with me everywhere I go.

I record my list of gratitudes in the back of this little book, and journal in the front of it, about things that arise throughout the day that feel uncomfortable or challenging. It fits into my purse, or into my computer case when I am traveling, so that I can record daily, any gratitudes as I experience them, and journal at will.

If experiencing and expressing gratitude is something that you find challenging to do at this time in your life, for whatever reason or reasons, as I did so many years ago when I was first introduced to the gratitude journal concept, I encourage you to take a look at a wonderful website: www. ThankGodI.com. I, personally, became affiliated with the organization behind the website's framework. And the theme of everything that is offered by the organization, and the many book titles that will be released, is the *Healing Power of Gratitude*. Nothing can move you faster to a place of inner peace and fulfillment than gratitude — and that is gratitude for all that is right now, ever has been, and ever will be. If you have signed up for my **Special Report** at: www.marilynjoyce.com, then watch for more information on this subject, as well as some wonderful inspirational stories. *If you have not signed up yet, what, in Heaven's name, are you waiting for?*

Something I love that came from Louise Hay:

> "I am forever grateful for all of the delightful and wonderful experiences
> that have come to me this year.
> I am so pleased with where I am, and I eagerly look forward to the future."

AN ATTITUDE OF GRATITUDE + BELIEF =
MORE OF EVERYTHING

Believe It . . . Achieve It . . . You Can Make It Happen!

"The longer I live, the more I realize the impact of attitude on life. Attitude to me is more important than facts. It is more important than the past, than education, than money, than circumstances, than failures, than success, than what other people think, say or do. It is more important than appearance, gift, or skill. It will make or break a company . . . a church . . . a home. The remarkable thing is we have a choice every day regarding the attitude we will embrace for that day. We cannot change our past . . . The only thing we can do is play on the string we have, and that is our attitude. I am convinced that life is 10% what happens to me and 90% how I react to it. And so it is with you . . . we are in charge of our attitudes."

—Charles Swindoll

Isn't it fascinating to watch children as they play? Nothing is impossible in their young minds. They believe they can do, have, or be anything they want to do, have or be! Dreams are as real as everything that is around them. There are no limits—only possibilities! And then a few years later we meet these young folks and notice that all, or most, of those dreams have been replaced with fear, doubt, limiting ideas and beliefs about themselves and their lives. What happened to all those dreams and possibilities? What changed their positive, optimistic, self-confident, never fail attitude, to one of hopelessness, pessimism, fear, doubt, lack and limitation?

They forgot the secret—what you think about, and focus upon, is what you achieve. And you have the choice in any given moment what you want to think about. I know. I know. You are up to your eyeballs in debt, and there is always too much month left at the end of your money. Or just trying to get through each day is a challenge in itself, due to overwhelming fatigue, or worse, a diagnosis of some kind of illness. Or maybe you're worried about getting older and losing your looks, health, or partner. We spend most of our lives thinking, worrying and talking about all of the things we don't want in our lives. And very rarely do we even contemplate what we do want.

"If you look at what you have in life, you'll always have more. If you look at what you don't have in life, you'll never have enough."

—Oprah Winfrey

We seem to have forgotten that universal truth that whatever we think about expands. So, if we constantly think about not being able to pay our bills, guess what. That's what we get more of—not being able to pay our bills. If we constantly think about why our business is not growing, then we get more of our business not growing. If we constantly think about how afraid we are to talk to people, then we get more fearful of talking to people. On the other hand, if we constantly think about how abundant and prosperous we are, then we will become more abundant and prosperous. If we constantly think about the motivated customers that want our products and services, we get motivated customers buying our products and services. If we think about the awesome people that are joining our business, we get awesome business associates joining us in our business. If we constantly think about how we attract open, vulnerable and happy people, then we attract more open, vulnerable and happy people. It's truly that simple! Well, there's a bit more to it . . .

Are you moving away from _____*, or moving towards* _____*?*
You fill in the blanks!

So, let's say you are ill with some disease, maybe cancer, fibromyalgia, or heart disease. The illness is not what is important here. My question to you, as it is to all of my clients, is this: *Are you moving away from the illness, or moving towards health?* Think about that. Do you get it? You can ask yourself the same question about anything in your life? Are you moving away from debt, or towards abundance and wealth? Are you moving away from toxic relationships, or towards healthy, fulfilling relationships? Are you moving away from depression, or towards joy, happiness and peace? Are you moving away from an unhealthy diet and lifestyle, or towards a healthy nourishing diet and lifestyle? Get it yet?

Well, let's really think about this question. If you are moving away from something, what are you actually doing? Are you not still focused on what you don't want, dragging it along behind you? Still attached to this thing you want to get rid of, and all of your thoughts on how to avoid it at any cost? Are you not investing a lot of thought and energy on what you need to do to get away from it—a lot of negative, unfulfilling energy wasted on FEAR—False Expectations Appearing Real? Are you not focused on what may happen if the illness does not get healed, or the toxic relationship goes from bad to worse, or the debt collectors come knocking on your door, or repossess your car, or your house goes into foreclosure?

How Does All Of That Make You Feel?

Yuk! Heavy, overwhelmed, buried in fear and hopelessness, right? And the more you focus on this, the worse you feel, and the worse it all gets! Carrying the baggage around behind you of what you don't want will only serve to block the flow of what you truly desire. And what you focus on expands! This is a universal truth.

Now, lets take a look at the other side of the coin: moving toward what you really want. If you move toward your desires, what are you actually doing? Where is your focus? Is it not on what you want versus what you don't want? *And when you focus on what you really want, how do you feel?* Great, right? You feel full of optimism, excitement, and joy at the possibilities. Remember, those young kids at play? Don't you feel a lot like they felt before they learned the behavior of fear (False Expectations Appearing Real) — before they learned about the concept of lack and limitation, and began to believe it!

When you consider that less than 1% of the world's wealth, for example, is controlled by less than 3% of the world's population, you have to ask yourself what they are doing differently from the masses — that other 97% that are always struggling with their lack of health, wealth, and fulfilling relationships. Well, in a nutshell, they did not buy into the big lie. That lie that says there is a limit to the good you can have in this world. That same lie that says you are not good enough, smart enough or strong enough to do what you want to do, to have what you want to have, and to be who you want to be.

The Universal Law Of Attraction

You can be tremendously healthy! You can be wildly wealthy. And you can enjoy amazing relationships built on love, trust, commitment, and joy. You just have to be aware of, and believe in the *secret*, The Universal Law of Attraction. Determine what you truly desire, and focus completely on that, with the vision of that desire directly in front of you, exactly as you desire it to be, as if it is already realized, and do this with all of the feeling and emotion you will feel when you have it. And then thank God and the Universe for the outcome you desire as if you have it right now. We have all watched world-class athletes achieve amazing feats. But have you stopped to consider why they won when another did not? It is all in the vision of winning with all of the emotion they can create within themselves, as though they have already achieved it! The appropriate actions manifest from their focused joyful intention, meeting and co-creating, with the universal flow of creation. Nothing more! Nothing less! This is a winner's attitude:

Intention + Focus + Emotion + Action = WIN / SUCCESS

"The Law of Attraction attracts to you everything you need,
according to the nature of your thought. Your environment and
financial condition are the perfect reflection of your habitual
thinking. Thought rules the world."
(I would simply add deep emotional belief to the mix.)
—Dr. Joseph Edward Murphy, Surgeon

So, move toward your desire or goal, knowing that it is yours right now. And acknowledge, but give no energy to, the fact that there is simply a bit of a time lapse between your joyful, intentional thought of achieving it, and your realization of that desire. Make a decision to focus on that desire or goal, and the way it makes you feel. And then take any action, towards that goal or desire, that you are guided to take. Over time, as you consistently practice this way of being, and internalize this process, so that it becomes a way of life to focus on the thoughts that feel good and bring you joy, and then follow your inner guidance as to the appropriate action, you will notice that good things happen more and more frequently, and that your desires begin to manifest almost instantly.

Sounds too simplistic? Sounds too good to be true? Well, during my journey with cancer, I was convinced, at one point, that I had no hope—that what I was being told was the reality. One and a half to two weeks to live! I was buying into that lie, that perception of reality. Remember that everything is simply someone's perception of what is real. How do I know this? Have you ever sat down with family members and discussed a certain event that really stands out in your mind? Only to discover that either the other members of your family had no recollection whatsoever of that event, or they had completely different pictures of that scenario! If you take a specific situation and ask 10 people to share their experience of it, you would likely hear 10 completely different versions of the same event. Try it and see what happens. It's all about perceptions—and like your thoughts, you can change them in an instant—if you are aware of them!

I know I am spending a lot of time on this subject. However, my personal belief (perception) is that this specific chapter can change your life forever if you get it! We all waste precious time, energy and money on fears and perceptions, that get us nowhere. We focus most of our resources on what we don't want. We rarely create a strongly felt vision for our lives as we truly would like to design them. And then we become victims to every circumstance that we perceive stands in our way. And the step that will immediately change this is so simple it's shocking! *Change your mind to change your outcome! Change your mind to change your life!!*

Wait! There's More . . .

Okay, you say, so you've done that, and still you achieve none of your desired results. Yes. There is more to it. It would be like the behavioral modification programs so often used in an effort to affect change. They just don't work — at least not long term. There are some other serious steps to take before change can happen. You can't just introduce a behavioral modification to a negative thought by having the thought, dismissing it, and creating a new one, and know that this will work from now on. What about one of those really bad days, when you seem to, proverbially, wake up on the wrong side of the bed? Everything that could go wrong seems to do just that! What's your reaction? You got it! That old victim habit just screeches into home plate, and you are right back to the same old stinkin' thinkin'. And then it's time for an attitude adjustment! Well, before you can do that, the answer is to get to the root of the problem — your deep-rooted beliefs about the circumstance or yourself.

What Kind Of Window Are You Seeing Your World Through?

We all have a unique, personal, individual window, or contextual framework of thought, through which we view our world. That window is made up of attitudes, beliefs, ideas and opinions. All of these work together in the development of our values (see the chapter: *The Aging Mountain Theory & Process* for the lists of *Values & Qualities*). And then our values contribute to our perceptions (our perceived reality) of what is happening around us and to us. These perceptions lead to our judgments about the various situations that occur throughout our day, and about the people we meet. And then these judgments are expressed as our behaviors toward each and every situation and person in our lives. These behaviors prompt our actions. And finally, of course, from our actions we observe our results. Can you see why changing our behavior usually results in only short-term success? We are not even close to the root causes of our actions at the point of behavior patterns!

Contextual Framework for Individual Thought
=
The Window Through Which You See Your Own World

Attitudes + Beliefs + Ideas + Opinions

→ Values

→ Perceptions

→ Judgments

→ Behaviors*

→ Actions

→ Results

*Let's take an example that many of us are familiar with. You want to lose weight. So, according to the behavioral modification programs, you have to stop buying the foods that trigger over-eating. So, with none of this food around, the premise is that you will not eat it. Five days into your program you are doing really well, and are committed to staying on the program until you reach your goal weight. On the sixth morning you get a call from your closest friends, who are celebrating their 25th anniversary. They are inviting you to their huge, spur-of-the-moment party to celebrate. You can't say no! After all, they are your closest friends. And they would be absolutely mortified if you did not show up for such an important occasion and celebration.

So, off you go to the party, committed to staying on track with your program despite the festivities. You reason that there must be food there that you can eat. Until you get there! Everything is on your forbidden list! Oh my goodness! What will you do? Well, now your mind kicks in with the old programming. One night can't hurt — after all I have been committed for 5 days. I deserve to indulge. I have been good — never cheated. And what can I do after all — all of this delicious food and it's not my fault if I can't stay on track tonight! Can you see what happened here? *Behavioral change didn't work!* It is a very surface change. It does not address the deep underlying issues. We need to get to the root of what we are doing in every instance in our lives.

And that, my friends, is our set of attitudes, beliefs, ideas and opinions that have been developed from day one, throughout our day-to-day connections and activities over our entire individual lifetimes. And that resulting set of values has become the basis for every decision we make in our lives! In order to actually stick to any program or regime, we have to get to the depth of the decision-making process — our individual context of thought, or window through which we see the world. We must change our attitudes, beliefs, ideas, and opinions about each item in our lives that we want to change. So, with the weight issue, we need to look at what our attitudes and beliefs are about weight and about ourselves in relationship to our weight, and where those beliefs, attitudes, ideas and opinions originated. If we think we do not deserve to be slim, our attitude will definitely reflect that thought. So, we need to evaluate where that belief, attitude or idea originated. And then change it!

For example, if you feel that you are always going to be fat because your whole family is, it is unlikely that changing your behavior will have a lasting impact. However, if you realize that your whole family has a weight issue, and that this does not have to be your belief about yourself, and attitude towards yourself — instead you create a belief that you are slim underneath the temporary padding — and express an attitude of gratitude for your true slim body — and then move towards being slim with everything you visualize, feel and do — you will wake up one day to your true slim self!

Please do not doubt this. At the age of 20 I weighed in at 250+ pounds! That's right — 250+ lbs! Now close to 60 years of age, no one would ever guess that this had been the case, except those who knew me then. I changed my belief about being a fat person who could not live without desserts and butter, to one that believes, and expresses the attitude, that I was destined to be slim for the rest of my life. The same thing was true of my journey with cancer. I chose not to believe that it was the end, and visualized moving towards health, expressing an attitude of gratitude daily for wellness, and only seeing and feeling, several times a day, what I wanted — absolute and complete health and vitality (versus what I did not want — ill health and death). That very vision and belief, synergistically propelled by my attitude of gratitude, led me towards making the right choices for health and vitality. No energy was spent on what I feared or did not want! None!!

> *"There are only two ways to live your life.*
> *One is as though nothing is a miracle.*
> *The other is as though everything is a miracle."*
> Albert Einstein

So, if you not are getting a particular result that you say you want, trace backwards from that specific result, through the chart above, to get to the root (your attitudes, beliefs, ideas, and opinions) of your outcome, and determine what amongst them is not serving your highest good in that particular instance. And change it! Now! And, of course, read on. There's more good news ahead. Just what radio frequency are you tuning into?

"The Secret" Is Really Not A Secret!

We are so very blessed today with special tools to help us on this path of conscious awareness and development, providing the means by which we can move toward fulfillment in every area of our lives. One of my favorite tools is the film (an extremely entertaining and fully engaging documentary) entitled *"The Secret"*. This movie is all about fulfilling your deepest desires easily and gracefully. Truly, everywhere you look and listen, the message today, and in this film, is the same, and it's clear. It's all about what you think about—and what you think about expands.

Basically, everyone everywhere who is successful is saying this very same thing—Change your thoughts to change your life. If you want to improve the quality of your life you have to change the quality of your thoughts. And if the questions you ask yourself and others are not giving you the right answers, then ask different questions. Let me share a truly insightful strategy, for changing your mind in an instant, which I recently had the good fortune to experience firsthand. I had already watched the movie, *The Secret*, so I had been reminded of the Universal Law of Attraction, and focusing on what you want, which makes you feel good, versus what you don't want, which makes you feel bad.

What Radio Station Are You Listening To?

I was invited, this past summer, to participate in a very challenging ropes course, at one of the most heavenly — and I mean *heavenly* — places I have ever visited. It is called EarthTeach Forest Park, just outside of Ashland, Oregon. There were only 30 participants, all leaders in their own right, and only a few of us prepared for what we were about to experience. I will not share all of the details because that is not what this chapter is about. What I will share is the first evening's discussion and the huge impact it had on my life. The facilitator, on our first evening, asked us what we hear when we listen to the FM radio. Then he asked what we hear when we listen to the AM radio.

Well that was easy! On FM radio, the news is generally upbeat, focused on the good things we want more of, the music is great, and the whole experience is very pleasant, uplifting, fun, and often inspirational. On the other hand, AM radio is generally all about the bad news, sensationalizing what is wrong, and not working, with a focus on what we don't want. It is often victimizing people, communities or countries, and is overall, depressing.

Okay so where am I going with this? Well, the facilitator pointed out that most of us are tuned in regularly to our AM radio. You know that negative little voice that constantly reminds us of our inadequacies, our shortcomings, our uncertainties, and all of the things we say we don't want! Now you know how fast you can change that dial when you have the radio on, and you don't like the AM programming? Guess what. You can change that dial in your mind just as quickly! Don't believe me? Remember, I told you I was going to share a firsthand, life altering realization with you that I had while at EarthTeach. I know, after you have read what follows, you'll want to check out the various programs yourself, sponsored by The Way Foundation, at www.earthteach.org, or call 541-482-4572. And I encourage you, from the deepest part of myself, to do just that. The experience will, dramatically and powerfully, impact your life!

My Personal Triumph On The Mountain . . .

Well, on with the story. The next morning we headed out to the exquisite mountain where all of the more physically oriented parts of the program were taking place. I could not believe my eyes when I saw the first activity. We each had to climb a tree pole many feet into the heavens – and you know how tall those evergreen trees grow – and then traverse across a log from one tree pole to another several feet away. I choked! So, instead of rushing to be first on that pole, I watched and waited.

Finally the moment of truth arrived. It was my turn to face my fears and do it anyway, as the cliché goes. So, all harnessed up, I stepped up to this towering tree pole, and began to climb. Halfway up the pole, which felt like miles up that darned pole, I heard my niggling mind chatter. "Who do you think you are? You're no spring chicken, girl! There is no way you'll ever get to the top and walk across that log to the other tree!" And then, "God, I am so tired, I'll never make the rest of the distance. I'm just not strong enough to do this. Why did I ever agree to come here in the first place? I'll never do this again!" *And then it hit me!* My AM radio had fully kicked in. And it was making me feel *really* bad!

What happened next was extremely powerful. At that fateful moment, I remembered what we had heard the night before, and immediately switched stations. That's right! Immediately I switched, in that very instant of realization, to my FM station. *I changed my attitude in an instant!* And I repeated to myself, "I can do this. I have everything within me that I need to do this. God, give me the strength to finish this with grace and ease." Over and over again, throughout the rest of the experience . . . And I felt *great!*

The rest was history—at least for me. I reached the top, headed across the log, arrived at the other tree pole, hugged it, stepped away from it, declared my love for God, the Universe, and everyone who was watching from far below—AND JUMPED! According to those tiny little people staring up at me—from all those many feet below, my journey was a flawless continual flow from the bottom of the first pole where I started, right to the jump out from the log into the air for the descent to the ground. How did that happen? I, simply, changed my thoughts in an instant from what I did not want, which made me feel terrible and fearful, to thoughts that empowered me and made me feel great.

The Solution is Easy

So, I encourage you to go, right now to www.thesecret.tv and buy the movie. It will be one of the best investments you will ever make in your life and in your business. I do not make a penny of profit from sending you to this website! I completely believe, with all of my heart and soul, that this movie will change your life! On a call I participated in recently, Joe Vitale (one of the *Secret* teachers), who, a few years ago was homeless, and is now a multi-millionaire, doing only what he loves and living his dream life—living **THE SECRET**—encouraged all of us on the call (and there were several hundred callers on that call!) to watch *The Secret* everyday, for 7 consecutive days! He said it would change the very structure of our DNA—and our lives would never be the same again! I have seen amazing results in my patients, friends and associates who have actually followed this recommendation. I guarantee that this works! I never suggest anything that I have not personally used and incorporated into my own life and the lives of my clients and friends.

So what are you waiting for? Do it NOW! The only time you have is Now, the Present! Your present from the universe—today is your gift. I am, after all, from the 60's! So I grew up with certain ideas that have significantly shaped my thoughts and my life—even if I have forgotten to remember them from time to time! A human frailty I suppose. Anyway, a book by Ram Dass, entitled **Remember, Be Here Now**, is still on my shelf today! Not as much, today, for the content, as for the title. And it goes hand in hand with a cliché I love: Yesterday is like a cancelled check, tomorrow like a promissory note—but today is cash in hand, spend it wisely. In other words, focus on today. And do remember, that the quality of your thoughts and actions today, including, and just as important, a deep seated attitude of gratitude for all that you have right now, will determine the quality of your life tomorrow!

Okay, a brief summary of this whole perspective is simply that the secret to anyone's success in any area of his or her life doesn't have much to do with what you do, but it has everything to do with what you think — and how you feel about what you think — your attitude! If you develop the habit of thinking predominately about the things you desire, instead of the things you don't desire, you will attract, by the Universal Law of Attraction, everything you desire. The key is to remember that whatever you think about expands. And there is always a feeling or attitude attached to that thought!

Remember that AM / FM radio I talked about earlier? Well, visualize your brain as both, a broadcasting station, and a receiving set, for all of the vibrations of thought around you. Every thought has its own vibrational frequency, and your attitude will, to a large part, determine that frequency. You can literally train your mind to think only about the things you desire, thereby tuning into the FM Station (upbeat attitude) that will allow those things to be received by you. Don't get discouraged if your thoughts sometimes go south. Like a physical fitness program and the reconditioning of your body, it will take some time to re-condition your mind to consistently think this way. But stick with it. The rewards are definitely worth it! So what do you think? Time for an *attitude* overhaul?

And here's a thought I'll leave you with. You know how we always hear the statement: "I'll believe it when I see it!" Well, how about this instead? "I'll see it when I believe it!" Feel the difference? It's all about attitudes!

A wonderful resource for a deeper exploration of the power of the attitude of gratitude in our daily lives is www.ThankGodI.com. There are plans to launch a series of books filled with inspirational stories, by people just like you and me, who have learned the power in their lives, of an attitude of gratitude in facing, and overcoming, some of the most challenging experiences life confronts us with. There will certainly be something for everyone in one of the more than 100 titles scheduled to be produced.

THE RULES FOR THE ROAD

It's actually pretty simple. If you want to be healthy and alive, you have to get foods with a life of their own into your body. So the following rules for the journey towards health and a vibrant life are very logical. We will begin on a positive note, with a list of only the Do's.

1. **Select the freshest foods you can find!** As food sits for long periods of time it becomes:

    a. stale with poor flavor, texture and appearance,
    b. rancid if it contains oils (grains, nuts, seeds),
    c. depleted of nutrients which are destroyed by exposure to oxygen in the air.

2. **Focus on fresh vegetables and fruits, raw non-toasted, un-roasted grains and cereals and legumes (beans, peas, lentils).** Each of these food groups contain their own specific forms of essential fiber, as well as essential vitamins, minerals, anti-oxidants and phytochemicals which fight free radical damage at the cellular level.

3. *Look for reliable sources,* either within your area, or by mail order, for **organic produce and grains,** and use these as much as possible in your daily menus. *Seek out the local or closest farmers' market* and shop there for produce.

4. **Use the simplest, shortest cooking methods possible** when preparing your food in order to insure optimum retention of nutrients. In other words, steam vegetables only to the point of el dente, grill fish and chicken until just done, steam rice or grains until tender and then remove from heat immediately. Gently simmer on low heat versus rapidly boiling on a high heat.

5. **Aim to eat at least 50% of your vegetables and fruits in their raw form.** This preserves the vitamins, minerals and active enzymes, which may be destroyed by heat and water during the cooking process. Your body requires a full profile of all of these nutrients, which work together, when in proper balance, to create the potential for every metabolic function within the body to take place.

6. **Eat the skins of your produce items (fruits and vegetables) whenever possible.** Many of the essential nutrients are right under the skin. To avoid contamination from the multitude of pesticides used in commercial farming, it is best to choose organic produce. And always, whether commercially, or organically, grown, wash all produce very thoroughly before eating.

7. **Choose whole vegetables and fruits over their juices.** The fiber that is discarded in the production of the juice is very high in vitamins, minerals, antioxidants and phytochemicals (plant chemicals), all of which are essential in the prevention of disease and illness. The juice contains only a portion of what is available in the whole food!

8. **Season foods with natural condiments,** such as fresh herbsfresh garlic, onions, lemon or lime juice, peppers, organic and ethnic vinegars, vegetable flakes and powders, and spices.

9. **Include a wide variety of foods in your diet.** This insures a better balance of essential nutrients. What one food lacks, another contains!

10. **Reduce your intake of fats, especially saturated fats.** These include fats from dairy products and most animal protein sources, other than fish and seafood.

11. **Use methods of cooking that do not require the addition of fats,** or substitute the fats with vegetable broth, water, or fresh lemon juice.

12. **Include small amounts of fats in your diet that are from plant oil sources,** focusing on pure virgin olive oil, Udo's Blend oils, avocados, sesame oil, and other cold-processed oils. Use them uncooked, in dressings, for salads and steamed vegetables. The general rule is to maintain, approximately 20% of the day's calories from these natural uncooked fats.

13. **Steer clear of any fats which are of a trans-fatty acid nature, or which incorporate hydrogenation in the processing.** These include:

    o   the wide array of margarines
    o   salad dressings
    o   mayonnaise

- o   most commercial nut butters (e.g. peanut butter)
- o   roasted nuts and seeds
- o   packaged and frozen baked goods, cookies, crackers
- o   snack foods and snack bars
- o   canned, packaged and frozen entree items
- o   powdered, canned, refrigerated or frozen coffee whiteners
- o   powdered flavored coffee mixes
- o   non-diary creams and dessert toppings

In other words, check the label for the words *hydrogenated,* or *partially hydrogenated,* or *palm oil,* or *coconut oil,* or *any other oil that is listed as hydrogenated.* Leave it on the shelf or in the case. These do not spell good health!

14. **Reduce or eliminate your consumption of meats, especially red meats (i.e. beef, lamb, and even pork.)** These meats are high in marbled saturated fats. Apart from the health risks associated with high fat intake, as indicated throughout the research, the fat of the animal is also where the toxic byproducts of metabolism, and the hormonal injections for faster growth, are stored.

15. **Choose fish or the leaner cuts of poultry,** i.e. **the** chicken or turkey breast *with the skin removed, in place of red meats.* If using ground turkey meat, select the skinless boneless breast of the turkey and ask the butcher to grind it for you.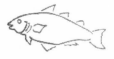

16. **Game meat provides a very lean and tasty alternative** to our higher fat domestic protein sources. These include rabbit, hare, muskrat, deer, moose, caribou, bear, wild goose, grouse, pheasant, turtle, frog legs, rattlesnake and eels, just to mention a few.

17. **Limit your intake of animal meats to a maximum of 3 to 5 servings per week,** with the focus on the leaner varieties, especially fish, and game meat. Fish and game meat are generally higher in a type of oil, commonly referred to as omega-3 oil, which according to large bodies of research, is beneficial in the reduction of the incidence of heart disease, various cancers, arthritis, Alzheimer's, etc.

18. **Select the plain, unflavored, nonfat and low fat versions of dairy products,** such as milk, cottage cheese, ricotta cheese, buttermilk and yogurt. Look for the lower fat varieties, now available, of firm

cheeses. Or better still, *try some of the new soy cheeses in the dairy section* of the grocery store or health food store.

19. **Increase your consumption of legumes as a high fiber, low fat, high calcium and iron, source of protein.** Included are soybeans and soybean products, such as tempeh, tofu, miso, and soymilk. Other varieties of legumes: chickpeas (garbanzo beans), pinto beans, white and red kidney beans, Roman beans, split peas, lentils, black-eyed peas, etc.

20. **Include at least 2 cups of plain, nonfat yogurt, kefir, or acidophilus milk daily** for their immune-enhancing properties. Select only those brands which list the specific cultures, and list them as *Live Cultures.*

21. **Reduce or eliminate the intake of potential toxins.**

Tobacco: whether firsthand or secondhand, cigarette smoking has been associated with illnesses and diseases too numerous to list here.

Alcohol can lead to illnesses of the liver, kidneys, bladder and overall elimination systems of the body. It increases free radical damage and lowers your resistance to snacking on high fat, high sugar refined foods.

Pesticides on our fresh produce may have hazardous effects on our overall health and immune systems. It is advisable to wash all produce upon purchase, even if it is organically grown. Add ½ cup of white vinegar to a basin of clean purified water, and soak produce, other than berries and leafy greens, for several minutes, and then rinse thoroughly in two sinks of clear water. Let dry on towels and then refrigerate.

Additives and preservatives added to our food sources may prove over time to have deleterious effects on our immune systems and general well-being. With the increasing consumption of packaged, processed preserved foods we are also seeing a parallel in increasing numbers of allergy sufferers, and general lethargy and restlessness among our children and adolescents. Is there a connection? Why take the risk?

Here are two well-known and potentially dangerous additives that have been extensively scientifically researched, and in the news, often:

Nitrites: includes many of the meat analog-based products, such as vegetarian forms of bacon, ham, hot dogs, bologna and deli sliced meats, as well as the actual processed meats from an animal source.

Sulfates and sulfites: includes dried fruits and other dried food products. Limit wine consumption, especially red wine, for this reason as well.

22. **Minimize risky foods.** These include:

    o   fatty meats
    o   salty foods
    o   sugar-laden desserts, chocolates and sweets
    o   pickled foods, especially those produced with white, distilled vinegar
    o   salt-cured meats and foods
    o   smoked meats, cheeses and other foods
    o   nitrite-cured meat products and other foods
    o   burned or well-done foods, including and especially those cooked on a barbecue

23. **Daily intake of fluids should include at least 6 to 8, 8 ounce glasses of water.** The diet in this book is high in natural fiber, which absorbs, like a sponge, many times its own weight in fluids. Without adequate fluid intake, you can become severely constipated, as well as experience flatulence (gas) and bloating.

    Water is required for every major function of the body, including carrying nutrients to where they are needed, as well as carrying wastes and toxins out of the body. Water is also necessary for proper functioning of the digestive juices and the digestive tract, so it may assist in prevention of indigestion. However, a rule of thumb is to drink water before a meal, but not during a meal.

    If you are ill, it is advisable to increase your fluid intake, to prevent dehydration which can result from diarrhea, vomiting, high fevers or hyperventilation.

24. **Regular daily exercise is essential for** *maintaining a healthy weight,* **and for maintenance of an efficient, fully functioning and energized body.** However, *gentle exercise,* done consistently, is the key to long term benefits. This includes natural forms of exercise, such as walking, swimming, climbing stairs (versus taking the elevator or escalator), bicycling, dancing, yoga and sexual activities.

Love your body with exercise. Gentle exercise is nurturing and soulfully nourishing. Punishing forms of exercise are breaking down tissue that then has to be rebuilt! *If you are ill, you do not have the extra stores* for any additional rebuilding, over and above the extra demanded for basic maintenance!

25. **Respect and love this wonderful machine: Your Body!** Listen to it! Be alert to any signals of *dis-ease,* indicating that something is not working right in the body. These can include pain in a part or parts of the body, indigestion, heartburn, constipation, diarrhea, flatulence, vomiting, fatigue, anxiety, irregular hair or nail growth, excessive fluid retention, or bloating, just to mention a few.

26. **Surround yourself with positive loving people.** Create around you the kind of loving community you desire, including friends, a personal coach, people who are doing with their lives what you say you want to do with yours; in general, people who will inspire and motivate you to stay on track.

27. **Include a quiet relaxation period in your daily life.** You only need 15-20 minutes per day of yoga or Tai Chi, or simply sitting quietly with calming music. And please: **Remember to breath** throughout the day; *breathing + exercise = oxygen flowing = energy!*

28. **Develop a daily attitude of gratitude,** living every day filled with gratitude in every area of your life, which, in turn, most effectively enhances your life's outcomes:

    a. **Write 5 things, large or small**, that you are grateful for each day in a journal. Focusing on the good in our lives miraculously produces more of the same!

    b. **Use positive "self-talk" and "visualization", along with** *feelization,* to achieve success in anything you decide to do. Positive "self-talk" and visualization are the keys to success. Add to that, the experience of *the feeling* of having accomplished what you desire, and you are truly on your way to success. Research has shown that athletes who see themselves as winning, and who internalize the feeling of what it will be like as they cross the finish line first, or jump the highest jump, or perform the most highly rated dance on ice, etc. are the ones who achieve their most desired goals.

c. **Live in the moment.** Remember, the past is like a canceled check, and the future like a promissory note, while the present is your cash in hand. It's the only thing you can depend on, so spend it wisely.

d. **See the funny side of life.** Laugh a lot. Laugh at yourself. In his book, *Anatomy of an Illness*, Norman Cousins profoundly demonstrates the healing power of humor.

e. **Honor yourself for a job well done.** It is very important to reward yourself for all of your accomplishments, and to celebrate your successes. This arouses a positive sense of self, a sense of worthiness, and the internalized thought that, "my word is law for me!" This positive energy then inspires success in other endeavors in our lives, including the overcoming of an illness.

f. **Remember, you have choices.** Get rid of the *"should, could, would"* mentality! Make choices that are in alignment with your dreams, desires, goals and personality. Stop *"shoulding"* on yourself!

29. **Take responsibility for your own life.** No one else has as much invested in your life as you do. Learn as much as you can, about what you can do to become healthy, or to maintain optimal health. Learn to discern! Don't take everything at face value. Ask questions. Go to the source. Awareness and knowledge, balanced with some wisdom and a generous dose of discipline, are the cornerstones of a healthy life.

30. **Live in integrity with yourself.** In life, do what you love to do. Be true to yourself about who you are, what you like and don't like, how you want to live your life, where you want to live your life, etc. Do not live your life to please others, *doing what you think others expect you to do*, and *presenting the image you think others want to see.* You are cheating yourself of the life you deserve. And furthermore, continually living with an underlying feeling of discontent will eventually erupt in an illness.

So to sum up what you have just read:

a. Incorporate a specific time daily (at least 5-10 minutes) for deep breathing practices, learning to first exhale completely before continuing with a deep breathing pattern.

b. Select the highest quality, most natural, organic, whole foods you can get.

c.   Minimize the amount and type of food preparation used, with 50% of your food being eaten in a raw state, especially vegetables and fruits.

d.   Drink at least 6-8 glasses of water daily, as well as your other beverages.

e.   Add a good measure of natural, gentle exercise, about 20-30 minutes daily.

f.   Take time out every day (at least 10-15 minutes) to just be still, and to rest, relax, rejuvenate, and eventually to learn to meditate. (This may require some practice, since most of us are programmed to believe that this step is a luxury that we don't have time for — big mistake!).

g.   Work on developing and maintaining a healthy, optimistic, *loving* attitude, towards yourself, as well as others and the world around you.

In time you will move through your life with Ease, Confidence, Peace of Mind and Health.

The Dilemma

To laugh is to risk appearing a fool.
To weep is to risk appearing sentimental.
To reach out for another is to risk involvement.
To expose feelings is to risk rejection.
To place your dreams before the crowd is to risk ridicule.
To love is to risk not being loved in return.
To go forward in the face of overwhelming odds is to risk failure.
But risks must be taken because the greatest hazard in life is to risk nothing.
The person who risks nothing does nothing, has nothing, is nothing.
He may avoid suffering and sorrow,
but he cannot learn, feel, change, grow or have.
Chained by his certitudes, he is a slave.
He has forfeited his freedom.
Only a person who takes risks is free.

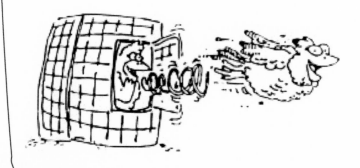

2. CULINARY STRATEGIES AND TOOLS FOR SUCCESS

WHAT NOT TO LOOK FOR IN THIS SEGMENT
OF THE BOOK

What you will not find in this segment of the book are a lot of numbers relating to the calorie counts in the foods and recipes, the sodium levels, the amount of available fiber, the level of sugar, or the number of fat grams provided. The reason is simple!

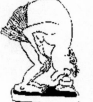

If you are eating according to the recommendations outlined throughout this book, especially those listed under *Rules for the Road,* you will never need to be concerned about how much of the potentially harmful items you are consuming.

It is the canned and packaged, processed and frozen, convenience foods, which have been prepared with large amounts of hydrogenated or partially hydrogenated fats (trans fats), increased levels of salt, MSG (monosodium glutamate) artificial sweeteners and simple sugars, as well as white refined flours. These white flours, regardless of the grain of origin, are devoid of the fiber found in the husk of the grain, the part removed during the milling process.

Natural foods, organically grown, and as fresh as you can find them, are nutritionally in tact, with both soluble and insoluble fibers, enzymes, natural oils in minimal amounts, low sodium levels, and naturally occurring sugars, in a more balanced and nutritionally sound base of the *vitamins, minerals and phytochemicals* so necessary for all of the biochemical and metabolic functions of a healthy body!

The preparation processes used in the menus and recipes are as simple as possible, and as minimal as possible, in order to preserve the greatest amount of the original nutritional value of the foods!

So throw away the calculator, calorie charts and fat gram books! Start simplifying your life NOW! Most importantly — it's a new adventure, so HAVE FUN!

LET'S DRINK TO OUR HEALTH!

Probably one of the most common questions I get asked by my clients and patients is *"What can I drink?"* Of course this question makes sense when you look at what most people drink every day without a thought towards its detriments or benefits to their health.

 What are the usual fluids included in the average diet? Here's the list:

♦ regular coffee
♦ regular decaf coffee
♦ specialty coffees, i.e.: latte, espresso
♦ flavored instant coffee
♦ cola drinks, regular and diet
♦ flavored sodas, regular and diet
♦ sports drinks
♦ energy drinks
♦ antioxidant drinks
♦ instant powder drinks
♦ hot chocolate
♦ ovaltine, flavored
♦ black teas
♦ wine
♦ beer
♦ distilled liquors
♦ fruit flavored beverages
♦ reconstituted fruit juices
♦ fruit juices, regular and sweetened
♦ instant chicken or beef broth, packages or cubes

Does this look like your daily selection of beverages? Well these are the ones I am going to recommend that you *eliminate, avoid, or drastically reduce!*

Are you now asking the question, *"What's wrong with these drinks?"* And, after all, haven't you been told that fruit juices are a healthy substitute for caffeine-based drinks? And that diet sodas are a great alternative for the diabetic, or the dieter?

Well let's take a good look at these commonly consumed beverages for a moment!

Caffeine, found in coffee, even decaffeinated coffee, cocoa, chocolate, regular black teas, cola drinks, other carbonated beverages, and many over-the-counter and prescription medications, has been associated in much of the scientific literature with many of the degenerative illnesses we know today. Even the chemicals used in the processing of the coffee beans may prove to be harmful to our health.

Sugar is found in very large amounts in most regular sodas. As there is absolutely no nutritional value in basic white sugar other than calories, loading up with all of sugar's empty calories, results generally, in a major deficit of the more nutrient-dense calories from wholesome foods.

If the aim is to provide only those foods which will do the most to enhance the health of our body, then there is no room in the diet for foods which not only, do not benefit the body, but may also have serious negative implications to our overall health!

The same is true of *alcoholic beverages*. They are high in calories, and provide no nutritional support in the development and maintenance of health. Also, note that *all alcoholic beverages carry a warning about potential health problems*. However you probably have little concern, if you are consuming no more than the recommended 1 serving per day for women or 2 servings per day for men.

Sulfites, which are used extensively in the preservation of wines, in North America, may have adverse side effects for those with allergies to this substance. Natural wines, prepared and aged properly, do not require preservatives!

Fruit juices *are often listed as a substitute for fresh fruit. Logically, how can that be?* Fresh fruit has a skin on it which contains fiber and carries many nutrients right under its surface. That skin certainly does not make it into the juice! Nor does the juice contain any of the fiber or the non-water soluble micronutrients of the flesh of the original fruit. *So again we get calories without benefits!* However, there is one exception, whole food fruit and vegetable juices made in a Vita Mix Machine. (For more information on whole food juices, go to www.marilynjoyce.com and sign up for our *Special Report.*

Sodium is, only required by the body in very small amounts—about 500 milligrams per day. North Americans tend to ingest five to ten times that amount, with about ¾'s of it coming from processed, packaged, canned and bottled foods and condiments, and sodas. This high sodium intake decreases the ability of our kidneys' to reabsorb calcium. For clarification here, we lose about 20-40 milligrams of absorbed calcium for every gram (1000 milligrams) of sodium consumed. So, it is recommended that we aim for a maximum of 2300 milligrams of sodium or less per day, and between 1300 (over 50 years of age) and 1500 milligrams daily for people with high blood pressure. And one teaspoon of regular table salt contains about 2400 milligrams of sodium.

Sodium is also used in the carbonation of most soft drinks and sodas. Most people are very aware of the sugar content in these drinks, but express great surprise about the high sodium content. Again, **Read the Label!** And to add insult to injury, carbonated drinks especially colas, are basically *calcium thieves*. There is significant evidence to suggest that soft-drink consumption in general, and phosphoric acid-containing cola drinks specifically, are associated with lower bone mass. To make up for the compromised ability of the kidneys' to reabsorb calcium due to the high sodium intake (necessary for the carbonation process), the carbonated molecules then, virtually steal calcium from your blood stream. The blood, in turn must replenish its calcium supply directly from your bones, in order to support muscle and brain function!

Salt, or sodium chloride, is in the news regularly, in relationship to high blood Pressure, strokes, cardiovascular disease, and in general, most of the degenerative illnesses that exist today. However, if you follow the recommendations in **INSTANT *E.N.E.R.G.Y.*™**, this should not be an issue for you! An excellent alternative to regular table salt is *"Real Salt"*. See the *Food Products* chapter.

There is a trend amongst people watching their weights, or limiting their sugar or caffeine intake, to substitute with beverages such as chicken or beef broth. Whether from a can, package, or bouillon cube, **Read the Label!** Generally these broths are loaded with **salt and MSG (monosodium glutamate)**. The fact that a large percentage of the population has a negative reaction to MSG, anything from a dull roar of a headache to actual convulsions, negates any of its flavor-enhancing qualities.

Artificially sweetened drinks and products are not recommended. Researchers are continually finding more scientific evidence to support the belief that the sweeteners being used today may have potentially harmful, long-term effects, such as the development of carcinogens in our bodies. Artificial sweeteners are toxic elements in our bodies. They should never be included in the diet of pregnant women, children or teenagers due to possible irreversible cell damage.

NutriSweet, Equal and Aspartame *are all different names for the same artificial sweetener.* Aspartame should be avoided at any cost! The accumulation of formaldehyde in the brain has been observed in recent studies in Europe. This accumulation of formaldehyde, a known carcinogenic substance, damages your central nervous system and immune system and results in genetic trauma. The sad news is that the FDA concurs with this, but believes that we do not consume enough to warrant concern! Excuse me!

No other food additive in history has had more complaints from the public. Aspartame has been linked to brain tumors, fibromyalgia, MS, lupus, seizures and a long list of other central nervous disorders. Possible side effects of aspartame include wheezing, coughing, nose and throat irritation, asthma, dizziness, headaches, migraines, panic attacks, irritability, nausea, vomiting, intestinal discomfort, skin rashes, nosebleeds, and nervousness. Aspartame has even been linked, in research, to depression and manic episodes. I ask you, does this sound like a healthy alternative to sugar?

Saccharin *was the first artificial sweetener to be widely available.* Sweet 10 (saccharin), Sweet'N Low, and other saccharin-based sweeteners, are still used in some prepared foods, gum, and over-the-counter medicines. Though the cancer warnings no longer appear in the US, many other countries have banned its use due to the potential for bladder cancer. My father, an avid, and I mean avid, saccharin user from as far back as I can remember — he never listened to me! — died of bladder cancer. This poison will never rest on a shelf in my pantry, far less make it into the bodies of anyone who visits or stays with me.

Splenda *is the trade name for sucralose,* and it is basically chlorinated sugar molecules. In my opinion, it may be made with sugar molecules, but it is not sugar! What happened to eating real food? Why are we always willing to make ourselves guinea pigs for the next man-made fake "product", disguised as a "food"? *Chlorine is a known carcinogenic agent!* What part of this picture are you not getting? We filter our water to get rid of the chlorine. We buy natural coffee filters in order to avoid filters bleached with chlorine. We avoid white flour products in order to avoid chlorine-bleached flour. I guess I am missing something here. In the name of "hoping" to lose a few pounds, *we kill ourselves with poisons.*

Well, there's no question that you won't have to worry about those extra pounds — if you're not here to bother! Perhaps a little bit of history will help to clarify what we may be dealing with here. In 1976, in the search for a new pesticide formulation, British scientists accidentally discovered a synthetic compound, which we now refer to as sucralose. Yes, the sucralose molecule is comprised of sucrose, which is sugar. However, three of the hydroxyl groups in the molecule have been replaced with three chlorine atoms. Because the bonds holding the carbon and chlorine atoms together are very similar to a chlorocarbon — and most pesticides are chlorocarbons — several independent researchers warn that sucralose may, in fact, have much more in common with pesticides than actual sugar. So, ingestion of sucralose may result in similar health challenges to those observed in the growing body of research evaluating the effects of the ingestion of pesticides.

Pesticides are among the many chemicals that have been identified as what we call endocrine disruptor chemicals (EDC's). These compounds appear to mimic the action of hormones when absorbed by humans, and interfere with the essential inner workings of our cells. Because the endocrine system influences all aspects of our health and well-being, including cognitive function, thyroid and metabolism, digestion and hormonal balance, and even our reproduction, and it is an extremely sensitive system, we may be setting ourselves up for some serious health challenges as our bodies attempt to break these compounds down and release them. See Chapter: *Rules of the Road.*

If you need a little sweetness in your life — added to your oatmeal, to your tea or coffee, or sprinkled on some berries, why not try something natural — organic sucanat (natural sugar cane crystals), pure maple syrup, natural honey right from the farm, agave syrup, or stevia. The herb stevia, Stevia rebaudiana is a natural sweetener that has been used for more than 400 years without any negative side effects. Stevia is 200-300 times sweeter than sugar, and has been the sweetener of choice in Japan for at least 20 years. Something to think about . . .

So, to sum up the negative components of our overall drinking habits in North America, and perhaps universally, **we consume far too much caffeine, sugar, salt, MSG, artificial sweeteners and the chemicals added for preservation and shelf-life**. And unfortunately most of what we drink, apart from providing a lot of empty calories with potentially harmful side effects, does not contribute any fiber, and at most, only minimal health-giving nutrients!

As I stated at the beginning of this book, this is primarily a **How-To** manual, rather than a **Why** manual. Because of the particular focus of **INSTANT**

E.N.E.R.G.Y.™, I have just *briefly* touched on a few of the many reasons why you should avoid the above beverages. There are many books available with a detailed focus on the whys. You will find some of these listed in the *References & Resources* section of this book. And again, sign up for our FREE *Special Report* at www.marilynjoyce.com. We will be covering all of these topics in much more details in future issues.

Now, let's look at the abundant variety of healthy, potentially beneficial, and delicious beverages available in the marketplace. There is absolutely no reason to feel deprived! Take a look:

◆ pure, filtered water
◆ mineral water
◆ sparkling waters, low sodium
◆ spring water, low sodium
◆ Club Soda, low sodium
◆ Crystal Geyser drinks
◆ organic fruit nectars, e.g. peach, pear, apricot, etc. (has more pulp and fiber, and the micronutrients clinging to the fibers, than regular juices)
◆ organic apple cider
◆ herbal teas, leaves or bags, e.g. those by Good Earth, Celestial Seasonings, Great Eastern Sun (Japanese organic Kukicha teas). **Read the Label!** Herbal teas are **not black teas with fruit or flower flavorings added!** Many large, commercial companies have this type of flavored tea available. *Avoid in the name of your health!*
◆ herbal teas for therapeutic purposes, e.g. constipation, runny nose, nausea, etc., produced by companies such as Traditional Medicinals and God's Herbs'.
◆ iced herbal teas, made either with regular brewed tea, chilled and iced, or with the new teas which can be brewed in cold water, e.g. those by Celestial Seasonings.
◆ white tea
◆ Chinese green tea, from China
◆ ginger tea, made with the natural root, or tea bags (see recipe)
◆ rosehip tea, leaves or bags
◆ red clover tea, leaves
◆ nettle tea, leaves
◆ mint tea/peppermint tea, leaves or bags
◆ alfalfa tea, leaves or bags
◆ ginseng tea, made with the natural root, or tea bags
◆ V-8 juice, low sodium

♦ tomato juice, low sodium
♦ organic coffee beans, use sparingly; buy whole beans, freshly grind as needed, and refrigerate to preserve freshness; oils in coffee beans become rancid when exposed to oxidation (contact with oxygen in the air).
♦ organic decaffeinated coffee beans, use sparingly; refrigerate, freshly grind as needed.
♦ Postum, a grain-based coffee alternative; can also make Postum latte, by using heated soymilk, almond milk or organic low fat milk.
♦ Cafix, a grain-based coffee substitute; can also make Cafix latte by using heated soymilk, almond milk or organic low fat milk.
♦ Teeccino, a carob and grain based coffee substitute; can also make Teeccino latte by using heated soymilk, almond milk or organic low fat milk.
♦ Organic Miso Soup mixes
♦ **Juice Plus+ Complete®,** a natural, identity preserved soy, whole food based, high protein, nutrient loaded, GMO free, powder; can be used alone in water, or with soy milk or almond milk, or in a variety of health drinks. (Check out the outrageously delicious **Complete®** recipes in *"I Can't Believe It's Tofu!"* by Dr Marilyn Joyce at: www.icantbelieveitstofu.com. There's one whole section of recipes incorporating this super mix.)

Note: *Be Creative and have fun with your beverages!*

♦ Mix different varieties of herbal teas to create your own flavors of hot or iced teas.
♦ Club soda or mineral water can be added to fruit nectars.
♦ A Virgin Mary can be made by spicing up tomato juice or V-8 juice.
♦ Sparkling beverages can be added to iced tea to perk it up with the bubbles.
♦ If you drink a little wine or beer, look for naturally prepared, without added sulfites.

FOODS TO AVOID AT ANY COST!

Anything fried

Bacon

Baked goods, commercial

Butter

Buttery crackers

Cheeses, non-organic whole milk

Cheeseburger, beef

Chocolate, dairy milk
and non-organic

Cream cheese

Doughnuts

Eggnog

Fat on meats

Fettuccini Alfredo, regular

French fries

Fried, battered chicken,
fish and meats

Hot dogs

Ice cream, commercial

Lard

Luncheon meats

Mayonnaise

Regular Miracle Whip

Margarine

Oils (except olive, flaxseed, sesame,
walnut, Udo's)

Organ meats

Pastries

Peanut butter

Pizzeria Pizzas

Potato chips

Salad Dressings, commercial

Sausage

Skin on chicken, turkey and fish

Whole milk products

GET THE SKINNY ON FATS . . .

Are you one of the millions who bought into the low, or no fat, craze that swept the Western world in the 1990's? Well, if you did, you were certainly not alone! Unfortunately, it was a recommendation founded on complete nonsense. We simply can't live without fats in our diet. Of course, I have to preface that comment with the words: healthy, all-natural, unprocessed, uncooked, unrefined, organic fats.

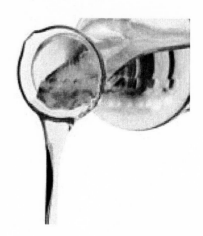

In this chapter my objective is to provide an overview of healthy versus unhealthy fats, and the best ways to get the optimum nutritional value from the fats you ingest. This will, in no way, be a complete guide to dietary fats and oils. There are such documents and books available, and I will reference a couple that you will gain great value from, should you decide to do more in depth personal research. My hope, though, is that you will gain enough insight from what you are about to read that, even without more research, you will have what you need to make much more informed decisions about what fats you will put into your mouth from this day forth. That is, of course, if you care enough about your health to do so! And I doubt you would be reading this book unless you did indeed care.

As with everything in life, balance is the key. We need a minimum of 15-20 % of our calories from fats — only natural, non-tampered-with fats! In their natural, unprocessed, or minimally processed form, fats serve many important functions in your body. The primary15 major functions are listed below.

They:

- ➤ Build, protect and maintain healthy cell membranes
- ➤ Construct and maintain healthy skin
- ➤ Provide fuel for every cell, tissue, gland and organ in your body
- ➤ Protect and repair your joints and connective tissue
- ➤ Aid in hormone and prostaglandin production
- ➤ Assist in proper nerve function

www.marilynjoyce.com

➢ Create energy and raise metabolism
➢ Stabilize blood sugar levels
➢ Help the your body burn fat
➢ Assist in oxygen transfer and recovery from fatigue
➢ Lubricate the body so that the cells can move freely
➢ Protect your body by buffering and neutralizing acids
➢ Transport fat soluble nutrients (vitamins A, D, E, K, etc.) throughout your body
➢ Increase absorption of other vitamins, minerals and phytonutrients
➢ Create the balance essential for an efficient immune system function

Not Enough Good Fats in Your Diet? Watch Out!

How many of you got caught up in that insane low to no fat diet craze in the 1990's? As many of my clients and patients discovered, this was a no-win game! For one thing, food tasted boring, bland and devoid of any real flavor. Secondly, you felt hungry a couple of hours after eating, and just never seemed to experience a sense of satiety (satisfaction) after eating. Well, that was just the beginning! Because, the overall lack of healthy fats in the diet, over even just a short period of time, eventually leads to the following very uncomfortable symptoms, just to name a few:

➢ Constipation
➢ Fatigue
➢ Indigestion, bloating
➢ Allergies
➢ Brittle nails
➢ Dry, brittle hair / hair loss
➢ Dry, flaky, itchy, scaly skin
➢ Poor nail growth / brittle nails
➢ Carbohydrate cravings
➢ Stimulant cravings
➢ Hormonal imbalances e.g. PMS, hot flashes, night sweats
➢ Mood problems / mood swings
➢ Short-term memory loss
➢ Anxiety / feeling "stressed out", overwhelmed
➢ Inability to concentrate / lack of focus
➢ Insomnia
➢ Infertility
➢ Poor wound healing
➢ Vision problems

Processed Fats versus Good Fats—What's the Difference?

Now, let's get something very straight here! *Processed* fats are not healthy alternatives. They are fats that are destroyed by the hydrogenation process, or any other heating process, to create a more stable fat that can sit on a shelf for a long time. Generally, any temperature above 118° Fahrenheit renders a fat unusable and toxic to the body. Some examples of processed fats include:

➢ Margarine
➢ Shortening
➢ Cooked meats, including bacon, and deli cold cuts
➢ Whole milk, butter and cheese (pasteurization uses very high heat!)
➢ Fried foods
➢ Hydrogenated and partially hydrogenated fats

The partially hydrogenated fats show up as what we now refer to as trans fats (see further in this chapter the section entitled: *Healing Fats Versus Poison Fats*), and are contained in the following foods:

➢ Commercial baked goods, cookies, cakes, pies, etc.
➢ Crackers
➢ Breads
➢ Peanut butter (and other hydrogenated nut and seed butters)
➢ Packaged cereals
➢ So-called "health" bars, including cereal bars
➢ Chips
➢ Canned and dehydrated products
➢ Roasted nuts and seeds
➢ Salad dressings and other commercial food toppings
➢ Mayonnaise
➢ Frozen foods: dinners, pizzas, soups, sauces, desserts, frosting, and ice cream

Are you getting the picture? The list includes almost anything packaged, processed, canned, frozen or treated in any way to change a natural whole food into something other than how it originally looked before anything at all was done to change it in even the slightest manner.

Essential Fats on the Other Hand . . .

Now, let's take all of this a step further. There are actually only two fats that are called essential fatty acids (generally referred to as EFA's), or essential fats, for short, and that is because they cannot be manufactured by the body. So they have to be provided by the food we eat. Those two essential fatty acids (EFA's) are omega-3 (n-3 or alpha-linoleic acid) EFA, and omega-6 (n-6 or linoleic acid) EFA. And they are called *essential* because your body has to have them in order to live and function normally. The body then converts the n-3 and n-6 EFAs into several n-3 and n-6 derivatives with important functions in the body. In fact, the best known derivatives of the n-3 (omega-3) EFA, which are, apart from being produced in your body, also found in fish, include eicosapentaenoic acid (EPA), used for hormone production (such as the eicosanoid hormones), and doxosahexaenoic acid (DHA), necessary for brain development and function, as well as vision.

Like everything else, a balance of these two nutrients is key to optimum health. And according to the tremendous amount of research done over the past 20 plus years by Erasmus Udo, PhD, a renowned expert on healthy fats and oils in the diet, a 2:1 ratio of n-3 to n-6 is indicated for optimum health. See his comprehensive book, *Fats That Heal, Fats That Kill* (Visit, explore, or buy the book, at his extensive website: http://www.udoerasmus.com/sitemap.htm.). And to further emphasize the benefits of reducing n-6 fats and increasing n-3 fats (ratio 4: 1, in this case), the results of the Lyon Diet Heart Study were very convincing. After 4 years, deaths by both heart disease and cancer were halved (De Lorgeril et al. Arch Inter Med 1998; 158: 1181-7).

N-3 (omega-3) deficiency is widespread today since it is extremely volatile. Apart from being easily destroyed during processing, it is also removed from foods in order to extend the shelf life of the particular foods and oils that contain omega-3 fats. Some of the symptoms of an n-3 deficiency include: low energy level, low metabolic rate, low thyroid and adrenal function, allergies, dry skin, leaky gut syndrome (LGS), weakness, retarded growth, poor muscle growth, learning and behavioral problems, depression, impaired healing, low testosterone, hyperactivity, tissue inflammation, edema (water retention), insulin resistance, sticky platelets (tendency to form blood clots in arteries), high blood pressure, poor vision, and the list goes on . . .

N-6 (omega-6) deficiency presents as dry eyes, dry hair and skin, itchy eczema-like skin conditions, brittle nails, fragile, thin skin, joint pain especially in the fingers, arthritic-like symptoms, skipped or irregular heart beat, hair loss, kidney malfunction, impaired glandular function, retarded growth, high cholesterol, impaired wound healing, fatty deposits in the liver, sterility, and miscarriage in women.

So, Where Do We Find Those Healthy Essential Fats?

Healthy fats are found in raw, organically grown—not roasted and salted or sugar-coated—nuts and seeds, such as almonds, walnuts, pecans, macadamia nuts, hazelnuts, cashews, brazil nuts, pistachios, flaxseeds, sunflower, sesame and pumpkin seeds, etc. They are also found in avocados, natural organic nut butters, olives, and extra virgin olive oils. They are __NOT__ found in extra light, or 100%, olive oil. Basically, if a label on a bottle of oil does not say unrefined, it has been processed, with the exception of extra virgin olive oil. Always look for cold-pressed or low heat expeller-pressed, oils, packaged in brown, green, or dark colored bottles, and preferably refrigerated. Buy in small quantities, store in the refrigerator, and use within a 2-3 months. Bottled oils can be frozen to preserve freshness for longer periods of time, since oils shrink rather than expand when frozen.

If you are a meat eater, or a part-time vegetarian, or a part-time vegan (no animal products whatsoever) who includes fish in your diet, you need to be aware of a few facts. We continually read about, and hear about, the benefits of including fish as part of our nutritional intake. However, not all fish are created equal. Apart from the potential mercury problem with some fish, not all fish are excellent sources of omega-3 fats. The best sources include high fat, cold-water fish such as wild salmon, sardines, herring, albacore tuna, ahi tuna, eels, kippers, mackerel, haddock, halibut and rainbow trout. Shellfish are generally not excellent sources of omega-3 fats. My personal choice would be to select fish from the Southern Hemisphere if possible—less risk of PCB's and heavy metal toxicity. To be sure that the fish you select is safe, go to www.nrdc.org/health/effects/mercury/protect.asp and click on *Mercury in Fish Wallet Card*. This parent site, www.nrdc.org/, is loaded with valuable information on protecting yourself, your family and the environment.

If you are a hunter and enjoy wild game meat, the good news is that the fat in these meats is an excellent source of n-3. This is likely due to the natural grasses and wild plants the animals feed on. *Grass-fed* beef also has a higher concentration of n-3 fats compared to conventionally raised cattle, including grain-fed beef, and cattle treated with growth hormones and antibiotics.

For years, I have been recommending the daily addition of 1 tablespoon of freshly ground, whole, golden flaxseeds, to a smoothie, or sprinkled on a salad or soup, or included in any other way that is not cooked. Flax is our richest plant source of n-3. And I firmly believe that this is a very healthy practice. Notice however, that I said freshly ground whole seeds! If flaxseeds are bought in packages already ground, it is very likely that you are getting a rancid product. The exposure of a larger surface area of the ground seeds to oxidation results in almost immediate rancidity, due to the extremely volatile (sensitive) nature of the seeds' pure oil when it is exposed to the oxygen in the air. The whole seeds, on the other hand, are very stable until ground.

And here's another point to consider. Research indicates that, just as in a whole food, versus consuming only one part (e.g. one nutrient) of a food, the same is true of whole seeds versus just consuming one part of them, such as the oil. There is a much wider array of nutrients available, as well as the synergy (i.e. the result or value is greater than the sum of the individual parts) of all of the nutrients in a whole food working in concert together. Cold pressed flaxseed oil is an excellent dietary source of the essential omega-3 fatty acids. However, research indicates that the lignans (fiber) in the flaxseeds are also essential. And the nutrients *attached* to the lignans are very important to your health as well. All of the nutrients in both, the oil, and the fibrous parts of the seed, work together synergistically.

That said, in the research on dietary fats, it is clear that an overabundance of n-3, from flaxseeds and other omega-3 supplements, can result in an n-6 deficiency. Essential fats compete for enzyme space in our cells. So, if you are getting excessive amounts of n-3 in relationship to n-6, the n-3 will crowd out the n-6, and lead to the expression of n-6 deficiencies. And as you have read above, the experience, of any, or even just a few, of these symptoms of deficiency, is not at all comfortable. That is why I now recommend, and include in my own nutritional program, Udo's Choice™ Ultimate Oil Blend, and Udo's 3•6•9 Oil Blend™. See the chapter on supplements & nutritional support products, *Dr Joyce Recommends* . . . , for more details about this oil blend.

Let me also repeat, that for more information on healthy versus unhealthy fats, you owe it to yourself to take a look at one of the most thorough books I have ever read on the subject, by Erasmus Udo, PhD, called *Fats That Heal, Fats That Kill*. You can also get a lot of great information at www.udoerasmus.com or www.fatsthatheal.com. The distributor for the oil blend is Flora, Inc. in the US at www.florainc.com or call 360-354-2110. In Canada, go to www.florahealth.com or call 604-436-6000.

Healing Oils Versus Poison Oils

I believe that we, the people, have unwittingly been slowly poisoned by the addition of a toxic substance (actually one of several, but we will focus on one right now) into our food supply for the past several decades. This substance tears your body down versus building it up. In fact, this substance does not occur naturally in nature, and is neither recognized, nor is it usable, by the human body. In fact, neither animals, nor insects, will eat it! This substance simply collects in and around your body's organs and fatty tissues. It blocks the healthy fatty acids and prevents them from performing their many beneficial functions (as outlined above).

What is this poisonous substance I am referring to? Trans-fatty acids! (Commonly known as Trans Fats.) They are basically deformed fat molecules that disrupt the functioning of healthy cells, by rendering the cell membranes inflexible and non-porous, preventing normal nutrient and waste transfer. Think about what would happen to you if you were not able to eliminate waste from your body. You would become very ill and die! Well, that is exactly what is happening, cell by cell, when we regularly eat Trans Fats. Your body's cells become sick and die! No nutrients can get into the cell, and no wastes can get out. They eventually suffocate and die! The health of your body – or lack of health – begins with each cell in your body, on the cellular level. Your body is simply the sum total of all of the cells in your body – good or bad!

Now, what is the basis of these deadly Trans Fats? Hydrogenated and partially hydrogenated fats! Trans Fats are created by adding hydrogen molecules to vegetable oils. The purpose of this process is to change the oil's liquid form into a solid form, at room temperature. Hydrogenation transforms once natural healthy fats into a saturated fat. These man-made fats have an indefinite lifespan, and therefore, allow foods to sit on shelves for a very long time without seeming to go rancid. They actually do go rancid (bad), but the average person can't smell the foul odor, or taste the bitter, despicable taste of the rancidity, because it is so well camouflaged by the hydrogenation process.

What are some of the documented adverse effects to your health from consuming hydrogenated and partially hydrogenated oils? Though there is a very long list, I will highlight a few of the most serious potential outcomes:

- ➢ Raises LDL (bad) cholesterol, and lowers HDL (good) cholesterol
- ➢ Raises serum cholesterol
- ➢ Interferes with absorption of essential fatty acids
- ➢ Causes free radical development, the underlying cause of degenerative illness
- ➢ Raises blood sugar levels and promotes weight gain
- ➢ Raises the risk, and accelerates the progression, of Type 2 Diabetes
- ➢ Causes high blood pressure
- ➢ Promotes heart disease

- Clogs artery walls, promoting atherosclerosis
- Impairs immune function
- Accelerates tumor growth
- Promotes various cancers, e.g. breast, prostate, colon
- Damages the cellular membrane, reducing absorption of necessary nutrients
- Reduces oxygen intake into the tissues
- Prevents elimination of wastes on a cellular level
- Causes liver disease
- Causes gallbladder disease
- Directly damages blood vessels
- Creates "sticky" blood — the cells stick together, reducing blood flow
- Impairs brain development in fetuses
- Increases the risk of low birth weight infants
- Reduces the volume and quality of breast milk
- Damages brain cells, impairing brain function
- Promotes ADHD (attention deficit hyperactivity disorder)
- Causes infertility
- Increases the risk of gum disease and tooth decay
- Promotes dandruff and acne

And the list goes on . . .

So, what do you think? Are those foods that are loaded with trans fats really worth all the above health risks? You may be asking, *"Just what can I do to avoid eating these villainous substances, when so many of the foods in the marketplace are loaded with them?"* Well, to start with, to seriously protect your own health and the health of your loved ones, read every label on every food you buy, and avoid, at all cost, any food that lists hydrogenated, or partially hydrogenated, fat as an ingredient.

½ Gram Rule — Here's Something to be Aware of When Reading Labels!

So, just in case you thought you were safe if you read the label and it seems to suggest that there are no trans fats in the food item you're contemplating buying, *think again*. The following question and answer is taken right from the FDA (US Food & Drug Administration) website. It is posted there, along with a lot of other questions with scary answers. This is truly a buyer "get informed, pay attention to your health, and beware of what is not written" world we live in. If you don't take the time to get educated, and then consistently practice what you learn, your health may drastically pay the price. *You can be sure that the government does not have your health interests at the top of its list!*. After reading what is written above about trans fats, you should find the following very insightful.

Q: Is it possible for a food product to list the amount of trans fat as 0 g on the Nutrition Facts panel if the ingredient list indicates that it contains "partially hydrogenated vegetable oil?" (Remember that partially hydrogenated fats are in fact Trans Fats!)

A: Yes. Food manufacturers are allowed to list amounts of trans fat with less than 0.5 gram (½ g) as 0 (zero) on the Nutrition Facts panel. As a result, consumers may see a few products that list 0 gram trans fat on the label, while the ingredient list will have "shortening" or "partially hydrogenated vegetable oil" on it. This means the food contains very small amounts (less than 0.5 g) of trans fat per serving.

And they think there is no problem with consuming this "small" amount in the packaged, processed foods we eat on a daily basis! Think about this for a minute. Say you ate 6 servings of one of these foods in a day — which is very easy to do if you get stuck into those corn chips (made with that "tiny" amount of trans fats) and salsa when you are famished after work. Then how many grams have you had? And how many times a week have you done something similar? I rarely see people eat only one serving of the addictive foods that are processed and prepared with even the smallest amount of trans fats. And every time you eat something processed with hydrogenated, partially hydrogenated, or fractionated oils listed in the ingredients, and there is a 0 grams listing for trans fats, you can bet it has at least the minimum amount that does not have to be listed on the label. Just something to think about . . .

The Rules for Choosing Healthy Fats & Oils?

Be aware that your first choice for healthy oils is *cold pressed*, which refers to oils obtained through pressing and grinding fruit, nuts or seeds with the use of heavy granite millstones or the more modern stainless steel presses, found in large commercial operations. Olive, sesame, peanut, and sunflower are a few of the healthiest oils obtained from cold pressing. Cold pressed oils retain all of their flavor, aroma, and nutritional value.

Expeller pressed oils are the next best choice. This is like cold pressing except that extreme pressure is added during the pressing to squeeze the oil from the fruit, nuts or seeds. This high pressure produces heat as high as 300°F through friction, so the oils produced with the expeller process can't be considered cold pressed. However, these oils do retain much their flavor, aroma, and nutritional value; just not to the extent of cold pressed oils.

Pretty much everything else out there has been completely refined by the use of chemical solvents in the extraction of the oil from its source, followed by boiling to remove most of the solvents. The oils are then degummed, bleached, deodorized, and heated again to very high temperatures. The final product has very little, if any, of the original flavor, aroma, or nutrients contained in the original seeds or fruit. In fact, the result is a product that has no health benefits whatsoever, simply a long shelf life.

Remember: All fats and oils are 100% fat and all oils are high in calories (about 120 calories per tablespoon) so they should always be consumed in moderation. Aim to include only the least processed fats and oils in your diet. Generally, I recommend about 2 tablespoons of oil each day — maybe 1 tablespoon of Udo's Choice Oil Blend added to a smoothie (see recipe in the chapter: *Dr Joyce Recommends . . .*), and another tablespoon of extra virgin olive oil, or cold pressed walnut oil, added to a salad dressing, or as a dressing on lightly cooked food, after the cooking process is complete.

NOTE: The minute that you cook oil to its smoke point (see the chart that follows), you have completely changed its molecular structure, and rendered it unhealthy.

Apart from this added oil, a daily nutritional program made up of a healthy balance and variety of fruits, vegetables, natural whole grains, a tablespoon of flaxseeds, and a handful of some raw nuts and seeds, should have you well covered in the essential fatty acid department. And steer clear of, or keep to an absolute minimum, saturated animal fats including, meat, butter, cream, whole milk and whole milk products, as well as those man-made, plastic-like trans fats we've just been talking about!

And just a little aside for all of you who continually ask me whether butter is better than margarine — YES! Tablespoon for tablespoon, margarine, in general, contains almost 10 times the amount of trans fatty acids contained in butter. Yes, butter does contain cholesterol and some saturated fat. However, humans have been eating butter for many, many thousands of years (as opposed to a few short decades of these sticky gummy man-made poisons, called Trans Fats). And a healthy body knows how to breakdown and use all of the components in butter.

There are two caveats here however: 1) Do not eat butter, without first getting the okay to do so from your doctor, if you have been placed on a diet restricting saturated fats. 2) Make sure that only organic butter is consumed. It should come from sources that have not used hormones or antibiotics in the raising of the cattle, and have used no chemicals in the production of the butter and other dairy products.

So, let's take a look at another important factor: the cooking of fats . . .

When fats are cooked there is what we call a smoke point, and it varies with each different fat. When the particular fat reaches its smoke point it begins to decompose, and is no longer a healthy addition to your diet, no matter how valuable it may have been in its original unprocessed form. Once the fat starts to smoke, or burn, and change color, even very slightly, this indicates that the fat is breaking down, and it generally emits a strong, harsh odor. It is believed that past the smoke point, the fat contains a large number of free radicals, believed to be the causative factor in the development of degenerative disease.

Several factors can contribute to a decrease in the smoke point of an oil. The length of time the oil has been heated, the temperature at which it has been heated, the number of times the oil has been used, the presence of salt or other impurities, whether or not it is a blended oil, and improper storage, can all result in a lowering of the smoke point. Unrefined oils, such as cold pressed and expeller pressed, usually have lower smoke points than the commercially refined hydrogenated oils. Generally, oils that are colorless, odorless, and tasteless are refined. Although it may not be necessary to know the actual temperature of the smoke points of various oils, it is important to know which oils and fats may be fairly safe to use for different cooking methods.

I want to be very clear that I personally don't advocate cooking with oils. From my very wide range of diversified cultural experiences, it is extremely clear to me that the healthiest populations on this planet do not cook their foods with fats and oils. They eat only unrefined oils, and they add the oils and fats for texture and flavor after the food is prepared and just prior to serving it. The reason that I have included the following chart is because I am constantly asked the same question: What oils can I safely use for cooking? This chart will serve as your guide. It would probably be a good idea to purchase a thermometer with which to check the temperature of your oils while you are cooking. Generally speaking, any temperature over 280 to 300°F will destroy the natural molecular structure of a healthy fat, as well as the nutrients inherent in the oil, no matter what the actual smoke point is. The smoke point is simply the stage at which the oil is going through a breakdown.

In the following chart, basically the oils that can be cooked at temperatures above 320°F have been refined, for the very purpose of cooking at higher temperatures, such as deep-frying, searing, sautéing, and pan-frying. Some of the oils that are listed below, for cooking under 320°F are unrefined oils, and are also available in refined forms. I have not included them, simply because I do encourage minimal cooking with oils. These refined oils with higher smoke points should be used sparingly, and only occasionally, if you truly care about your health.

Smoke Point of Various Oils and Fats

Type of Oil or Fat	Refined Smoke Point	Cooking Methods
Avocado Oil	520°F	Sauté, Pan-fry, Sear, Deep-fry, Stir-fry, Grill, Broil
Rice Bran Oil	490°F	Sauté, Pan-fry, Sear, Deep-fry, Stir-fry, Grill, Broil
Ghee (Indian Clarified Butter)	485°F	Sauté, Pan-fry, Sear, Deep-fry, Stir-fry, Grill, Broil
Tea (Camellia) Oil	485°F	Sauté, Pan-fry, Sear, Deep-fry, Stir-fry, Grill, Broil
Hazelnut Oil	430°F	Sauté, Pan-fry, Sear, Deep-fry, Stir-fry, Grill, Broil
Cottonseed Oil	420°F	Sauté, Pan-fry, Sear, Deep-fry, Stir-fry, Grill, Broil
Macadamia Nut Oil	390°F	Sauté, Pan-fry, Sear, Stir-fry, Grill, Broil, Baking
Lard	375°F	Sauté, Pan-fry, Sear, Baking
Almond Oil	350°F	Sauté, Pan-fry, Sear, Stir-fry, Grill, Broil, Baking
Coconut Oil	350°F	Sauté, Pan-fry, Sear, Stir-fry, Grill, Broil, Baking
Olive Oil (Virgin)	350°F	Sauté, Pan-fry, Sear, Stir-fry, Grill, Broil, Baking

Smoke Point of Various Oils and Fats

Type of Oil or Fat	Refined Smoke Point	Cooking Methods
Hemp Oil	330°F	Light sauté, Low-heat grilling, Low-heat baking
Vegetable	325°F	Sauté, Pan-fry, Sear, Baking Shortening
Corn Oil	320°F	Light sauté, Low-heat grilling, Low-heat baking, pressure cooking, sauces, salads
Grape Seed Oil	320°F	Light sauté, Low-heat grilling, Low-heat baking, pressure cooking, sauces, salads
Peanut Oil	320°F	Light sauté, Low-heat grilling, Low-heat baking, pressure cooking, sauces, salads
Pumpkin Seed	320°F	Light sauté, Low-heat grilling, Low-heat baking, pressure cooking, sauces, salads
Sesame Seed Oil	320°F	Light sauté, Low-heat grilling, Low-heat baking, pressure cooking, sauces, salads
Soybean Oil	320°F	Light sauté, Low-heat grilling, Low-heat baking, pressure cooking, sauces, salads
Walnut Oil	320°F	Light sauté, Low-heat grilling, Low-heat baking, pressure cooking, sauces, salads
Butter	300°F	Sauté, Pan-fry, Sear, Grill, Broil, Baking

Smoke Point of Various Oils and Fats

Type of Oil or Fat	Refined Smoke Point	Cooking Methods
Olive Oil (Extra Virgin)	250°F	Light sauté, Low-heat grilling, Low-heat baking, pressure cooking, sauces, salads
Canola Oil	225°F	Blend it with oils with higher smoke points for low heat cooking
Safflower Oil (Regular or High Oleic)	225°F	Light sauté, Low-heat grilling, Low-heat baking, pressure cooking, sauces, salads Blend it with oils with higher smoke points for low heat cooking
Sunflower Oil (Regular or High Oleic)	225°F	Light sauté, Low-heat grilling, Low-heat baking, pressure cooking, sauces, salads Blend it with oils with higher smoke points for low heat cooking
Flaxseed Oil		Never, ever cook with this oil
Udo's Oil Blend		Never, ever cook with this oil blend

The Healthy Dozen:
Top Tips for Buying, Storing and Using Healthy Oils

1. Buy oil in small quantities, in dark colored bottles, preferably organic if possible, and store in the refrigerator. Keep no longer than one year. Never buy refined hydrogenated and partially hydrogenated oils!
2. Always store flaxseed oil in the refrigerator, and use within 60 days.

3. Avoid cooking with fats. Why buy cold pressed and expeller pressed oils if you are just going to destroy them with high heat cooking methods?

4. Cook and stir-fry with broth, and then lightly drizzle oil over prepared foods, just before serving, for flavor and texture.

5. Make all of your own salad dressings from scratch (Try the easy and delicious recipes in the chapter on *Salad Dressings*), versus buying what I refer to as *death in a bottle*.

6. Use extra virgin olive oil, flaxseed oil, or walnut oil as the salad dressing base.

7. Add olives, avocados, nuts and seeds to salads instead of saturated animal fats, such as meat and cheese.

8. Throw out all oils, nuts, seeds and nut butters as soon as they develop even a slight odor, or a bitter taste—signs of rancidity due to oxidation.

9. Avoid processed, packaged, canned, or frozen prepared foods—most are loaded with trans fats! You saw the list of foods earlier in this chapter.

10. Add a tablespoon of freshly ground flaxseeds to a smoothie, a salad dressing, or sprinkled on soups, stir-fries, and cooked cereals.

11. If you eat fish, include only those listed earlier in this chapter.

12. Avoid all fried foods, especially deep-fried foods—choose foods in restaurants that have been broiled, grilled, lightly steamed, and raw.

For more tips on eating out and eating on the road, check out our *Special Reports* at www.marilynjoyce.com. Often the biggest challenges we face in limiting unhealthy fats in our nutritional program are encountered when we eat in restaurants or on the run.

SLASH THE BAD FATS

INSTEAD OF:	USE:
Bologna, Salami, Hog Dog	Sliced turkey breast Sliced chicken breast Marinated tofu slices Marinated and baked pork tenderloin Spicy tempeh slices
Bread Stuffing From Mix	Brown rice with seasoning Bulgur, Couscous or Oatmeal with seasoning
Butter, Margarine (as a spread)	Fruit preserves Olive oil spray Butter sprinkles
Butter, Margarine, Oils, Lard (in cooking)	Nonstick vegetable spray Vegetable broth or purified water Virgin olive oil, Sesame oil (sparingly)
Cream	Skim milk Evaporated skim milk 1% Low fat milk
Cream Cheese	Nonfat cottage cheese, blended Low fat cream cheese Low fat ricotta Low fat ricotta and low fat yogurt, blended
4% Creamed Cottage Cheese	Nonfat cottage cheese Low fat cottage cheese Low fat ricotta cheese

Cream Sauces for Pasta	Marinara, clam or tomato sauce
	    w/no meat
	Blended low fat yogurt, lemon, garlic
	    & Parmesan

INSTEAD OF:	USE:
Cheese, hard or semi-soft	Low fat cheese Nonfat cheese Part-skim mozzarella or ricotta Soy cheese
Chili Con Carne	Chili with ground turkey breast Vegetarian chili
Cold Cereals, commercial (flakes, puffs, crisps)	Alpen Muesli Grape-nuts, All-Bran Shredded wheat, regular and spoon size Wheetabix
Crackers, high-fat	Brown rice cakes Corn Thins, organic Crackers, fat free zero trans fats Whole wheat matzo crackers
Croissants, Doughnuts, Danish	Low fat wholegrain muffins Wholegrain bagels and low fat cream cheese Wholegrain English muffins, rolls
Egg noodles	Brown rice or wholegrain pasta
Fried Chicken	Baked or grilled chicken breast, no skin Sautéed chicken breast nuggets, in broth
Fried Fish	Grilled, baked, poached or broiled Salmon, canned in water Tuna, canned in water Broiled or boiled shellfish, occasionally
Granola Cereal	No added fat granola No added fat muesli Any cooked grains or grain combinations

INSTEAD OF:	USE:
Hamburger, beef	Turkey burger, ground breast meat Salmon burger Low fat soy or vegetable burger
Ice Cream	Frozen fruit or frozen fruit bars Nonfat frozen yogurt (occasionally) Blended frozen fruit and nonfat yogurt Juice Plus+® Complete popsicles
Margarine, Oil (in baking)	Use only 'No Trans Fat' and ⅓ to ½ the amount Applesauce Pureed Prunes
Mayonnaise	Low or nonfat mayonnaise Nayonaise Nonfat cottage cheese and yogurt, blended Plain low or nonfat yogurt with herbs Vegenaise
Milk Shakes, Eggnogs, Floats	Fresh fruit frappe Fruit nectars, whole fruit juices Low fat milk or soymilk health shake
Peanut Butter, Nut Butters	Flavored tofu, blended Legumes with lemon and garlic, blended Marinated tofu slices
Pizza, Cheese and Pepperoni	English Muffin (wholegrain) pizzas Vegetarian pizza on wholegrain crust
Popcorn, buttered	Air-popped popcorn w/butter sprinkles Air-popped popcorn w/all natural sprays Low sodium wholegrain pretzels
Scalloped Potatoes, French Fries	Baked potatoes with low fat yogurt topping Seasoned oven-baked potato wedges Baked sweet potatoes with low fat yogurt

INSTEAD OF:	**USE:**
Sour Cream	Plain low fat yogurt
	Blended nonfat cottage cheese & lemon juice
	Blended low fat ricotta and lemon juice
	Blended low fat buttermilk & low fat ricotta
Tortilla Chips, regular	Potato or tortilla chips, baked
	Raw vegetables
Vegetables in Butter or Cream Sauces	Steamed fresh vegetables with butter sprinkles
	Vegetables w/lemon or lime juice, or vinegar
	Vegetables w/yogurt or buttermilk dressing
	Vegetables w/homemade nonfat dressing
	Vegetables w/Bragg Liquid Aminos
	Vegetables w/sprinkling of Parmesan or Romano cheese
Whipped Cream	Whipped evaporated skim milk
Whole Eggs	2 to 1 whites to yolks
	3 ounces tofu and 1 large egg
Whole Milk	Fat fee milk
	Low fat milk
	Evaporated skim milk

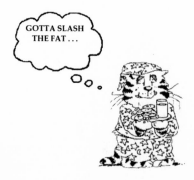

GOTTA SLASH THE FAT . . .

SNACK ATTACK!

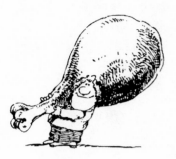

So you've got the munchies! And they're fierce! You're craving something — *anything* — to take the edge off! And all that you can think of, at this moment, are the foods I have recommended for you to avoid. After all, isn't that what we mean when we think of snack foods? *Aren't they the forbidden delights?* Those foods loaded with fats, sugars, salt and cholesterol? **WRONG!**

In light of the fact that most of us can't think straight when we're in the middle of a snack attack, I felt that it was only fair to provide a ready list of delicious, easy to prepare, and to have on hand, alternatives to the regular, much advertised variety of *"junk foods"* which are so available, and so eye-catchingly displayed, in the most obvious sections of your local grocery and convenience stores.

The following list is by no means the last word on snack foods! But it is a very good base from which to start when you can't move your thoughts past potato chips and sour cream dips, or pizza loaded with cheese and pepperoni, or a box of chocolate chip cookies, or a pint of Ben & Jerry's ice cream.

And remember, that apart from all of the suggestions outlined here, *we all have leftovers from time to time that can be eaten* as they are, or can be incorporated into other dishes, for tasty alternatives to the typical convenience snack foods available in every corner store in America. **Just think low fat, low sugar, low sodium, low cholesterol and high fiber!** And then make your wise choices accordingly.

In the *Food Products* chapter of this book, you will find listed some of the companies that produce healthy alternatives to the usual high fat, sodium-laden, heavily sugared, and cholesterol-loaded foods and condiments. Many of these products are available in your local supermarket, or health food store. If you can't find the products anywhere, write to, or call the company, for information on how and where to get them. Several companies actually have mail order services set up, so that no matter where you live, or how remote the area is, they will ship their products to you.

Now, on to the list of snack ideas. Here's to snack attacks!

Remember, this is a new adventure. Have fun with it! Copy this list and put it somewhere obvious so you can refer to it before you uncontrollably crunch and munch!

- ½ sprouted wholegrain bagel with preserves
- ½ sprouted wholegrain bagel with blended low fat ricotta cheese and fruit preserves
- air-popped popcorn, sprayed with all natural flavor sprays
- air-popped popcorn, seasoned with herbs
- air-popped popcorn, seasoned with garlic-flavored butter sprinkles
- applesauce and plain, low fat yogurt
- apple slices with low fat string cheese
- apple slices with nut butter e.g. almond, peanut
- apple slices with tofu cheese
- baked potato topped with nonfat refried beans and tofu cheese
- baked potato topped with salsa or Dijon mustard
- baked potato topped with low fat yogurt seasoned with herbs
- baked potato chips and seasoned low fat yogurt dip, or salsa, or the combination
- baked tortilla chips with salsa
- bean burrito with corn tortilla and nonfat refried beans
- blended frozen banana
- broiled nonfat grated cheese and sliced tomato on sprouted wholegrain toast
- brown rice heated, served with Bragg Liquid Aminos
- brown rice heated, and served with seasoned low fat yogurt
- brown rice leftover, with vanilla soymilk, fresh fruit, and a teaspoon pure maple syrup
- buckwheat heated, and served with seasoned low fat yogurt
- celery with curried nonfat cream cheese and chives
- cup-a-soup, or meal-in-a-cup, dehydrated, low fat, low sodium varieties
- fresh fruit, low fat plain yogurt and cinnamon whipped together
- frozen grapes or frozen chunks of mango, pineapple or papaya
- fruit frappe, with blended fresh fruit and ice cubes
- fruit nectar popsicles
- fruit, pureed and frozen in ice cube trays
- fruit slices with low fat yogurt dip, flavored with almond extract and pure maple syrup
- garlic whole wheat sourdough toast using all natural flavor sprays
- Juice Plus+® Complete popsicles

- leftover pasta and vegetables mixed together as a salad with nonfat dressing
- leftover steamed vegetables with seasoned low fat yogurt
- low fat granola bar
- low fat granola and soymilk
- low sodium whole grain pretzels
- marinated tofu slices on sprouted wholegrain bread or roll
- milkshake of low or nonfat milk or soymilk and frozen fruit
- millet heated, served with Bragg Liquid Aminos
- miso soup with tofu cubes and sliced green onions
- mulled organic apple cider
- nonfat frozen yogurt (sparingly)
- nonfat fruit juice-sweetened, cookies
- nonfat or low fat wholegrain or bran muffins
- nonfat wholegrain crackers and nonfat cottage or ricotta cheese
- nonfat whole wheat, wholegrain or rye crackers
- organic green salad with low fat dressing
- plain, low fat yogurt with fresh fruit
- potato salad with seasoned, low fat yogurt or buttermilk dressing
- raw vegetable strips (e.g., carrots, celery, broccoli, turnip, cauliflower, mushrooms, green and red peppers, cucumber, zucchini) with yogurt dip
- raw vegetable strips and salsa
- raw vegetables with nonfat refried beans
- rye crisps or rice cakes spread with low fat cream cheese (use sparingly)
- seasoned baked potato wedges
- seasoned blended chickpeas with whole wheat pita wedges
- soy or almond cheese and nonfat wholegrain crackers
- sprouted wholegrain toast with apple butter
- sprouted whole wheat toast with blended nonfat cottage cheese and applesauce
- tofu cheese and nonfat wholegrain crackers
- vanilla or chocolate, almond or soy, milk
- wholegrain breadsticks
- wholegrain English muffin pizza, using grated low fat cheese and tomato sauce
- wholegrain graham crackers

PRESCRIPTION FOR INDIGESTION

Whether healthy or ill, we all at times, due to lack of rest, overwork, or undue stress, experience that uncomfortable feeling of indigestion with the accompanying gas, after we've eaten a meal. This seems to increase as we get older, possibly due to a decrease over the years, in the amount of enzymes produced by our bodies. The problem definitely appears to be much more pronounced in someone dealing with a chronic illness, especially of the degenerative nature, such as cancer, A.I.D.S., heart disease, diabetes, etc. However there are several steps that can be taken to alleviate the problem.

1. **Eat only until you feel satisfied.** Beyond that puts added stress on your overworked body to digest and distribute or store the extra that it does not need at that time.

2. **Avoid eating when you feel anxious, uptight, worried or overly stressed.** Take the time to calm yourself, prior to eating, by using techniques such as deep breathing, yoga, relaxing music, or an unhurried bath with only the light of candles.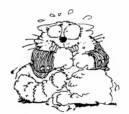

3. **Eat your larger meals earlier in the day, making the evening meal your lightest meal of the day.** This way the body gets the greater intake of food when it is less tired from the day's activities and therefore, most able to handle digestion.

4. **Changing the way you combine your foods at a meal may have an impact** on the way your body handles the intake. Because of different rates of digestion, some foods which are digested more quickly, such as fruits, do not mix well with more slowly digested foods, such as meats. This has made a big difference for many of my clients! *Here are some general guidelines:*

Bad Combinations:
- Starches with meat, fish, poultry, nuts, seeds, soybeans
- Any fruit with a starch
- Any fruit with a protein, e.g., meat, fish, poultry, nuts, seeds, soybeans
- Any fruits, except tomatoes, with any vegetables

- Acid fruits (citrus, pineapple) with sweet fruits (dried fruits, banana)
- Oils (vegetable oils, butter, margarine) with starches
- Melons (any variety) with any other foods
- More than 4 vegetables at a meal
- More than 3 fruits at a meal
- More than 1 protein food at a meal
- More than 1 starchy food at a meal

Good Combinations:
- Leafy greens with meat, fish, poultry, nuts, seeds, soybeans
- Vegetables with starches
- Grains with all legumes except soybeans
- 3 starchy vegetables (maximum), e.g., potatoes, squash, corn at a meal
- Leafy greens with oils
- Acid fruits (citrus, pineapple) with oils
- Sub acid fruits (e.g., apple, pear, grapes, mango, papaya, etc.) with oils

(See the *References & Resources Section* for recommendations on books, materials, and organizations that may be able to assist you.)

5. **Grated raw daikon radish, eaten as a relish** with a meal, has been used for centuries in the Orient, as a digestive aid. In it's raw state it is loaded with enzymes!

6. **Fresh ginger, grated into salad dishes, or added to cooked dishes,** not only adds a delicious flavor, but appears to stimulate more efficient digestion of the foods it is eaten with. *Ginger tea,* either hot or iced, (see recipe) is an excellent accompaniment to a meal.

7. **Fresh, natural, low fat yogurt which contains live cultures,** including *lactobacillus acidophilus and bifidus cultures,* as well as *lactobacillus bulgaricus and streptococcus thermophilus yogurt cultures,* creates a healthy environment in the colon, by killing unhealthy bacteria. **Yogurt, acidophilus milk, and kefir in the plain, low fat form,** facilitate digestion and increase resistance to infections. **Yogurt's active bacteria, and by-products of the bacteria's activity,** in the digestive tract and colon, have been reported to boost the immune system, to serve as natural antibiotics against infection, and to act

as suppressants of the activity in the colon that converts harmless bacteria into carcinogens. Be sure to purchase only organic varieties of these dairy-based foods to avoid hormones and antibiotics used in commercial farming.

For those who have chosen to follow a Vegan diet (no animal products) there are now a number of very delicious soy—based yogurts available.

8. **Lactose intolerance, due to a deficiency of lactase, a digestive enzyme, which digests lactose,** the milk sugar in milk and dairy products, can result in gas, cramping and diarrhea when the undigested milk sugar, reaches the colon. *Yogurt does not generally create a problem* for lactase deficient individuals. The active bacteria used in the preparation of yogurt, breaks down the lactose in the process.

9. **A sudden switch to high fiber foods,** especially whole grains and legumes, as well as an increase in raw vegetables and fruits, can result in the production of gas. Generally, this will lessen and return to normal after a few weeks*One strategy would be to implement a gradual increase in fiber intake,* to allow the colon time to adjust. Another strategy is to ensure that you drink 6 to 8 glasses of water of day.

10. **Swallowing air can create a severe gas problem.** This occurs while eating, drinking, chewing gum, smoking, belching or breathing deeply and rapidly with your mouth open, as during physical activity. *Take smaller bites of food, chew food slowly with your mouth closed, and <u>drink</u> liquids, not gulp liquids, before or after meals, not during meals.*

11. **Foods which seem to create a problem in their whole form** may be more digestible in a more broken down, more bioavailable form such as: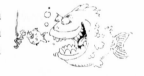

   a. ground up beans in hummus or vegetarian refried beans
   b. blenderized vegetables, used in sauces or smooth soups
   c. blenderized fruits in healthy protein drinks and frappes
   d. any of the above, blended with yogurt, acidophilus milk, buttermilk, kefir, or the live acidophilus culture itself
   e. the addition of fresh ginger root or fresh daikon radish to any of the above blended products may assist digestion and prevent gas

12. **The use of enzyme and probiotic supplements** about 15 minutes prior to eating a meal may ease or eliminate the problem. Start with a *basic papaya and pineapple enzyme supplement*, available in most health food stores, or *Beano*, available in most pharmacies, and many grocery stores. A wonderful, scientifically researched, probiotic that I recommend to my patients and clients, and personally incorporate daily, is *Bifidobacteria longum BB536*.

   In his book, *Food Enzymes: The Missing Link To Radiant Health*, Dr. Humbart Santillo, MH, ND and the creator of *Juice Plus+*® writes, "Enzymes are needed for every chemical action and reaction in the body. Our organs, tissues and cells are all run by metabolic enzymes. Minerals, vitamins, and hormones need enzymes to be present in order to do their work properly. Enzymes are the labor force of the body." For more detailed information you can go to the chapter: *Dr. Joyce Recommends* . . .

   And always seek the advice of a qualified health professional, e.g. a Registered Dietitian or a Medical Doctor, should the problem continue to occur.

13. **Drink adequate fluids daily.** At least 6 to 8, 8-ounce glasses every day! *Water is essential for every process or function within the body! Including Digestion.* For more information see the chapter: *Water, the Elixir of Life*.

14. **Specific, basic yoga exercises** can significantly alleviate the production of gas, or quicken its release from the body. See the *References & Resources* chapter for recommendations on magazines, journals, books, DVD's, and organizations that may be able to assist you. Also, listed in the same section, is a good contact for audio and videotapes: The Motivational Tape Company. For a quick and easy yoga routine that anyone can do anywhere, see the chapter: *Fit in Fitness*. And do check out the yoga DVD and CD featuring Susan Winter Ward, originator of Yoga for the Young at Heart, at: www.marilynjoyce.com.

NOTE: We would love your feedback on any of the recommendations you may have tried from this chapter. Or, for that matter, any other strategies you may have tried that have resulted in positive outcomes for you! Just email us at: info@marilynjoyce.com with any of your stories, insights, challenges, or major successes, so that we can share your valuable experiences with all of our *Special Report* subscribers. By the way, have you signed up for one of our news breaking, information-packed, *Special Reports* yet? You can join us at www.marilynjoyce. com; and www.icantbelieveitstofu.com. You will be very happy that you did!

SHOP FOR HEALTH
Stocking the Refrigerator and Pantry with Healthy Choices

The **Pyramid of _E.N.E.R.G.Y._** ™ that follows is based loosely on Maslow's Hierarchy of Human Needs, with the inclusion of healthy living foods. Regarding the food sections in this _E.N.E.R.G.Y._™ **Pyramid**, you will see that they are primarily filled with the most power-packed, natural, generally unprocessed foods available today! At most, the foods listed, contain only minimal amounts of added fats, sugars, sodium, caffeine, preservatives, food colorings, or cholesterol. If you select your foods from this chart, you will have no problem achieving optimum health with boundless energy.

To assist you with the _shop_ and _stock_ process, you will find, following the **Pyramid,** a comprehensive shopping list, which is broken down into the food groups from the **Pyramid,** plus sections for **Condiments and Flavorings,** for **Dried Herbs, Spices and Vegetable Seasonings,** for **Beverages,** and for **Miscellaneous Items.**

Remember that this is an _extensive list_, demonstrating the incredible variety of foods, beverages and seasonings available for the development and maintenance of your health! By no means do you have to immediately run out and buy everything listed on your first shopping trip. Start by purchasing the items you are most familiar with, or that appeal to you most. Then over time, experiment with the items listed that you have never tried before. You will find ideas, suggestions and recipes throughout this book for ways to use the various foods listed.

The most fun will be enjoyed by those who view this wholesome, natural way of shopping and eating as an exciting new adventure!

With respect to the multitude of fresh fruits and vegetables available, as much as possible _buy them in season_. This varies according to the area in which you live. If you are unsure about the seasonal breakdown where you live, you can contact the Department of Agriculture and they will send this information out to you. Your local library may also be able to provide you with further information, or resources for information, on this matter.

Avoid the myriad of canned fruits and vegetables throughout the vast expanse of the grocery store shelves. Apart from the high salt or sugar solutions saturating the products sitting in those cans, the amount of heat and handling involved in the canning process of those fruits and vegetables, has virtually destroyed most of the nutrient value and all of the active enzymes, resulting in a much less than satisfactory texture, taste and nutritional component. *Believe me, once you readjust your taste buds to the taste, texture and aroma of fresh produce, you will never open another can.*

The few canned or bottled products included in the following lists are those which are changed very little in the processing, in comparison to the preparation at home, which may be lengthy and/or time-consuming. *Choose bottles over cans whenever possible!*

PYRAMID OF E.N.E.R.G.Y.™

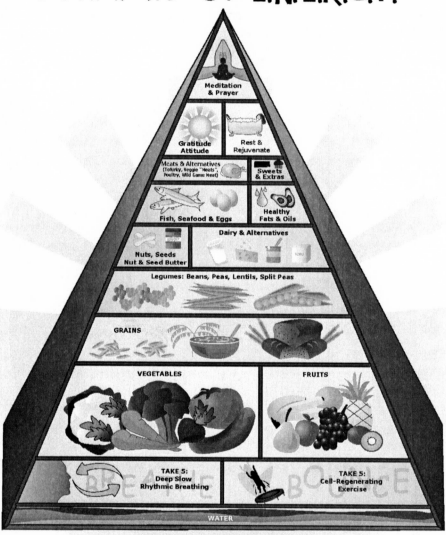

NOTE: For best results when using the food sections of this Pyramid of E.N.E.R.G.Y.™ begin by selecting more foods from the lower layers, with portion sizes and number of servings decreasing as you climb the Pyramid.

THE PYRAMID OF *E.N.E.R.G.Y.*™ SHOPPING LIST

Vegetable Group:
- [ ] Alfalfa Sprouts
- [ ] Artichokes
- [ ] Asparagus
- [ ] Bamboo Shoots
- [ ] Beets/Beet Greens
- [ ] Bok Choy
- [ ] Broccoli
- [ ] Broccolini
- [ ] Brussel Sprouts
- [ ] Cabbage
- [ ] Carrots
- [ ] Cauliflower
- [ ] Celery
- [ ] Chives, Fresh
- [ ] Cilantro
- [ ] Corn on the Cob
- [ ] Cucumber
- [ ] Daikon Radish
- [ ] Dark Green Lettuce
- [ ] Eggplant
- [ ] Endive
- [ ] Escarole
- [ ] Ginger Root
- [ ] Green or Yellow Beans
- [ ] Green Peas, Fresh
- [ ] Green or Red Peppers
- [ ] Hot Chili Peppers
- [ ] Kale
- [ ] Kolrabi
- [ ] Maitake Mushrooms
- [ ] Mixed Greens
- [ ] Mushrooms
- [ ] Okra
- [ ] Onions
- [ ] Parsley
- [ ] Parsnips
- [ ] Potatoes
- [ ] Radishes
- [ ] Red Lettuce
- [ ] Romaine Lettuce
- [ ] Rutabagas
- [ ] Salsa
- [ ] Scallions
- [ ] Sea Vegetables
- [ ] Shiitake Mushrooms
- [ ] Snow Peas
- [ ] Spinach
- [ ] Summer Squash
- [ ] Sweet Potatoes
- [ ] Swiss Chard
- [ ] Tomato Paste
- [ ] Tomato Sauce
- [ ] Tomatoes
- [ ] Turnips
- [ ] Vacuum-packed Tomatoes
- [ ] Watercress
- [ ] Winter Squash
- [ ] Yams
- [ ] Zucchini

Fruits:
- [ ] Apples
- [ ] Applesauce, Unsweetened
- [ ] Apricots, Fresh/Dried
- [ ] Bananas
- [ ] Blackberries
- [ ] Blueberries
- [ ] Cantaloupe
- [ ] Cherries
- [ ] Currants
- [ ] Dates
- [ ] Dried Peaches, Apples, Bananas
- [ ] Dried Tropical Fruits
- [ ] Figs, Fresh/Dried
- [ ] Granny Smith Apples
- [ ] Grapefruit
- [ ] Green Grapes

- Guava
- Honeydew Melon
- Kiwi Fruit
- Lemons & Limes
- Mango
- Nectarines
- Oranges
- Papaya
- Peaches
- Pears
- Persimmon
- Pineapple
- Plums
- Pomegranate
- Prunes
- Raisins
- Raspberries
- Red Grapes
- Star fruit (Carambola)
- Strawberries
- Tangerines
- Watermelon

Legumes: Beans, Lentils, Peas, Split Peas

- Canned Beans, Peas & Lentils
- Canned Chick Peas (Garbanzo Beans)
- Canned Vegetarian Chili
- Dried Beans, Peas & Lentils
- Edamame
- Lima Beans
- Refried Beans, Nonfat
- Tempeh moved from Meats
- Tofu moved from Meats

Bread, Cereal, Rice & Pasta:

- 7 & 10 Grain Cereals
- Air-Popped Popcorn
- All-Bran Cereal (no flakes or puffs)
- Bagels, Sprouted, Wholegrain
- Barley, Wholegrain & Pearled

- Breads, Rye, Pumpernickel
- Breads, Sprouted & Multi-grain
- Breads, Whole Wheat & Wholegrain
- Brown Rice, Short & Long Grain
- Buckwheat
- Bulgur
- Cornmeal, Yellow
- Cracked Wheat Cereal
- Crackers, Low & Nonfat, Wholegrain
- Cream of Wheat
- English Muffins, Wholegrain
- Essene Bread
- Granola, No Added Fat
- Matzo Crackers, Whole Wheat
- Millet
- Muesli, No Added Fat
- Noodles, Wholegrain
- Pastas, Vegetable & Spinach, Wholegrain
- Pastas, Whole Wheat & Wholegrain
- Pita Bread, Whole Wheat
- Pretzels, Whole Grain, Low Sodium
- Rice Cakes, Nonfat
- Rolled Oats, Old Fashioned
- Rye-Crisp Crackers
- Shredded Wheat
- Tortilla Chips, Baked
- Tortillas, Corn or Whole Wheat
- Triscuits, Low Sodium
- Wheat Bran, unprocessed
- Wheat Germ, unprocessed
- Weetabix
- Whole Wheat & Wholegrain Flour
- Wild Rice

Milk, Yogurt & Cheese:

- Acidophilus Milk, Low fat
- Almond Milk
- Buttermilk, Low fat
- Cream Cheese, Low fat
- Cheeses, Nonfat & Reduced Fat
- Evaporated Skim Milk

□ Kefir, Low or Nonfat
□ Mozzarella, Part Skim
□ Rice Dream Milk
□ Ricotta Cheese, Reduced Fat
□ Ricotta Cheese, Nonfat
□ Skim Milk, Nonfat & 1%
□ Soy Cheeses
□ Soymilk, Plain & Flavored
□ Yogurt, Low Fat, Plain

Sprouts:
□ Alfalfa Sprouts
□ Broccoli Sprouts
□ Clover Sprouts
□ Fenugreek Sprouts
□ Lentil Sprouts
□ Mung Bean Sprouts
□ Onion Sprouts
□ Pumpkin Seed Sprouts
□ Radish Sprouts
□ Soy Bean Sprouts
□ Sunflower Seed Sprouts
□ Wheat Berry Sprouts

Nuts, Seeds, Nut & Seed Butters:
□ Almond Butter
□ Almonds, Raw, Unsalted
□ Brazil Nuts, Raw, Unsalted
□ Hazelnuts (Filberts), Raw, Unsalted
□ Pecans, Raw, Unsalted
□ Pumpkin Seeds, Raw, Unsalted
□ Sesame Seeds, Unsalted
□ Sunflower Seeds, Raw, Unsalted
□ Tahini (Sesame Seed Butter)
□ Walnuts, Raw, Unsalted

Poultry, Fish, Wild Game,
    Lean Meats, Eggs:
□ Ahi Tuna
□ Buffalo Meat
□ Canned Salmon in Water
□ Canned Sardines

□ Canned Tuna in Water
□ Chicken Breast, Free Range
□ Eggs, Free Range
□ Fish, Deep Water, Wild
□ Ground Turkey Breast
□ Haddock
□ Halibut
□ Mackerel
□ Pork Tenderloin, Organic
□ Rabbit
□ Red Snapper
□ Salmon, Fresh
□ Sea Bass
□ Shellfish, sparingly
□ Turkey Breast, Free Range
□ Venison

Healthy Fats & Oils:
□ Avocados, Fresh
□ Butter, Organic (sparingly)
□ Flaxseed Oil, Cold Pressed
□ Nayonnaise
□ Olive Oil, Pure Virgin
□ Olives (sparingly)
□ Parmesan Cheese
□ Romano Cheese
□ Salad Dressings, Nonfat
□ Salad Dressings, Low fat
□ Sesame Oil, Cold Pressed
□ Udo's Oil Blend
□ Vegenaise
□ Walnut Oil

Sweets & Other Extras:
□ Agave Syrup, Organic
□ Blackstrap Molasses, C Grade
□ Fruit Nectars
□ Fruit Preserves
□ Honey, Organic
□ Maple Syrup, Pure
□ Sucanat, Organic
□ Stevia

Condiments & Flavorings:

- [ ] Bragg Liquid Aminos
- [ ] Butter Buds
- [ ] Capers
- [ ] Flavor Extract, Pure Almond
- [ ] Flavor Extract, Pure Lemon
- [ ] Flavor Extract, Pure Orange
- [ ] Flavor Extract, Sherry, Brandy
- [ ] Flavor Extract, Pure Vanilla
- [ ] Flavor Sprays
- [ ] Hot Pepper Sauce
- [ ] Mustard, Dijon
- [ ] Mustard, Stoneground
- [ ] Nutritional Yeast
- [ ] Seaweed, Kelp
- [ ] Seaweed, Nori
- [ ] Seaweed, Wakame
- [ ] Soy Sauce, Low Sodium
- [ ] Taco Sauce, Green
- [ ] Taco Sauce, Red
- [ ] Tamari Sauce
- [ ] Tabasco Sauce
- [ ] Vegetable Broth & Seasoning, Bernard Jensen's
- [ ] Vegetable Broth, Gayelord Hauser's
- [ ] Vinegar, Balsamic
- [ ] Vinegar, Cider
- [ ] Vinegar, Malt
- [ ] Vinegar, Rice
- [ ] Vinegar, Wine

Dried Herbs, Spices
& Vegetable Seasonings:

- [ ] Allspice, Ground & Whole
- [ ] Anise
- [ ] Basil Leaves
- [ ] Bay Leaves
- [ ] Bell Pepper Flakes, Dried
- [ ] Caraway Seeds
- [ ] Cardamom, Ground
- [ ] Cayenne Pepper
- [ ] Celery Seeds
- [ ] Chervil
- [ ] Chili Powder, Mild & Regular
- [ ] Chilis, Dried & Crushed
- [ ] Chilis, Dried & Whole
- [ ] Chives Dried
- [ ] Cilantro, Dried
- [ ] Cinnamon, Ground & Sticks
- [ ] Cloves, Ground & Whole
- [ ] Coriander
- [ ] Cumin, Ground
- [ ] Curry Powder
- [ ] Dill Seeds
- [ ] Dill Weed
- [ ] Fennel Seeds
- [ ] Fine Herbs
- [ ] Garlic Powder
- [ ] Garlic, Minced
- [ ] Ginger, Powdered
- [ ] Horseradish, Powdered/ Prepared
- [ ] Italian Seasoning
- [ ] Mace, Ground
- [ ] Marjoram
- [ ] Mint Flakes & Leaves
- [ ] Miso
- [ ] Mrs. Dash/Spicy Mrs. Dash
- [ ] Mustard, Dry
- [ ] Mustard Seeds
- [ ] Nutmeg, Ground
- [ ] Onion Flakes
- [ ] Onion Powder
- [ ] Oregano Leaves
- [ ] Paprika
- [ ] Parsley, Dried
- [ ] Pepper, Black
- [ ] Pepper, Red
- [ ] Pepper, White
- [ ] Peppercorns, Black
- [ ] Poppy Seeds
- [ ] Poultry Seasoning
- [ ] Real Salt
- [ ] Rosemary Leaves
- [ ] Rosemary, Ground

- Saffron
- Sage
- Salad Herbs
- Sesame Seeds
- Tarragon Leaves
- Thyme Leaves
- Thyme, Ground
- Turmeric
- Vegetable Flakes & Powders

Beverages:

- Cafix
- Chinese Green Tea
- Club Soda, Low Sodium
- Coffee Beans, Organic (sparingly)
- Crystal Geyser Fruit Drinks
- Decaf Coffee Beans, Organic
- Fruit Nectars, Unsweetened
- Ginger Tea, Root or Bags
- Ginseng Tea, Root or Bags
- Herbal Teas, Leaves or Bags
- Iced Herbal Teas
- Juice Plus+® Complete, Powder
- Mineral Water
- Mint Tea, Leaves or Bags
- Nettle Tea, Leaves
- Perrier Water
- Postum
- Red Clover Tea, Leaves
- Rosehip Tea, Bags or Leaves
- Spring Water, Low Sodium
- Sundance Sparklers
- Teeccino, coffee alternative
- Tomato Juice, Low Sodium
- V-8 Juice, Low Sodium
- Water, Pure, Filtered

Miscellaneous Items:

- Baking Powder, Aluminum-free
- Baking Soda
- Blue Green Algae
- Canned Soups, Organic
- Chlorella
- Cookies, Fat Free & Low Fat, Wholegrain
- Fig Bars, Fat free, Whole Wheat,
- Frozen Fruit Bars
- Imitation Bacon Bits, Organic
- Meal-in-a-Cup, Organic
- Nonfat Frozen Yogurt (sparingly)
- Nonfat Granola Bars
- Spaghetti Sauce (meatless)
- Spirulina
- Veggie Burgers

WHAT'S ALL THE FUSS ABOUT ORGANIC??

Just What Does "Organic" Mean Anyway?

With organic products sales increasing exponentially at an annual rate of 20%, consumers are obviously making some seriously different choices about what goes into their shopping carts these days. But what exactly does the term "organic" mean?

Organic refers to food that is grown and processed in a practical, systematic, and ecologically harmonious partnership with nature, using environmentally sustainable farming practices and renewable resources. Organic farmers rely on earth-friendly, natural pest control, nurtured and maintained rich soils, complimentary plant groupings, rotation of crops, seasonal planting, lunar cycles, and a genuine love and commitment for their land, what grows on it and their families' health and welfare.

It does not depend on the use of harsh, synthetic, toxic pesticides, fertilizers or herbicides. It does not depend on hormones, antibiotics, or genetic engineering. And it does not use seedlings or seeds that have had been DNA-altered by genetic modification to grow only once! Or, worse, have been enriched with pharmaceuticals! I wonder if that might explain our drug addicted youth today.

Organic foods are minimally processed with no artificial ingredients, preservatives or irradiation. When you choose organic foods you are assisting both, in the protection of your own health, and the ecology of the land. And apart from safer foods, that taste far better than conventionally grown foods, you are also contributing to the creation of a just and sustainable food system for today, and for future generations.

A Little History Goes a Long Way in Shaping Our Choices Later

I was very fortunate to have been taught valuable health lessons during my formative years, by two truly remarkable teachers. They fully understood and embraced the many practical reasons for, and the most efficient ways to produce, delicious, organic foods, while sustaining a healthy productive environment on a consistent basis. My grandparents grew almost everything they ate—and it was picked daily, at the peak of ripeness, as needed for each meal. They took incredible pride in every step of the production of the food that made it to their table. And the tremendous abundance of their garden fed many more than our immediate family! Everything was grown completely by natural, organic methods, together with a huge amount of love and care.

In fact, my grandfather's green thumb was the talk of the entire county — and beyond, I am sure. In his late 80's he was as handsome and as fit as most men in their forties today. And he thought nothing of walking 15-20 miles in a day just to help a neighbor out who was struggling to keep their garden growing. That was, of course, until my granddad saved their day! He often expressed his certainty that the new farming conglomerates beginning to surface throughout the country would be the death of humankind. Overall, my grandparents were very moderate in their approach to life, except that the food they ate had to be of the highest quality — with the understanding that a well-fueled body was capable of dealing with almost any challenge it may be confronted with. And what was most significant was how incredibly delicious the meals tasted, despite the absolute simplicity of preparation.

So the shock for me, as I grew into an adult and began purchasing my foods from the local supermarkets, was that nothing ever tasted like those meals I had enjoyed with my grandparents. And then, of course, I would revisit them, and re-experience that fresh picked flavor of foods grown with the highest of standards, no pesticides, no hormones or antibiotics in the animal products, and lots of loving care. Returning to my urban lifestyle, and tasteless fruits and vegetables, as well as far too many commercially processed packaged and canned foods, was always a disappointment. I did whatever I could to provide what I thought were nutritionally healthy meals for my family, but could never replicate what I had enjoyed as a child. Today, I sadly understand what we have done in the name of profit and greed, to render, what used to be healthy, delicious foods, into toxic, generally tasteless, pesticide-laced, time bombs waiting to explode when our bodies simply can't handle the ingestion of another millimeter of poisonous chemicals.

Tragically, I believe that we are only just beginning to get a glimpse of the terrible future that awaits our children and our grandchildren, if we do not soon awaken and stop this insanity! Prolonged ingestion of poisonous chemicals leads to accumulation of toxins in our bodies, and prolonged toxic build-up leads to obvious signs of illness, and prolonged illness often results in premature death! Babies and children, today, are bombarded from birth, with toxic chemicals in everything they eat, drink, breathe, wear, and clean themselves with. Perhaps even the things they touch, handle, and chew on, may prove, down the line, to be produced from materials that will leach out toxic elements at certain temperatures.

Furthermore, most of what kids eat and drink today would not have even been considered foods or beverages a few decades ago. And so much of the produce they eat today is so heavily contaminated with pesticide residues, that our children don't even have a clue what the original unaltered, unadulterated, naturally grown food tastes like. Research has actually found that children who switched to an organic diet had significantly reduced levels of pesticides in their bodies, scored higher on intelligence tests and were more physically fit than their counterparts, who were ingesting pesticide-laden produce.

So how can we re-create a healthy diet, and re-establish the practice of healthy food choices on a daily basis? The first step is to eat real organic food, grown naturally in healthy soils, using environmentally sustainable farming practices. Buying organic foods can significantly reduce our exposure to toxic chemicals. I know this is repetition, but what better teacher than repetition? The second step, since we may not always be able to buy organic foods, is to know which foods, grown conventionally, may have deleterious effects on our bodies due to the large amounts of extremely toxic pesticides used throughout their growth and production.

And here's something to think about! We know, from biochemistry, that it takes 90 to 120 days to change all of the red blood cells in our bodies. And we know, from psychoneuroimmunology, that as we replace the cells in our bodies, we replace them with a new cellular memory. That's great news! Because this also means that we can retrain our taste buds, through our new cellular memory, to crave the healthy, tasty foods that our bodies so desperately need in order to function optimally with unlimited vitality.

The Surprising Truth About Some Everyday Foods!

Though I could most definitely write an exhaustive list of foods here, I have selected, from my research, what appear to be the most important foods to buy organically. Several resources are also included in this section, so that you can continue your own research and education on this important subject.

10 Most Important Foods to Buy Organic

Following are 10 of the most frequently, and most heavily, pesticide-contaminated food products. Check out your local natural foods stores, food co-ops and farmers' markets.

1. Baby Food: Federal pesticide standards do not adequately cover infant foods—16 pesticides are detectable in most mainstream brands. And remember that those little bodies are very sensitive to pesticides, so either make your own or buy organic.

2. Strawberries: The single most heavily contaminated fruit or vegetable sold in the U.S., and virtually impossible to adequately wash. **Raspberries** fit here as well!

3. Rice: Herbicides and insecticides have consistently contaminated ground-water near rice fields in California's Sacramento River Valley.

4. Oats and Other Grains: With 6 to 11 recommended daily servings, you can't afford to ingest the excessive pesticides commonly used on grains. Read the labels! Buy organic, if not for yourself, for the sake of your children's health.

5. Milk and Dairy Products: To stimulate greater milk production, many conventional dairy companies routinely use the growth hormone rBGH, followed up with antibiotics to prevent infections often caused by the hormone. Known as BGH, rBGH, BST, and rBST, this genetically engineered hormone is banned in Canada and Europe.

6. Corn: 50% of all pesticides applied annually in the U.S. find their home in corn. And most of our corn is genetically modified to begin with! And remember that corn syrup comes from corn, so choose organic when buying it, or products containing it.

7. Bananas: The pesticides used during banana production include benomyl (linked to birth defects) and chlorpyrifos (a neurotoxin). And thiabendazole, which damages the brain and nervous system, is used to preserve the bananas on route to the Americas!

8. Green Beans: Mexican green beans are the worst offenders—9.4% of the crop is contaminated with illegal pesticides. Some of the pesticide line-up includes acephate, benomyl, chlorothalonil, and methamidophos. All of these damage the brain and nervous system, and cause birth defects.

9. Peaches: The FDA in the US cited above-average rates of illegal pesticide violations on conventionally grown peaches, on a consistent basis. **Nectarines** fit here as well!

10. Apples: Domestic apples have been found to be nearly as contaminated as strawberries.

According to the Environmental Working Group, other foods that may have dangerous levels of pesticides include spinach, pears, imported grapes, cherries, bell peppers and celery. Some of the foods they have listed as having the lowest levels of detectable pesticides include avocados, broccoli, cabbage, onions, asparagus, mangos, papaya, pineapples, kiwi and sweet peas.

Why Buy Organic?

Now, if what you have read above has not inspired you to buy organic, following are 10 major reasons to consider organic as the only option!! This wonderful document was a handout available at the Mrs. Gooch's Stores in Los Angeles. It seems to best sum up the variety of legitimate reasons for using organic foods regularly.

10 Reasons to Buy Organic

1. **Protect Future Generations:** "We have not inherited the earth from our fathers, we are borrowing it from our children." — Les Brown. The average child receives 4 times more exposure than an adult to at least 8 widely used cancer-causing pesticides in food. The food choices you make will impact your child's health in the future.

2. **Prevent Soil Erosion:** The Soil Conservation Service estimates that more than 3 billion tons of topsoil are eroded from the United States' croplands each year. That means soil is eroding 7 times faster than it is being built up naturally. Soil is the foundation of the food chain in organic farming. But in conventional farming the soil is used more as a medium for holding plants in a vertical position so they can be chemically fertilized. As a result, American farms are suffering from the worst soil erosion in history.

3. **Protect Water Quality:** Water makes up 2/3's of our body mass and covers 3/4's of the planet. Despite its importance, the Environmental Protection Agency (EPA) estimates pesticides (some cancer causing) contaminate the ground-water in 38 states, polluting the primary source of drinking water for more than ½ of the country's population.

4. **Save Energy:** American farms have changed drastically in the last 3 generations, from family-based small business dependent on human energy, to large-scale factory farms highly dependent on fossil fuels. Modern farming uses more petroleum than any other single industry,

consuming 12% of the country's total energy supply. More energy is now used to produce synthetic fertilizers than to till, cultivate and harvest all of the crops in the U.S. Organic farming is still mainly based on labor-intensive practices such as weeding by hand and using green manures and crop covers, rather than synthetic fertilizers, to build up the soil. Organic produce also tends to travel fewer miles from field to table.

5. **Keep Chemicals off Your Table:** Many pesticides approved for use by the EPA were registered long before extensive research linking these chemicals to cancer and other diseases had been established. Now the EPA considers that 60% of all herbicides, 90% of all fungicides and 30% of all insecticides are carcinogenic. A 1987 National Academy of Sciences report estimated that pesticides might cause an extra 1.4 million cancer cases among Americans over their lifetimes. The bottom line is that pesticides are poisons designed to kill living organisms, and can also be harmful to humans. In addition to cancer, pesticides are implicated in birth defects, nerve damage and genetic mutation.

6. **Protect Farm Worker Health:** A National Cancer Institute study found that farmers exposed to herbicides had 6 times greater risk than non-farmers of contracting cancer. In California, reported pesticide poisonings among farm workers have risen an average of 14% a year since 1973, and doubled between 1975 and 1985. Field workers suffer the highest rates of occupational illness in the state. Farm worker health also is a serious problem in developing nations, where pesticide use can be poorly regulated. An estimated one million people are poisoned annually by pesticides.

7. **Help Small Farmers:** Although more and more large-scale farms are making the conversion to organic practices, most organic farms are small independently owned and operated family farms of less than 100 acres. It is estimated that the U.S. has lost more than 650,000 family farms in the past decade. And with the U.S. Department of Agriculture predicting that ½ of this country's farm production will come from 1% of farms by the year 2000, organic farming could be one of the few survival tactics left for family farms.

8. **Support a True Economy:** Although organic foods might seem more expensive than conventional foods, conventional food prices do not reflect hidden costs borne by taxpayers, including nearly $74 billion

in federal subsidies in 1988. Other hidden costs include pesticide regulation and testing, hazardous waste disposal and clean-up, and environmental damage. Author, Gary Null says, "If . . . . you add in the real environmental and social costs of irrigation to a head of lettuce, its price can range between 2 and 3 dollars."

9. **Promote Biodiversity:** Mono-cropping is the practice of planting large plots of land with the same crop year after year. While this approach tripled farm production between 1950 and 1970, the lack of natural diversity of plant life has left the soil lacking in natural minerals and nutrients. To replace the nutrients, chemical fertilizers are used, often in increasing amounts. Single crops are also much more susceptible to pests, making farmers more reliant on pesticides. Despite a 10-fold increase in the use of pesticides between 1947 and 1974, crop losses due to insects have doubled — partly because some insects have become genetically resistant to certain pesticides.

10. **Taste Better Flavor:** There's a good reason why many chefs use organic foods in their recipes — they taste better! Organic farming starts with the nourishment of the soil, which eventually leads to the nourishment of the plant and, ultimately, our own palates and our bodies.

Where on Earth Can I Find Organic Foods & Products?

The question I am sure many of you are asking is how and where do you buy organic foods and products consistently? Here are some simple steps and tips that I have shared over the years with my clients and patients.

1. Look for stores, markets, farmers' markets, and *produce stands in your area,* that specialize in, and advertise, organic products. Some of these markets include: Whole Foods, Henry's, Wild Oats, Trader Joe's, as well as many independent health food stores. *And support your local farm stands, buying their fresh, in-season, organic produce.*

2. Check out CSA (Community Supported Agriculture) programs in your own community, and *organic food co-op's.* Some direct mail suppliers online include: DiamondOrganics.Com, KidsOrganics. Com, and Charansprings.com.

3. If you have no such stores or markets in your area, then go to your local store and ask the produce manager what they have that is

organic. A tip from *The Great Boycott*, an organization dedicated to putting a stop to this rampant use of pesticides, is to fill your cart with everything else you plan to buy (preferably earth-friendly products), *and then* to approach the manager with this request.

4. Express gratitude for the availability of these foods and products in the store, assuring that you will continue to shop there as long as they carry these products.

5. When inquiring at outdoor and indoor markets, especially farmers' markets, about whether foods are organic or not, *be discreet*. Get to know the farmers or managers first. Be friendly and enthusiastically chat about life. Then, the more politely you inquire about the foods and products they sell, the more likely you are to get an honest answer. Simply ask how they grow their produce, what kinds of chemicals they use, what proportions and how the soil is cared for.

6. *Spread the word:* about the best places to shop for these healthy products, to everyone you know who is concerned about their health. More consumers buying the products, keeps the products coming into the store.

7. Write and/or call the mega-companies and food giants and ask them to use more organically grown raw materials in their products. One voice may not make a difference. But thousands of small voices add up over time. Look at all of the more wholesome food stores popping up all over the country these days!!

For more information, an excellent resource is: www.foodnews.org/index. php. It provides a guide that lists 43 commonly eaten fruits and vegetables, and the various numbers of pesticides found in each. For the tremendously informative National Green Pages, go to www.coopamerica.org. Here you can find out about almost anything regarding organics, fair trade purchasing, investing in a sustainable environment, as well as how to build your own healthy home and community from the foundation to completion. And since it is my mission to educate and inspire people to become optimally healthy, and maintain the highest level of vitality and zest for life, please do drop by www.marilynjoyce.com, and subscribe to our *Special Report.*

What we have covered here is only the very tip of a huge iceberg! You owe it to yourself and your family to become fully informed as quickly as possible. For further information, go to the *Organic Resources* chapter.

A Final Note:
Who's Producing & Using Those Darn Pesticides Anyway?

Okay, so who are the culprits who place financial greed ahead of the world population's health? And what are some of their products to avoid at any cost if we want to recreate a healthy planet?!! Are you ready for this?

The Top AgroChemical (Pesticide) Companies in 2006

The following companies are profiled:

– Arysta Life Sciences
– BASF
– Bayer
– Cheminova
– Crompton (now Chemtura)
– Dow AgroSciences
– DuPont
– FMC
– Hokko Chemical Industry Co Ltd
– Ishihara Sangyo Kaisha (ISK)
– Kumiai Chemical
– Makhteshim-Agan Industries (MAI)
– Monsanto
– Nihon Nohyaku
– Nippon Soda
– Nissan Chemical
– Nufarm
– Sipcam-Oxon
– Sumitomo Chemical
– Syngenta

Since when did pharmaceutical companies become the pros on agricultural matters? Am I missing something here? Drugs? Food? It seems to me that this is a strange combination . . .

All of these companies are behind the speedy implementation of genetically engineered food crops. Why create such foods? Well it sure isn't for our health! These crops are being developed in order to withstand tremendous levels of sprayed toxic herbicides. If you have read what I have included above you will understand the seriousness of this situation. *In the name of profit for the few, the majority of us may die due to the toxic poisoning of our air, water and soil—our entire environment!! This is not a joke!!*

If you are interested in stopping the destruction of our environment and creating a healthier future for our children, one of the best steps to take is to find out more about the products produced by these companies, so that you can avoid purchasing them. For more information regarding this subject visit:

> ➤ The Institute for Responsible Technology at: www.seedsofdeception.com
> ➤ The Alliance for Bio-Integrity at: www.biointegrity.org
> ➤ The Pesticide Action Network North America at: www.panna.org.

And to learn which foods are genetically modified and how to protect yourself visit:

> ➤ www.GeneticRoulette.com (part of The Seeds of Deception website)
> ➤ The Organic Consumers Association at: www.organicconsumers.org.
> ➤ The Center for Food Safety at: www.centerforfoodsafety.org

I realize there are many other organizations that you can check out in your quest for the truth. These are simply a starting point to jump start your own research in your journey towards better health for you, your family and the environment.

So, again, *why choose organic foods*? Well, simply, it's alive, vibrant—not dying! When you bite into a live, organic food, your body immediately responds energetically. It is as if your mouth and body were shouting "Hurray! This is what we have been looking for!" So, go ahead. Take the challenge. Try it yourself. Bite into a commercially grown apple. Then bite into an organically grown apple. Which one tastes deliciously alive and vibrant?

Be healthy. Stay healthy. Eat organic . . .

SO WHAT'S ON A LABEL?

The fact is that if you are eating in the fashion outlined in the section entitled "Rules for the Road," you will not need to be so attentive to labels on packages. **Fresh vegetables are fresh vegetables no matter how you slice or dice them!** Except to seek out those which are certified organic, as well as truly *fresh*, there is little else to look for.

The same is true of fresh fruits!

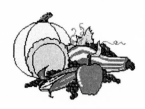

And, except for the wide array of available packaged breads, which may or may not be wholegrain, **a raw, unprocessed, whole grain is exactly that:** *a raw, unprocessed, whole grain*. Just be sure it is *fresh*, and packaged in an *airtight container*. The germ in the whole grain contains oil, which becomes rancid quickly if exposed to oxygen in the air, or if the grain is sitting too long on the shelf. A good rule of thumb is to *buy only amounts that you will use within one to two months*, and *keep them refrigerated* if possible. Definitely keep them in tinted airtight containers away from direct light or sunlight.

Inevitably, if you follow and utilize the **INSTANT *E.N.E.R.G.Y.*™** shopping list, you will be buying some packaged and canned products. However, even those items, included in the list, have been carefully examined and selected, with the objective of providing speed and convenience without sacrificing optimum nutrition and health. And *as long as about 80% of the foods you eat are not from packages and cans*, and those foods which are from packages and cans are from the shopping list, not only will your total fat intake be low, *it will reflect a very low intake of saturated and hydrogenated fats, as well as cholesterol*, all of which appear to be primary suspects in relationship to raised blood cholesterol levels, heart disease, stroke, cancer, obesity, osteoporosis and arthritis.

Note: See "Read Your Labels" in the chapter *Let's Wake up To the Health of Our Children,* for my top 12 worst ingredients in packaged and processed foods.

Much of the information included on the new food labels, on canned and packaged products, relates to what percentage of the RDI (Reference Daily Intake) you will be getting when you eat a specific amount of that particular item. The RDI's are based on minimum daily requirements for known vitamins and minerals, and maximum recommended allowances for fats

(30% of total daily calories), cholesterol (300 mg) and sodium (3300 mg), for **most** normal, healthy people to maintain their health.

But, remember I said earlier in this book, that *when our focus is on eating whole foods in their natural state, we do not need to be counting a lot of numbers and making a lot of calculations.*

And since we are aiming for optimal health, *we are **not** focusing on minimum requirements to maintain health.* Especially if we are not healthy to begin with, and must first build up our health to a level which then readies us for a maintenance program.

Furthermore, I'm suggesting, also, that you strive to keep your *total fat intake* **below** *20% of your total daily calories* (that's about 40 to 50 grams), and your *total sodium intake* **below** *2000 mg per day.* This is easy to do, without any calculations, following the **INSTANT *E.N.E.R.G.Y.*™** plan!

However, there are a few things that are important to be aware of when reading labels. These items are written below as a checklist to assist you at the point of shopping. Good luck!

☑ **Check the serving size!** If you eat twice as much as the amount listed as a serving size, then you have to realize that you are also getting two times the amount of fat listed, as well as the salt, sugar, and cholesterol.

☑ **Check the total calories.** A calorie is a unit of energy that measures how much energy a food provides to the body. And the number of calories listed on a food label indicates the number of calories found in one serving.

☑ **Look at the calories from fat and the total fat grams!** A basic rule of thumb is to avoid any foods with more than 3 grams of fat per serving. At 9 calories per gram of fat, this would account for 27 of the total number of calories in a serving. If you have equivalent to 2 servings of an item with 3 grams of fat per serving, then you will get 54 calories from fat.

Now take this a step further! If an item has 500 calories per serving, and lists the calories from fat at 330 calories per serving, you can find the percentage of fat in the product by dividing the 330 calories from fat by the total number of calories in the serving which is 500, and then multiply by 100 to arrive at the percentage of calories from fat in one serving. So, in this case the result is 66%. If we are recommending an upper limit of 20% of our food intake as fat, this food item is way out of line!

The equation for calculation of % fat in an item is:

Total calories of fat X 100 = % Calories from Fat
Total calories

☑ **When a label boasts that a product is, for example, 90% Fat Free, 10% Fat, this refers to percent fat by weight, not percent fat by calories.** If we have 50 grams of sliced luncheon meat at 90% Fat Free, 5 of those grams are from fat. That's the 10% fat! However, at 9 calories per gram of fat, we have 9 calories X 5 grams, which is 45 calories. If this product has 100 calories, and 45 of them are from fat, we see that 45% of the calories come from fat. So it is obvious that the percent by weight (10% in this example) can be very different from the percent by calories (45%).

☑ **Understand Food Label Claims About Fat. Reduced fat** means that the product has 25% less fat than the same regular brand. **Light** means that the product has 50% less fat than the same regular brand. **Low fat** means the products has less than 3 grams of fat per serving.

☑ **If a food is listed as fat free, sugar or sodium free, or free of calories,** this indicates that only negligible amounts, or absolutely none, of that particular element listed as **"free"** is available in the food.

☑ **Be wary of terms such as "light", "lite" and "low".** These descriptions are somewhat elusive, carrying more than one meaning. It is always best to check the total number of grams or milligrams, in the product, of the specific nutrient in question, e.g., fat, sugar, sodium or cholesterol.

☑ **Be aware, when buying wholegrain bread,** that unless it says specifically "whole wheat," "100% wholegrain," "100% whole wheat," or "Stoneground wholegrain," it is not what you are looking for! *Wheat flour is white flour.* If the bread is brown in color, it is likely molasses or brown sugar that has been added for that purpose. READ THE LABEL!

☑ **Let's examine what the term Total Carbohydrate means.** Listed in grams, this number combines several types of carbohydrates (sometimes called carbs) including dietary fibers, sugars, and other carbohydrates. Healthy carbohydrates are most abundant in whole grains and whole grain products, fruits, vegetables and legumes. Unhealthy carbohydrates are found in snack foods, candy, sodas, white flour based pastas, breads and baked goods. These are often referred to as "empty calories" because they have next to no nutritional value. Each gram of carbohydrate has 4 calories.

☑ **The "sugars" number is not necessarily accurate!** Although naturally occurring sugars, e.g. fruit sugars and milk sugars are included, the longer-chain sugars, which can account for up to 2/3's of some corn syrups, are omitted.

☑ **Furthermore, there are many names for sugar, besides the word "sugar"!** Basically whenever you see a word on the label which ends with "ose", you can be fairly certain that it is a sugar! To assist you in deciphering sugars in products, I am including a list of terms you may see on a label:

Brown Sugar	Invert Sugar
Corn Syrup	Mannitol
Corn Syrup Solids	Molasses
Dextrose (simple sugar)	Natural Sweeteners
Fructose (fruit sugar)	Raw Sugar
Glucose	Sorbitol
High-Fructose Corn Syrup	Sucrose (cane sugar) or Sugar
Honey	

☑ **And let's go a step further and list the artificial sweeteners, which are to be avoided!** Remember, only the most natural foods in their most natural states are to be consumed. And artificial sweeteners are anything but natural! So AVOID them.

aspartame includes NutraSweet & Equal
saccharin includes Sweet' n Low
acesulfame K includes Sweet One & Sunette
sucralose is "Splenda"

☑ **Now, a word about protein.** The label lists the amount of protein in a single serving and is measured in grams. The general rule is a daily intake of 10 to 20% of our calories from protein. Our skin, muscles and immune system are predominately made up of protein. Foods high in protein include legumes, nuts and seeds, soy products, fish, eggs, dairy products, poultry, and animal meats.

☑ **Choose monounsaturated fats and polyunsaturated fats over saturated fats.** And select the least processed, cold-pressed (especially avoid heat processed) varieties, as much as possible.

☑ **Avoid anything listed as** *"hydrogenated, partially hydrogenated or trans,* fats or products using *vegetable oils which are saturated fats* such as coconut oil or palm oil, palm kernel oil, or cocoa butter.

☑ **Avoid hard fats such as lard, margarine, and butter.** Select butter sprinkles instead! Or try the all natural flavor sprays! See *Get the Skinny on Fats* chapter.

NOTE: As you incorporate more wholesome wholegrain products and fresh organic produce into your diet, you will begin to more fully appreciate their wide variety of unique natural flavors. And, in turn, your need for flavor enhancers e.g. butter and fatty spreads will diminish. **We only require flavor enhancers to make up for the lack of the original flavor remaining in depleted, over-processed, fabricated foods!**

☑ **For the % Daily Value (DV) listed on the food label,** you are being told how much of (in other words, what percentage of) the recommended daily total you will be consuming just from that one food. The basic rule of thumb is: *"If a food has 20% or more of the DV for a particular nutrient, e.g. sodium, it is high in that nutrient. If it has 5% or less of a particular nutrient, it is low."* So to *insure a healthy diet; look for foods with a DV of 5 or less for fat, saturated fat, cholesterol and sodium.*

☑ **All ingredients on the label are listed in descending order according to weight.** So, if sugar is the first ingredient in the list, you can bet it makes up the bulk of the product. Therefore, the last item listed makes up the smallest amount of the product by weight.

☑ **As a general guideline for some key dietary components,** below you will find listed approximate daily recommended quantities, as based on the USDA Food Guide and the DASH Eating Plan for a 2000 calorie diet:

Protein	91-108 grams
Carbohydrates	271-288 grams
Total Fat	48-65 grams (I recommend a lower fat intake.)
Saturated Fat	10-17 grams (Again, I recommend less fat.)
Monounsaturated	Fat 21-24 grams
Trans Fats	0 grams (Notice it is zero!)
Cholesterol	136-230 milligrams
Sodium	1500-1779 milligrams
Fiber	30 grams

This checklist addresses some of the important points to consider for anyone who is very serious about taking charge of his or her own health. *Awareness is the first step* towards making healthy choices. However, **"Awareness without Action" is nothing!** So let's get **active! Read the labels!**

The next step, however, is to go through your cupboards and toss out anything not included in the **Pyramid of E.N.E.R.G.Y.™ Shopping List**. Then stock your shelves and refrigerator with only those foods listed, varying the produce and fish choices each shopping day, and according to season. **Armed with the label information outlined here,** you are now prepared to analyze the items on the shopping list which are packaged or canned.

This may represent a big change in eating habits and lifestyles for many of you. Like any new practice, career, relationship or project, it takes a little getting used to. You may stumble along the way, even fall completely off the wagon. **Whatever you do though, don't beat yourself up!** Remember, you're like a baby learning to walk. It takes time, and a lot of uncertain and unsteady steps, to get it right!

I know, because I've been there and I've done that!! And occasionally, now and then, I give myself permission to eat something higher in fat than I would normally consume. It does the soul and the psyche good to break the pattern a bit. However, I am also reminded at those times, of how much better I feel when my diet is wholesome and natural! Believe me, as time passes, so do the temptations and unhealthy desires. You never want to give up that healthy, alive feeling! Even for a second!

SO WHAT'S IN A SERVING?

According to the USDA, one serving looks like this:

Fats, Oils and Sweets:

Limit calories from these, especially if you are trying to lose weight, or balance your blood glucose levels.

Fruits:

♦   1 piece of fruit
♦   1 wedge (½ cup) of melon
♦   ¼ cup of dried fruit
♦   2/3 cup of fruit nectar
♦   ¾ cup fresh-squeezed juice (use rarely)

Milk, Yogurt and Cheese:

♦   1 cup of plain low fat yogurt
♦   1 cup of acidophilus milk
♦   1 cup of low fat milk
♦   1 cup of soy, almond, or rice milk
♦   1 ½ to 2 ounces nonfat cheese
♦   1 ½ to 2 ounces almond, tofu or soy cheese

Protein: Poultry, Fish, Meat, Eggs, Dried Beans and Nuts

♦   2 ½ to 3 ounces of cooked, skinless turkey or chicken, esp. breast
♦   2 ½ to 3 ounces of cooked lean game meat
♦   3 ounces of cooked lean fish
♦   ½ cup of cooked beans
♦   2 tablespoons of almond butter (equal to ⅓ serving of meat)
♦   1 large egg (equal to ½ serving of meat)
♦   ½ cup of low or non fat cottage cheese

Vegetables:

♦   ½ cup of raw, chopped vegetables
♦   ½ cup of cooked vegetables
♦   1 cup of leafy raw vegetables

www.marilynjoyce.com

Note: Eat the maximum number of vegetable servings recommended on the Pyramid of *E.N.E.R.G.Y.* ™ every day!

Whole Grains: Bread, Cereal, Rice and Pasta

- 1 slice wholegrain bread
- ½ cup cooked rice or pasta
- ½ cup cooked cereal
- 1 ounce of ready-to-eat cereal
- 1 sprouted corn or wheat tortilla

Recommendations:

- 1 to 2 tbsp total, daily, used in cooking or as part of a salad dressing
  (You will get the most value using oil in an uncooked form!)
  See the chapter, ***Get the Skinny On Fats*** for the safest cooking oils.
- 1 to 2 tbsp of sweeteners and fruit preserves, total, daily
- 1 tbsp of Parmesan or Romano, total, daily
- ¼ of an avocado 2 or 3 times per week
- 1 cup of organic coffee, maximum per day

A WELL-EQUIPPED KITCHEN IS
AN EFFICIENT KITCHEN

Most of us, in an effort to simplify our lives, have kitchens full of equipment and appliances we never use. On one hand, we are very blessed to have so many options available to us. On the other hand, we are cursed! Much of the equipment which was created with the ease of preparation of food in mind, has the added, less attractive feature, of much more work to cleanup after use. So the equipment sits on our shelves, or in our cupboards, until we finally give it away or throw it out!

Taking this into account, the list of items suggested for inclusion in your kitchen, are generally the most user-friendly pieces of equipment and appliances I have been able to assemble over the years. On my own journey to efficiency I've made many mistakes and accumulated many useless pieces of equipment that rarely, if ever, got used.

Therefore, the versatility, as well as ease of cleanup, became important factors in the decision to buy, or not to buy, a particular appliance or piece of equipment.

The following is a basic, but comprehensive, list of those items which have proven, over time, to be the most useful and most versatile items available. When you simplify your food intake, it leads to a simplification of everything else you do in the kitchen as well.

The description of a particular piece of equipment was included only where it was thought to be necessary.

Non-Electrical Equipment

- 1 set of good quality sharp knives, including utility, paring, slicing and chef's knives
- 2 collapsible steaming baskets, stainless steel
- 2 or 3 cutting boards, preferably dishwasher-safe, plastic, marble, non-porous surface
- 2 sets of measuring spoons
- 2 sets of dry and liquid measuring cups
- 3 to 4 ice-cube trays for freezing pureed fruit, nectars, stocks, water
- Apple wedger
- Baking pans, cookie sheets**
- Baster

- Broiler pan and broiler pan rack
- Can opener, heavy duty non-electric for easy cleaning after each use
- Canisters, airtight, for grains, pastas, legumes, flour, teabags and loose tea, etc.
- Citrus reamer for juicing
- Colander
- Dish Drainer
- Egg-separator, to separate whites from yolks
- Fat separator
- Food scale for weighing foods, e.g. fish, poultry and meats
- Food thermometer
- Garlic press
- Gold Coffee filter
- Jar Opener
- Hand grater
- Kitchen scissors
- Kitchen timer
- Melon baller
- Spatulas, spoonulas and scrapers, regular and slotted
- Oven Thermometer
- Paper towels on mounted holder
- Pastry brush
- Plastic wrap and food storage bags
- Popsicle forms for fruit nectar, or pureed fruit, pops
- Pot holders, close to stove, oven, toaster-oven
- Pots and Pans: 8" & 12" skillet, 1Qt & 2Qt saucepans, large Dutch oven pot, oven-safe skillet**
- Pressure cooker, for long cooking foods, follow manufacturer's directions
- Pyrex oven casserole dishes with lids
- Salad spinner
- Scoops for frozen yogurt, vegetables, coleslaw, etc.
- Sherbet glasses for serving yogurt desserts or fruit salad desserts
- Soup ladle
- Stock/Soup Pot
- Spaghetti lifter
- Tea strainers for loose tea leaves and herbs
- Tongs
- Vegetable brushes for scrubbing vegetables
- Vegetable masher
- Vegetable peeler
- Wire mesh sieve or strainer

- ◆ Wire whisks for blending sauces and dips
- ◆ Wok, nonstick or stainless steel
- ◆ Wooden spoons

** Choose cast iron, stainless steel, enameled iron or glass. Avoid all non stick pans

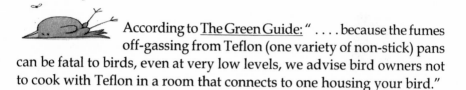

According to The Green Guide: " . . . . because the fumes off-gassing from Teflon (one variety of non-stick) pans can be fatal to birds, even at very low levels, we advise bird owners not to cook with Teflon in a room that connects to one housing your bird."

Electrical Appliances:

- ◆ Blender — a more powerful motor is more versatile.
- ◆ Blender, handheld — especially useful when traveling.
- ◆ Citrus juicer — a quick and easy way to juice a lemon or a lime for various uses. A good idea is to use some of the pulp as well, for fiber and bioflavinoids.
- ◆ Coffee-maker — If you drink coffee, grind *organic* coffee beans and prepare the coffee with a good machine to prevent over-cooking it. A coffee-maker can also be used to make herbal teas and keep them hot.
- ◆ Coffee mill — for grinding grains, almonds, organic coffee beans, flaxseeds and whole spices.
- ◆ Crockpot or other slow cooker — takes 3-½ to 4-½ hours on high setting, and 6 to 9 hours on low setting. Meal can be cooking while you're at work. The taste of some herbs and spices changes in slow cooking, so you may need to adjust types and amounts. Cut vegetables into small, uniform pieces and layer them at bottom of the pot with rest of ingredients on top. It is almost impossible to overcook in a crockpot. Do not remove the lid during cooking!
- ◆ Food Dehydrator — an easy way to dry foods at home, naturally without preservatives.
- ◆ Hot-air popcorn popper — fast and easy fluffy, popcorn in minutes. Shake hot popcorn and seasonings together in a brown paper bag or spray the popcorn with all natural flavor sprays.
- ◆ Microwave oven — optional. An efficient way to reheat foods, but rarely produces a good quality food when used for cooking. If you get one, look for a microwave with a 650 — to 700-watt output. To learn the pro's and con's of microwave food preparation, subscribe to our **INSTANT *E.N.E.R.G.Y.*™ *site*** at www.marilynjoyce.com

- Mini-chopper / Mini-food processor.
- Rice cooker / Vegetable steamer — simplifies the cooking of rice, grains and vegetables. Easy to use and easy to clean. Follow the directions that come with it!
- Toaster oven — great for open-faced grilled low fat cheese sandwiches, heating leftovers, toasting large slices of bread, bagels, and rolls, heating tortillas and pita breads, making mini-pizzas, baking potatoes, cooking casseroles, making low fat nacho plates, etc. Saves on energy bills!
- Vita-Mix machine, "the lawnmower for food." It mixes, blends, chops, grinds, grates, crushes, purees, liquefies, freezes and cooks food in seconds. In juicing, nothing is thrown away. Cleanup is a snap! The fastest, easiest, and most versatile machine to use, it insures the maintenance of an optimum level of the nutrients originally available in the food. It has almost replaced my blender, coffee grinder, hot plates, chopper and crockpot. For more information on the Vita Mix machine, go to www.marilynjoyce.com, and see the *Equipment* Chapter.
- Yogurt maker — best way to get high quality yogurt at a good price. Use certified raw milk or soymilk, and high grade live cultures.

As you can see, **I have not included in my list, a food processor or a juicer, other than the citrus juicer.** For me, the Vita Mix machine efficiently takes the place of both of these appliances, as well as several others on the list. If you don't have a Vita-Mix machine, but you do have a food processor, by all means use it. The work involved in the cleanup resulted in my own food processor being sold at a yard sale. Also the finished food product just didn't compare with that of the Vita-Mix machine.

As far as a juicer is concerned, it is an expensive way to throw away all, or most, of the fiber present in our foods, and the nutrients clinging to that fiber! During my own illness, it was not until I began to drink whole food juices, made in the Vita-Mix machine, with nothing thrown out, that my health began to improve dramatically. Obviously there was something in the part of the food I was throwing away, when I used the juicer to make juice that my body required to get well.

The juices, made in the Vita-Mix machine, are finer in texture and more emulsified, but of course thicker, since every part of the food is included. Simply add more liquid (e.g. water, fruit nectar, vegetable broth, low sodium vegetable or tomato juice, etc.) to thin it down to the consistency you prefer. **Once you get used to the taste and consistency of juices made from whole foods, you will never desire the alternatives again!**

Finally, in order to have the most efficient kitchen, it is important to have everything you use within easy reach. **Equipment stored in the cupboard rarely sees the light of day!** So have your equipment and utensils where you can see them and get to them quickly and easily. Keep frequently used utensils in a decorative jar close to the stove and work center of your kitchen. Mount small appliances to the wall or under the cupboards.

Until one is committed there is hesitancy, the chance to draw back, always ineffectiveness. Concerning all acts of initiative (and Creation), there is one elementary truth, the ignorance of which kills countless ideas and splendid plans: that the moment one definitely commits oneself, then providence moves too. All sorts of things occur to help one that would otherwise never have occurred. A whole stream of events issues from the decision, raising in one's favor all manner of unforeseen incidents and meetings and material assistance, which no man could have dreamt would have come his way. I have learned a deep respect for one of Goethe's couplets:

> *Whatever you can do, or dream you can, begin it.*
> *Boldness has genius, power and magic in it.*
>
> — *Goethe*

W.N. Murray
from The Scottish Himalayan Expedition

3. EPICUREAN DELIGHTS

30 MENUS FOR BREAKFAST

MENU 1 ♦ Vibrant Fruit Salad ♦ Plain Low Fat Yogurt ♦ Lemon Zinger Herbal Tea	MENU 11 ♦ High Protein Breakfast Shake	MENU 21 ♦ Berrie Good Kasha ♦ Plain Low Fat Yogurt
MENU 2 ♦ Raspberry Delight (meal in a glass)	MENU 12 ♦ Fresh Peaches, Sliced ♦ Nonfat Cottage Cheese ♦ Fat-free Wholegrain Crackers	MENU 22 ♦ Poached Egg/Salsa ♦ Nonfat Refried Beans/ Grated Low Fat Cheese ♦ Corn Tortillas
MENU 3 ♦ Low Fat Granola ♦ Vanilla Soymilk ♦ Fresh Fruit in Season	MENU 13 ♦ Hot 10-Grain Cereal ♦ Low Fat Plain Yogurt ♦ Ripe Banana/Raisins	MENU 23 ♦ Low Fat Banana Apricot Loaf ♦ Low Fat Cottage Cheese and Applesauce Spread
MENU 4 ♦ Honeydew Melon ♦ Wholegrain Toast ♦ Almond Butter	MENU 14 ♦ French Toast ♦ Pure Maple Syrup ♦ Bananas and Strawberries	MENU 24 ♦ Toasted Tempeh and Alfalfa Sprout Sandwich ♦ Nayonaise/sliced Tomato
MENU 5 ♦ Brown Rice Pudding ♦ Ripe Banana	MENU 15 ♦ Wholegrain Bagel, Toasted ♦ Reduced Fat Cream Cheese ♦ Fresh Lox ♦ Tropical Fruit Salad	MENU 25 ♦ Breakfast Bulgur
MENU 6 ♦ Spoon-sized Shredded Wheat ♦ Vanilla Soymilk ♦ Prunes and Apricots, Soaked	MENU 16 ♦ Authentic Muesli ♦ Plain Low Fat Yogurt	MENU 26 ♦ Scrambled Tofu and Tomatoes ♦ Wholegrain Bagel ♦ Butter and Garlic Flavor Spray
MENU 7 ♦ Fresh Orange ♦ Poached Free-Range Egg ♦ Sprouted Wholegrain Toast ♦ Fruit Preserve	MENU 17 ♦ Weetabix ♦ Berries and Bananas	MENU 27 ♦ Brown Rice Delight ♦ Plain Low Fat Yogurt

MENU 8	MENU 18	MENU 28
♦ Millet Fantasy ♦ Plain Low Fat Yogurt	♦ Oatmeal Pancakes ♦ Applesauce ♦ Pure Maple Syrup (optional)	♦ The Green Machine Shake
MENU 9	MENU 19	MENU 29
♦ Hot Oatmeal, Soaked ♦ Soymilk or Low Fat Yogurt ♦ Fresh Applesauce	♦ Fruit Smoothie ♦ Potato and Egg Scramble ♦ Dark Pumpernickel Bread ♦ Fruit Preserves	♦ Fruity Yogurt ♦ Low Fat Wholegrain Muffin
MENU 10	MENU 20	MENU 30
♦ Fresh Fruit Salad ♦ Scrambled Egg and Tofu ♦ Rye Toast and Fruit Preserves	♦ Wholegrain English Muffin ♦ Ricotta Cheese and Fruit Spread ♦ Ginger Tea	♦ Crazy Mixed-Up Grains ♦ Apple and Strawberry Sauce

Noteworthy Facts

Do not skip Breakfast! It is the meal that breaks the fast and raises and maintains your blood sugar level throughout the morning. You need protein, carbohydrates and fats! Fruit, or coffee, alone, won't do it!

1. Eat only breads listed as *100% Whole Wheat, or 100% Wholegrain, or Stone-ground.* **Read the Label!** The first ingredient should <u>always</u> be *whole wheat flour,* or another whole grain flour, not just *wheat flour,* which is simply white, over-processed, flour. Better still, buy sprouted whole grain breads. They are much more nutrient dense than regular whole grain breads.

2. Leftover brown rice, wholegrain or vegetable pasta, or other grains, from the previous lunch or dinner, can be modified for breakfast.

3. Blended organic tofu is a good substitute for yogurt, and generally easier to digest than regular milk, especially for someone experiencing lactose intolerance.

4. One serving of cooked rice or grains, as listed in the breakfast menus on the previous page, is 1 cup, which relates to 2 servings in the *So What's In A Serving* chapter. You can increase or decrease portion size according to your needs.

5. Fresh fruit and plain, low fat yogurt combinations can be prepared the night before for a breakfast on-the-run, or for a brown bag breakfast or lunch. Carry nonfat granola toppings separately and sprinkle on top just prior to eating, to maintain crispy texture.

6. Muffins are great for a brown bag breakfast or lunch! But if you buy prepared or packaged muffins, choose those *with no more than 5 grams of fat* and a 100% wholegrain base. *Sugar should not be one of the primary ingredients!* (Refer to *So What's On A Label chapter*.) **Avoid** muffin mixes; they are generally higher in sugars and fats than a healthy diet warrants.

7. Use *All Natural Flavor Sprays*, or Butter Buds, on toast, or in egg dishes.

8. If you are truly on the run, have a flight to catch or have a long car drive ahead of you and can't stop to make breakfast, choose from the **Healthy Snack Bars** listed in the *Food Products* chapter.

30 MENUS FOR LUNCH

MENU 1 ♦ Split Pea Soup ♦ Fresh Organic Salad Mix ♦ Nonfat Dressing	**MENU 11** ♦ Lentil Vegetable Soup ♦ Rye Krisp Crackers ♦ Greens and Tomatoes with Dressing	**MENU 21** ♦ Fresh Fruit Platter ♦ Nonfat Cottage Cheese ♦ Nonfat Wholegrain Crackers
MENU 2 ♦ Chicken Pita Sandwich ♦ Plain Low fat Yogurt Smoothie	**MENU 12** ♦ Turkey Burger with Dijon Mustard ♦ Whole Wheat Burger Bun ♦ Tomato and Onion Slices	**MENU 22** ♦ Lively Chef's Salad ♦ High Omega-3 GLA Dressing ♦ Whole Wheat Garlic Toast
MENU 3 ♦ Tuna Salad Sandwich ♦ Fresh Orange	**MENU 13** ♦ Mediterranean Potato Salad ♦ Fresh Fruit Smoothie	**MENU 23** ♦ Vegetarian Chili ♦ Baked Tortilla Chips ♦ Carrots, Celery and Green Peppers
MENU 4 ♦ Baked Potato with Skin ♦ Vegetarian Refried Beans ♦ Yogurt and Salsa Topping	**MENU 14** ♦ Eggless Egg Salad Sandwich ♦ Spinach and Mushroom Salad ♦ Peach Nectar	**MENU 24** ♦ Bean Burritos with Diced Vegetables ♦ Mixed Greens and Cherry Tomatoes with Garlic Balsamic Dressing
MENU 5 ♦ Turkey Loaf on Whole Wheat Kaiser Roll ♦ Tomato and Red Onion Slices	**MENU 15** ♦ Low fat Cheese and Avocado Pita Pocket with Sprouts ♦ Fresh Low fat Banana Yogurt	**MENU 25** ♦ Chickpea Spread (Hummus) ♦ Sprouted Whole Wheat Pita ♦ Zucchini Salad with Spicy Dressing
MENU 6 ♦ Nonfat Cottage Cheese with Peach, Chopped ♦ Nonfat or Low fat Bran Muffin	**MENU 16** ♦ Turkey and Tomato on Rye ♦ Raw Vegetable Sticks with Yogurt and Salsa Dip	**MENU 26** ♦ Curried Lentil Soup ♦ Tempeh Sandwich on Sprouted Wholegrain Bread
MENU 7 ♦ Minestrone Soup	**MENU 17** ♦ Curried Brown Rice Salad	**MENU 27** ♦ Crabmeat Salad

◆ Garlic Pumpernickel Toast ◆ Fresh Pear	◆ Cucumber and Tomato Raita ◆ Iced Ginger Tea	◆ Baked Potato, Hot ◆ Steamed Broccoli and Cauliflower
MENU 8 ◆ Wholegrain English Muffin Pizzas ◆ Tossed Green Salad ◆ Nonfat Mustard Vinaigrette Dressing	**MENU 18** ◆ Wholegrain Pasta ◆ High Protein Marinara Sauce ◆ Mixed Green Salad with Dressing	**MENU 28** ◆ Citrus Rice and Bean Salad ◆ Low fat Creamy Cole Slaw
MENU 9 ◆ Pasta Salad ◆ Sprouted Wholegrain Bagel ◆ Green and Red Seedless Grapes	**MENU 19** ◆ Steamed Broccoli, Cauliflower and Carrots with Yogurt Dressing ◆ Whole Grain Roll w/Flavored Spray ◆ Pineapple and Mango Frappe	**MENU 29** ◆ Vegetable-Tofu Medley ◆ Brown Rice with Bragg Liquid Aminos ◆ Cucumber and Tomato Raita
MENU 10 ◆ Marinated Tofu and Sprout Sandwich ◆ Fresh Cantaloupe Half	**MENU 20** ◆ Almond Butter, Tomato and Sprouts on Sprouted Multi-Grain Bread ◆ Miso Soup with Tofu Cubes ◆ Home-Blended Low fat Vanilla Yogurt	**MENU 30** ◆ Salmon Dill Sandwich on Sprouted Wholegrain Bread ◆ Fresh Fruit Salad

Noteworthy Facts

Re-read the notes pertaining to the Breakfast menus!

1. Generally breads are listed in these menus as Wholegrain, versus a specific type, so that you have choice. **Try different varieties to find your own favorites.** As much as possible, **avoid white breads,** including sour dough. Look for breads which begin the listing of ingredients with 100% Wholegrain or Stoneground. Wheat flour is the same as white flour, so don't be fooled by terminology! Whenever possible, buy sprouted versions of all bread products.

2. Lunch is a great time to use up leftover grains, rice or whole grain pasta in transportable salads. Simply add:

   a. leftover or fresh steamed vegetables
   b. fresh raw vegetables
   c. leftover chicken or turkey breast

    d.   leftover fish or shellfish

    e.   nonfat or low fat seasoned dressing of choice. See **Dressings** chapter.

3.   To make garlic toast there are several possible ways, ranging from Lower fat to Low fat to No fat.

    a.   Combine ½ cup olive oil, ½ cup softened butter and 2 cloves of minced garlic (or to taste) and whip in blender. It keeps well in refrigerator for about 1 week. Spreads easily. Use sparingly!

    b.   Spray toasted bread, bagel, or English muffin with all natural oil spray and then spritz with Garlic juice, see *Food Products* chapter.

    c.   Shake butter sprinkles and garlic powder, onto hot toast. For an extra flavor boost, sprinkle grated low fat cheese onto the garlic toast and grill briefly under the broiler to melt the cheese.

4.   **Meat-based lunches are limited in the menus,** providing for an increased intake of high fiber forms of protein, such as the combination of grains and beans (legumes).

Remember: *the meat group includes not only beef, pork, lamb and game meats, but also chicken, turkey, and fish.* All of these are *flesh foods*, but game meats, fish, turkey and chicken are generally lower in fat especially if the skins are removed.

30 MENUS FOR DINNER

MENU 1
- Baked Chicken Breast
- Baked Potato w/Low Fat Yogurt Topping
- Steamed Broccoli with Butter Sprinkles
- Frozen Grapes

MENU 11
- Turkey Loaf w/Mustard Yogurt Dressing
- Steamed Broccoli with Lemon
- Garlic Whole Wheat Sourdough Bread
- Spiced Apple Cider

MENU 21
- Wholegrain Spaghetti
- Tofu-Mushroom Marinara Sauce
- Garlic Whole Wheat English Muffins
- Frozen Grapes and Banana Chunks

MENU 2
- Vegetable and Bean Chili
- Steamed Brown Rice
- Mixed Greens and Tomatoes with Buttermilk Dressing
- Frozen Banana and Date Delight

MENU 12
- Light Whole Wheat Macaroni & Cheese
- Red and Green Cabbage Slaw
- Pumpernickel Rolls
- Fresh Fruit Salad

MENU 22
- Baked Potatoes
- Tuna and Seasoned Yogurt
- Steamed Asparagus w/Butter Sprinkles
- Fresh Cantaloupe

MENU 3
- Fettuccine Alfredo for Health
- Caesar Salad with Nonfat Caesar Dressing
- Fresh Apple and Pear Slices

MENU 13
- Potato and Lentil Soup
- Romaine, Watercress and Tomato Salad with Dressing
- Nonfat Wholegrain Crackers
- Orange Sections

MENU 23
- Salmon Burger on Whole Wheat Kaiser Roll
- Three Bean Salad
- Apricot Dream

MENU 4
- Baked Potatoes
- Steamed Broccoli, Cauliflower and Carrots
- Seasoned Yogurt & Tofu Topping
- Peaches and Blueberries with Garnish of Nonfat Granola

MENU 14
- Turkey Burger on Wholegrain Roll
- Tomato and Onion Slices
- Sweet Potato and Raisin Yogurt Whip

MENU 24
Evening With Friends:
- Vegetable Platter
- Baked Tortilla Chips
- Variety of Dips
- Wine Spritzers/Fruit Spritzers

MENU 5
- Salad Bar Dinner
- Nonfat Dressings
- Heated Wholegrain Rolls with Flavor Spray

MENU 15
- Sweet Potato and Vegetable Casserole
- Spinach and Tomato Salad with Honey—Lemon Dressing
- Raspberry-Banana Frappe

MENU 25
- Tofu-Vegetable Frittata
- Creamy Cabbage Slaw
- Wholegrain Bagel w/Flavor Spray
- Pineapple-Almond Whip

MENU 6	MENU 16	MENU 26
◆ Steamed Bulgur w/Nonfat Yogurt ◆ Curried Vegetables and Imitation Crabmeat ◆ Cucumber and Tomato Raita ◆ Blended Frozen Bananas w/Raisins	◆ Pasta and Vegetable Medley ◆ Mixed Green and Red Lettuce with Balsamic Dressing ◆ Heated Low fat Oatmeal Muffin with Blended Fruit Topping	◆ Steamed Bulgur ◆ Curried Chickpeas and Onions ◆ Broccoli-Cauliflower Salad ◆ Berry-Ricotta Surprise
MENU 7	MENU 17	MENU 27
◆ Turkey Chili ◆ Steamed Brown Rice ◆ Spinach and Mushroom Salad with Vinaigrette Dressing ◆ Whipped Peaches and Almond Yogurt	◆ Kitchen Sink Salad with Salsa-Yogurt Dressing ◆ Whole Wheat Sourdough Bread ◆ Brown Rice Pudding with Peaches	◆ Wholegrain Pasta Primavera ◆ Mixed Green Salad w/Herb Dressing ◆ Whole Wheat Garlic Toast ◆ Fresh Fruit Salad w/Apricot Sauce
MENU 8	MENU 18	MENU 28
◆ Tri-Color Vegetable Pasta and Vegetable Salad (Hot) ◆ Tomato and Cucumber Slices with Nonfat Dressing ◆ Melon Wedge	◆ Baked Turkey Breasts ◆ Seasoned Baked Potato Wedges ◆ Nippy Dijon Coleslaw ◆ Whipped Vanilla & Strawberry Yogurt	◆ Baked Red Snapper with Gingery Pineapple Sauce ◆ Seasoned Buckwheat Groats ◆ Steamed Kale with Lemon and Butter Sprinkles ◆ Cantaloupe Frappe
MENU 9	MENU 19	MENU 29
◆ Fresh Baked Trout ◆ Baked Potato with Yogurt Topping ◆ Mixed Greens w/ Lemon Dressing ◆ Whipped Prunes and Almond Yogurt	◆ Curried Brown Rice, Salmon and Vegetable Salad ◆ Marinated Tomato, Onion and Cucumber Slices ◆ Mango and Papaya Frappe	◆ Salmon Loaf with Mustard Sauce ◆ Creamy Potato Salad ◆ Romaine and Tomato Salad with Lemon-Ginger Dressing ◆ Tropical Fruit Yogurt
MENU 10	MENU 20	MENU 30
◆ Fish or Chicken Fajitas ◆ Corn Tortillas ◆ Mexican Brown Rice ◆ Grapes and Melon Slices	◆ Spicy Beans and Vegetable Stew ◆ Steamed Millet ◆ Carrot and Celery Sticks ◆ Tofu-Yogurt Almond Pudding with Raspberry Puree	◆ Steamed Brown Rice ◆ Spicy Potatoes, Broccoli and Black-eyed Peas ◆ Raw Veggie Platter with Buttermilk Dip ◆ Date and Almond Whip

Noteworthy Facts

1. The Lunch and Dinner menus are interchangeable. **Remember:** *Choice* **is the key!**

2. The preparation time may take longer in the beginning. But as you become more familiar with this way of eating, and get a handle on the recipes and recipe ideas, you will find your speed picking up. *As you know, you have to crawl before you can walk!*

3. Where a grain is listed as part of the meal, feel free to substitute with any grain you desire, or any prepared grain you have on hand that you want to use up. You can also mix together a variety of grains that you have leftover from previous meals, and create a whole different flavor.

4. Though *I do not recommend cooking with a microwave,* it can be a convenient way to reheat foods, such as grains, potatoes, vegetables or meats, leftover from previous lunches or dinners. Please limit your use of the microwave since the jury is still out.

5. In an effort to maintain the aspect of choice as much as possible, salad dressings have not been fully specified for every salad throughout the menus. You can choose from the variety included in the *Salad Dressing* chapter. You may also choose to substitute one of your favorites for those which have been specified in the menus. Just be sure the dressing you choose is nonfat or very low fat.

6. An acidophilus-based topping on a main course item, or an acidophilus-based dessert (such as yogurt with live cultures), is incorporated into almost every dinner meal, with the purpose of increasing healthy bacteria in the colon, which in turn, will result in less infections due to a *much stronger, more resilient and healthier Immune System.*

7. Where breads and rolls are listed in the menu, be adventurous! Try different types, varieties and brands. See the notes under Lunch menus for ways to make garlic toast or other flavored breads or toasts.

8. It is not imperative that you eat the specific vegetables listed in the menus. Simply substitute another vegetable of similar color, texture or variety for the one listed. There is one exception! *Where tomatoes are listed, it is wise to include*

them, as the Vitamin C in the tomato enhances the iron absorption of the other foods listed in that meal.

9. Steamed vegetables may not initially appeal to you in this basic form. However, high fat sauces are not the best solution. Some ideas for dressing up your vegetables include:

    ♦ flavor sprays
    ♦ butter sprinkles
    ♦ lemon juice
    ♦ Parmesan or Romano cheese (sparingly)
    ♦ Mrs. Dash, Spicy Mrs. Dash, other herb and spice blends
    ♦ Bragg Liquid Aminos
    ♦ Tamari sauce
    ♦ seasoned yogurt
    ♦ salsa
    ♦ seasoned vinegars *(avoid white distilled vinegar!)*
    ♦ a fresh cilantro and lime combination
    ♦ mustard and buttermilk, or yogurt blends
    ♦ uncreamed horseradish
    ♦ hot sauces, e.g. Tabasco, Louisiana Hot Sauce, and Jalapeno pepper sauces.

10. If you have a tendency to eat too much at meals, it may be helpful for you to begin your lunch and dinner meals with a broth-based soup, that can be made simply by adding about 1 tsp-1 tbsp of a base to a cup of hot or boiling water. Some base ideas include:

    ♦ Bragg Liquid Aminos
    ♦ Gayelord Hauser's All Natural Instant Vegetable Broth
    ♦ Bernard Jensen's Vegetable Broth and Seasoning Powder
    ♦ Red Miso Paste
    ♦ Hatcho Miso Paste
    ♦ Marmite vegetable paste

All of those listed are natural, wholesome products without added salt, sugar or MSG. They can be used as a *hot beverage* to replace coffee, or as a *soup base*, or as a *seasoning* in cooked or raw foods.

Other seasonings, chopped vegetables, tofu cubes, or leftover grains or beans, can be added to these soup blends to give a real zingy flavor, or more sustenance.

www.marilynjoyce.com

11. It is wise to make up a large amount of some of your favorites, e.g. the soups, stews, chilis, or meatloaves, as these are very versatile items that lend themselves to a multitude of different meal combinations. For example, the turkey chili:

   - chili and brown rice
   - sloppy joe on wholegrain roll
   - chili over vegetable pasta
   - chili and grains mixed, as a casserole, with low fat cheese topping
   - chili burritos on corn or whole wheat tortillas
   - baked potato topped with chili and nonfat or low fat cheese
   - thinned with vegetable stock, and rice and vegetables added, for soup

   This is your opportunity to be creative. Give it your best shot!

12. Beverages, other than fruit frappes, have not been listed with the meals. If you look under the chapter *Let's Drink to Our Health,* which lists the wonderful variety of drink and beverage possibilities, you can try them all to determine which ones you enjoy the most and will continue to use. Remember, variety is the spice of life, so don't get stuck in a rut, using only one or two of the choices. *There is no excuse for boredom with such a selection!*

13. *Remember!* Drink your beverages before you eat, or 30 minutes to an hour after you eat. Water during your meal will dilute your digestive enzymes that your body naturally produces. You will have less effective digestion and poor assimilation of the nutrients from the food you eat.

QUICK AND EASY RECIPES AND
FOOD PREPARATION HINTS

The goal of the following recipes is to provide the highest level of nutrition, with the most enjoyable flavor, in the least amount of time. Generally, only items which require a minimum number of steps in their preparation are included. Overall, my philosophy is, *if it can't be done in 5 minutes, it won't be done by me!*

Throughout this section the objective has been to provide all of the information necessary to make incorporation of the 30-day menus, for breakfasts, lunches and dinners, a snap. Apart from the actual recipes for the specific menu items, wherever appropriate, further suggestions and ideas are included to assist you in widening the variety of options you have. Some recipes actually lend themselves to the substitution of particular ingredients, with other ingredients, which in turn can result in a different flavor or texture, or both.

Also, if you do not like a particular ingredient in a specific recipe, either omit it or substitute it with something else. For example, if a shake recipe calls for a banana, and a banana is the one fruit you detest, change it to a fruit you love, such as a peach or a pear. Remember what I said about being adventurous! And now, with all of the right foods stocked in your cupboards and refrigerator, preparing healthy meals **will** be a snap. So go for it and have lots of fun doing it!

In order to ease your shift towards a less meat-oriented diet, the directions for buying, storing and preparing the various grains and legumes, have been presented in user-friendly chart forms, that you can copy and attach to your refrigerator with a magnet, for easy reference. For your interest, some pertinent nutrition information is also included.

With respect to the amounts and types of seasonings used in the recipes please understand that these are only suggestions. Nothing is carved in stone! Because everyone's taste buds are different, you may want to experiment to find your own most desired flavors. **This is your opportunity to be the creator!** Start with what is recommended in the specific recipe, and adjust it until you get it the way you want it. And remember that fresher herbs and spices are more potent in flavor than those which have been sitting on your shelf for awhile, so use less.

One suggestion I will share with you that I have personally found to be of real valuable, is that of saving any changes you make to a recipe, or any experiments you try, that are successful. Just jot those changes down on the page beside the particular recipe. That way, when you come back to that recipe, you won't be thinking in your head, "I know I made a great addition (or subtraction) here that we all loved, but what the heck was it?" Instead, whenever you use that recipe, your changes will be right at your fingertips! You won't have to go through the trial and error stage again and again. And you won't have to waste time searching through all of your stickies, or loose scraps of paper for those notes you made that you thought you'd never forget! You know the notes I'm talking about? Those little pieces of paper that just seem to get gobbled up by your desk or workspace!

And a final note:

If you want to find a particular recipe in a hurry, look it up in the **Recipe Index** at the end of the book. In the **Table of Contents** page, at the front of the book, it will be listed under the heading that best describes the menu item, e.g., Salad Dressings, Marinades, Breakfast Entrees, etc.

So let's get started!

On your mark, get set . . .

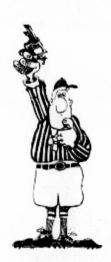

THE SCOOP ON BEANS AND LENTILS!

Shopping Tips:
- Buy large packages of dried beans.
- Buy canned beans with natural preservatives, (organic if available) for convenience.
- Try different types of beans — be adventurous!
- Generally 1 lb. of dry beans equals 2 cups, or 6 cups cooked.
- One 16 ounce can of beans equals 2 cups cooked.

Storage Tips:
- Avoid storing at high temperatures and humidity.
- Store in cool, dry, dark place.
- Keep in air-tight and moisture-proof jars or containers.
- Drain cooked beans while hot; store in refrigerator or freezer.
- Drain and rinse canned beans before storing.
- Drained liquid can be stored separately; add to beans later.
- Dry beans properly stored keep indefinitely.
- Cooked beans keep up to 1 week in refrigerator.
- Cooked beans keep up to 1 year in freezer.

Nutrition Points:
- Combined with whole grains, beans are a good protein source.
- Complex carbohydrates contribute to sustained energy levels.
- High dietary fiber maintains a healthy colon and digestive tract.
- B vitamins protect the nervous system and turn food into energy.
- Iron builds healthy red blood cells.
- Potassium is important for regulation of body fluid balance.
- Calcium and phosphorus form basis of strong bones and teeth.
- Copper, magnesium, manganese, and zinc are for metabolic processes.
- Beans are low in fat, cholesterol and sodium (unless canned).

Cleaning Beans:
- Wash dry beans thoroughly, removing bad beans and objects.
- Drain and rinse canned beans thoroughly to reduce sodium.

Soaking Dry Beans:
- Overnight: Add 6 to 8 cups cold water to 1 lb. of beans. Let stand overnight at a cool room temperature. Drain and rinse, discard the soaking water.
- Quick soak: Add 6 to 8 cups hot water to 1 lb. of beans. Bring water to a boil and cook for 2 to 3 minutes. Set pot of beans aside, covered, for 1 to 2 hours.

Cooking Beans:
- Drain and rinse soaked beans after either soaking method.
- Place beans in a large pot and cover with 6 cups hot water.
- Simmer beans until they are tender, keeping the pot lid tilted.
- Essential to flavor are long, slow cooking and low temperatures.
- Add water as necessary to keep beans covered while cooking.

Bean Facts:
- Cooking too fast at high temperatures splits the skins.
- Hard water or high altitude increase soaking and cooking times.
- A tablespoon of olive oil added during cooking reduces foaming.
- Acidic ingredients slow down cooking, so add tomatoes, lemon or lime juice, vinegar, wine, etc. at end of cooking.
- Baking soda results in a loss of vitamins, so avoid using it.
- Salt toughens bean skins and slows cooking, so add when beans are almost tender.
- Lentils, red, brown or green, do not require presoaking.
- For convenience, soak and cook a double batch of beans, and freeze ½ of it for future use.

- The flavor of any seasonings added during cooking, develops more fully if beans are prepared the day before.
- Beans and lentils can be added to salads, soups, stews, stir-fries, and casseroles, or made into dips and sandwich spreads.
- Drained liquid from cooked beans can be used as a base for soups or stews, to steam vegetables, or added to casseroles.
- Mashed beans can be used to thicken soups and stews.

Cooking Times:

♦	Azuki (adzuki) beans	1 ½ - 2 hours
♦	Black beans	2 - 2 ½ hours
♦	Black-eyed peas	30 - 45 minutes
♦	Chick-peas	3 - 4 hours
♦	Great Northern beans	2 ½ - 3 hours
♦	Green peas, whole	60 - 75 minutes
♦	Kidney beans	2 - 2 ½ hours
♦	Lentils	40 - 60 minutes
♦	Lima beans	40 - 75 minutes
♦	Marrow beans	2 ½ - 3 hours
♦	Navy beans	2 - 2 ½ hours
♦	Pea beans	3 - 3 ½ hours
♦	Pinto beans	2 - 2 ½ hours
♦	Red beans, small	3 - 3 ½ hours
♦	Roman beans	2 - 2 ½ hours
♦	Soybeans	3 - 3 ½ hours
♦	Split peas	45 - 60 minutes
♦	White beans, small	3 - 3 ½ hours

** These are approximate times only. Generally beans are done when the skins begin to break and the beans are tender throughout. Check for tenderness by biting into a bean.

THE SCOOP ON GRAINS!

Shopping Tips:
- Buy only fresh grains, as high fat content in germ of whole-grains turns rancid quickly.
- Buy from stores and mail-order houses with a high turnover.
- Small amounts bought as needed, is the rule of thumb.
- Purchase vacuum-packed or sealed packages instead of scooping and bagging your own from a large open container.

Storage Tips:
- Keep in air-tight and moisture-proof jars or containers.
- Store in a cool, dark place preferably the refrigerator.
- Stored properly and in the refrigerator most will keep up to 6 months.
- Stored properly but in a cupboard, most will keep up to 2 months, unless in a hot climate, or a hot season.
- Store cooked leftover grains in air-tight container up to 3 days in refrigerator, or up to 6 months in freezer.

Nutrition Points:
- Combined with legumes, grains are a good protein source.
- Complex carbohydrates contribute to sustained energy levels.
- High dietary fiber maintains a healthy colon and digestive tract, and contributes to lowering of blood cholesterol.
- B vitamins protect the nervous system and turn food into energy.
- Magnesium assists muscle and nerve functions, and regulates blood pressure.
- Iron builds healthy, oxygen-rich red blood cells.
- Zinc is essential for wound-healing and proper immune function.
- Vitamin E is a natural immune-system booster.
- Grains are low in fat, cholesterol and sodium.

Cleaning Grains:
- Always rinse whole-grains in cool, running water before cooking.
- Bulgur and couscous are exceptions; they turn soggy if rinsed.

Cooking Grains:
- Couscous and bulgur are fluffier when soaked in boiling water for about 15 to 20 minutes, instead of cooking.
- For other grains, bring water to a boil and add the grain.
- Bring to simmer, cover and cook for appropriate amount of time.
- Avoid stirring while cooking; it makes most grains sticky.
- Cornmeal (or polenta) is cooked uncovered and stirred often.
- General Rule, 2 cups water to 1 cup dry grain, except cornmeal at 4 cups water, and brown rice and barley at 3 cups water.

Grain Facts:
- Flavor of most grains, especially millet, is enhanced by roasting lightly in a dry skillet prior to cooking.
- Use vegetable broth or juice, or fruit nectar or juice, instead of water for cooking.
- Add chopped onions and garlic during cooking process.
- Leftover grains can be used as the base for a salad, added to soups, stews, and casseroles, made into healthy puddings, added to protein shakes, or eaten as is with a dressing.
- Grains can be ground to a finer texture or a powder, in a coffee mill or blender, and used to coat fish or chicken.
- Ground dry grains can be used to thicken soups, stews, sauces, and dips, or added to health drinks.
- Prepare "cooked" <u>ground</u> grains, individually or mixed, by soaking ground grains briefly (about 20 minutes) in hot water, or lemon juice, or a combination of both; then serve.

Cooking Times:

◆	Barley	1 - 1 ½ hours
◆	Brown Rice	30 - 45 minutes
◆	Buckwheat (kasha)	15 - 20 minutes
◆	Bulgur (cracked wheat)	15 - 20 minutes
◆	Cornmeal (polenta)	15 - 20 minutes
◆	Couscous	10 - 12 minutes
◆	Millet	20 - 30 minutes
◆	Oatmeal	7 - 15 minutes
◆	Quinoa	12 - 15 minutes
◆	Wheat Berries	1 ½ - 2 hours

**These are approximate times only. Follow directions on the package. Cook or soak the grain until desired consistency. It is best to let the grain sit covered for a few minutes after cooking. Then fluff with a fork.

COOKING WITH HERBS AND SPICES
(Seasoning Without Salt)

Apart from the individual herbs and spices listed here, there are many herb and spice *blends* available, which are also handy to have in your spice cupboard. The label on the bottle or container outlines the many uses for the particular blend. Be adventurous and try some of them. Some are listed in the **Food Products** chapter.

However, some points to remember when purchasing individual herbs and spices, or the blends:

a. Buy only small amounts of each item to insure freshness and full flavor enhancement. Keep only 6 months, at most 1 year, and then discard.

b. Buy organic whenever possible. At the very least, shop for herbs and spices in ethnic grocery stores, where they are often at their freshest!

c. Avoid irradiated herbs and spices! The label on packaged seasonings will tell you if they are. You can find excellent quality herbs and spices in Whole Food, Health Food and Food Specialty Stores.

d. With the blends, avoid anything with MSG or excessive amounts of salt, if any.

e. To interchange fresh herbs for dried, use 3 to 5 times more fresh than dried.

f. Allow the flavor of herbs and spices in salad dressings to develop, by letting the mixture sit for at least 15 minutes prior to serving.

g. For long-cooking soups, stews and sauces, add the seasonings during the last 30 minutes of cooking. Prolonged cooking dissipates flavor.

h. To reduce salt intake, substitute strong, flavorful seasonings such as garlic, onion, black pepper, cayenne pepper, chili powder, curry, cumin, basil, or oregano.

i. To release the flavor of dried herbs, crumble them before adding to the dish.

j. Toasting whole spices briefly in a heavy, dry skillet just before using them, intensifies their flavor.

k. Many herbs and spices are very powerful, so go slow. Experiment until you find the amount that's right for your taste buds!

l. If you add too much to a particular dish, doctor the dish with unseasoned grains, rice, extra potatoes, or more of all of the ingredients. Or serve the dish chilled!

Name	Culinary Uses
Allspice	casseroles, curries, rich soups, carrots, tomatoes, squash, eggplant, sweet potatoes, marinades, desserts, fruit pie, pumpkin pie
Anise	soups, stews, casseroles, fruit salads, vegetable salads, poultry, breads, cakes, cookies, applesauce, apple pie
Bay Leaf	marinades, soups, stews, stuffings, sauces, fish, poultry, tomato juice, tomato soup, sauces for cooked greens, dressings for raw greens, meat, roasts
Basil	tomatoes, tomato sauces, eggs, cheese dishes, dips, curries, soups, salad dressings, sauces, marinades, vegetables, fish, poultry, game meats, appetizers, pizza, Italian cooking, Mediterranean cooking
Capers	sauces, gravies, salads, salad dressings, canapés, tomato dishes, eggplant dishes, fish dishes
Caraway	cabbage, carrots, green beans, potatoes, sauerkraut, cabbage soups, borscht, goulash-type stews, breads
Cardamom	marinades, curries, cabbage, fish, poultry, pork tenderloin, coffee, spiced punches, pies, cakes
Cayenne	egg dishes, cheese dishes, fish, salads, soups, sauces, stews, curries, dressings, Mexican cooking. (**NOTE:** Helps to prevent flatulence from gaseous vegetables.)
Celery Seed	soups, stews, salads, stuffings, vegetable dishes, potato salad, coleslaw, egg salad, tuna salad, fish dishes, game meat dishes, breads
Chervil	cream soups, stews, sauces, salad dressings, egg salads, chicken dishes, fish dishes. **NOTE:** Loses flavor when used in cooking.
Chicory	salads, coffee substitute

<u>Name</u>	<u>Culinary Uses</u>
Chives	cold soups, salads, dips, eggs, yogurt, potatoes, cabbage, vegetable dishes, fish dishes, chicken dishes. **NOTE:** Loses flavor when used in cooking
Cinnamon	eggplant, squash, tomatoes, carrots, apples, chicken and game meats cooked with fruit, pork tenderloin, cakes, pies, spiced beverages
Cloves	marinades, pickled fruits, pickled vegetables, cakes, cookies, spiced beverages
Coriander	marinades, curries, fish, game meat dishes, relishes, yogurt desserts, pickles, spicy punches, coffee, cakes, breads
Cumin	rice dishes, curries, dips, spaghetti sauce, chilis, salads, sauerkraut, yogurt dishes, tofu dishes, spicy vegetables, spicy game meats, Indian cooking, Mexican cooking
Curry (a blend)	rice dishes, curries, dips, yogurt dishes, spicy vegetables, spicy fish, chicken or game meats, lentil dishes, Indian cooking, Oriental cooking, ginger dishes
Dandelion	lentils, omelettes, soups, salads, sandwiches, vegetables, breads, coffee substitute, jellies
Dill	soups, sauces, salads, vegetables, potatoes, carrot salads, cucumbers (especially pickled), green beans, cabbage, sauerkraut, fish (especially salmon), shellfish, yogurt, eggs, cottage cheese, rice dishes
Fennel	soups, stews, sauces, salads, vegetables, sweet potatoes, spicy game meats, fish, oily fish, seafood sauces, pizza, breads, cakes
Fenugreek	curries, stews, spice mixtures, chutneys, yogurt puddings, baked goods, breads, sweet sauces
Garlic	marinades, dips, salad dressings, soups, sauces, salads, egg dishes, cheese dishes, vegetable dishes, fish, poultry, Italian cooking. **NOTE:** ¼ tsp. of garlic powder = 1 small clove of garlic

Name	Culinary Uses
Garam Masala (a blend)	soups, stews, dressings, vegetable stews and dishes, seafood dishes, tofu dishes, yogurt dips, yogurt drinks
Ginger	marinades, curries, ginger tea, salads, horseradish dips, cocktail sauces, mustards, relishes, salad dressings, appetizers, oily fish, clams, seafood, Oriental cooking
Horseradish-uncreamed	dips, cocktail sauces, mustards, relishes, salad dressings, appetizers, oily fish, clams, seafood
Lovage	soups, stews, sauces, casseroles, chowders, omelettes, salads
Marjoram	soups, stews, stuffings, sauces, salads, eggplant, tomatoes, Brussels sprouts, carrots, spinach, zucchini, mushrooms, squash, fish, fowl, pork tenderloin, egg dishes, cheese dishes, Mediterranean cooking
Mint/Spearmint	cold soups (especially fruit), fruits, beans, carrots, eggplant, peas, potatoes, spinach, yogurt dishes, strong-flavored fish, cheese dishes, cheese balls, teas, beverages, desserts
Mustard	soups, stews, sauces, dips, salad dressings, cheese dishes, eggs, potato dishes, onion dishes, tofu dishes
Nutmeg	eggplant, squash, tomatoes, carrots, applesauce, chicken and game meats cooked with fruit, cheese dishes, spicy punches, cookies, pies, breads
Onion	marinades, soups, stews, sauces, dips, salads, stuffing, vegetable dishes, egg dishes, cheese dishes, fish, poultry, game meats
Oregano	soups, stews, salads, stuffings, tomatoes, tomato sauces, peppers, summer squash, zucchini, beans, eggs, pasta dishes, pizza sauces, pork tenderloin, game meats, Italian, Greek and Mexican cooking
Paprika	soups, stews, chilis, Hungarian goulash, sauces, eggs dishes, cheese dishes, potatoes, pasta dishes

Name	Culinary Uses
Parsley	soups, stews, sauces, salads, stuffings, vegetable and salad garnish, tomato dishes, potato dishes, cheese dishes
Pepper	all purpose spice, preservative (especially for meats)
Poppy Seed	marinades, dressings, stuffings, fruit dishes, yogurt desserts, cottage cheese blends, breads, cakes
Rosemary	marinades, sauces, stews, gravies, pea soup, beans, carrots, squash, peas, cauliflower, rice dishes, poultry, fish, pork tenderloin, fish and poultry stuffing, vegetable dishes, breads
Saffron	rice dishes, poultry dishes, fish dishes, breads, cakes, Spanish cooking e.g. Paella
Sage	soups, chowders, stews, sauces, stuffings, eggplant, onions, tomatoes, lima beans, omelettes, herb cheese, fish, game meats, pork tenderloin, duck, coffee and tea substitute
Savory	soups, stews, salads, stuffings, beans, green peas, pea soup, oily fish, game meat dishes, pork tenderloin
Tarragon	egg dishes, omelettes, Béarnaise sauce, tartar sauce, fish, poultry, salad dressings, vinegar, French cooking
Thyme	creamy soups, clam chowder, stews, sauces, stuffings, beans, beets, carrots, mushrooms, onions, potatoes, tomatoes, summer squash, green vegetables, fish, poultry, game meats, pork tenderloin
Turmeric	curries, rice dishes, salad dressings, dips, egg dishes, tofu dishes, Indian cooking
Vanilla/Mexican	shakes, yogurt desserts, sweet yogurt dips, rice dishes, rice
Vanilla	Vanilla pudding, breakfast grains, sweet sauces, milk drinks and milk desserts

VERSATILE TOFU: THE CULINARY CHAMELEON

Tofu is one of those rare foods that can be added to virtually any dish to enhance the protein content, without adding a distinctive flavor of its own. It simply takes on the flavors and seasonings of anything it is cooked or prepared with.

Tofu, also called *bean curd*, is a protein-rich food, which is low in calories, sodium, and fat, especially saturated fat, has no cholesterol, and is relatively inexpensive. It comes in several versatile forms, from **soft or silken**, to **firm**, to **extra-firm**, making it an excellent product for thickening, extending, adding to soups, stews, salads, egg or vegetable dishes, or as a main dish item.

In recipes calling for cream, cream cheese, cottage cheese, ricotta cheese, or eggs, tofu can be substituted. *A one-to-one ratio is a good substitution standard.*

This wonderfully versatile food can be cubed, diced, crumbled or pureed. It can be an obvious ingredient in a recipe, or camouflaged by the other ingredients or flavors.

You will find several recipe ideas in this book. But apart from actual recipes, there are many quick-fix possibilities which incorporate tofu for the purpose of increasing the protein content, and therefore, the sustained satiety value (satisfied feeling after eating) of a meal; a meal which may otherwise have left you feeling hungry an hour after eating it.

So here's a list of suggestions! Try them. And then create your own!

1. Blend ½ cup of soft tofu into a healthy breakfast shake, or a milk shake.

2. Blend soft tofu, plain yogurt, fruit and maybe a teaspoon of pure maple syrup together into a dessert pudding.

3. Blend or mash, soft or firm tofu into savory or sweet dips.

4. Marinate ¼ inch thick slices of firm or extra-firm tofu, in a blend of tamari sauce, garlic, ginger, minced capers, green onions and organic cider vinegar, overnight, and then:

   a. Use as a sandwich base, with lettuce, alfalfa sprouts and tomatoes
   b. Cut into cubes to toss into a chef's salad

c. Add to scrambled eggs, egg salad, or omelets
d. Add to potato salad or potato-based casseroles
e. Cut into cubes and toss over brown rice, or other grains
f. Serve as a main dish entree with steamed vegetables
g. Place a slice in a baked potato, and top with a yogurt and chive dressing
h. Use as a base for a pita pocket sandwich with a thin hummus dressing
i. Toss cubes into a basic miso broth
j. Crumble or finely dice, the tofu slices over steamed vegetables

5. Add cubes of tofu to vegetable or bean, soups or stews, to increase protein content after soups or stews are finished cooking. ***DO NOT COOK TOFU!***

6. Add cubes of firm tofu, or mashed soft tofu, to any casserole dish.

7. Mash soft tofu into basic non-meat marinara sauce for added sustenance. Add after cooking is completed.

8. Chop firm tofu into marinara sauce for a chunkier texture. Add after cooking is completed.

9. To top a baked potato, puree ½ cup of soft tofu, and blend with juice of 1 lemon and 1 tbsp. chives.

10. Serve slices of extra-firm tofu with low sodium soy sauce, or Bragg Liquid Aminos, for breakfast, or lunch on wholegrain toast.

11. For a creamy vegetable soup, blend tofu with reheated leftover vegetable soup.

12. For a cold, creamy fruit soup, blend tofu, vanilla soymilk, frozen berries and a banana together, and sprinkle cinnamon on top of each serving.

Another food, which deserves honorable mention here, is tempeh. It is also a very versatile high-protein cultured food, made from soybeans and sometimes grains. Though most tempehs are flavorful to begin with, they adapt very well to many of the suggestions outlined above for tofu, especially the more savory combinations.

This unique food is also adaptable to the use of marinades. Tempeh, like tofu, can be marinated in the combination of ingredients outlined in Suggestion #4, and served in the various ways listed for marinated tofu.

Tempeh is available in a variety of flavors. So don't be shy! Try them all to find the flavors you most enjoy. Experiment with different ways of serving this nutritious alternative to meat. *Your body will thank you for giving it such high-powered nutrition without all of the additional saturated fats and chemicals present in most of our meat-based products.*

NOTE: For one of the most comprehensive guides available on ***tofu, and soy foods*** in general, go to: www.icantbelieveitstofu.com. You can download, **"I Can't Believe It's Tofu!"** my best selling, unique and innovative nutrition and recipe book, in just seconds. It is absolutely loaded with the most delicious, easy-to-prepare, 1 to 5 minute tofu and soy recipes you will ever find anywhere! And you will not believe that you're eating tofu! While you're there, why not go ahead and sign up to receive our free *Special Report, "Tofu Wizard 4 Fun & Health."* Can't wait to see you there!

30 QUICK TOPPINGS FOR
BAKED POTATOES, BROWN RICE, WHOLE GRAINS

1. Low fat, plain yogurt with chives
2. Low fat yogurt and salsa — equal parts
3. Nonfat vegetarian chili topped with nonfat grated cheddar cheese
4. Steamed broccoli and cauliflower over potato, topped with low fat yogurt
5. Heated marinara sauce and soft tofu, blended and sprinkled with Parmesan cheese
6. Nonfat vegetarian refried beans, or any seasoned beans, blended until smooth
7. Chopped onions, mushrooms, and tuna
8. Lentil and vegetable soup, topped with a dollop of low fat yogurt
9. Salsa topped with grated low fat cheese, and melted under the broiler
10. Low fat yogurt and low fat ricotta cheese blended, with chopped dill and chives added
11. Equal blend, with either a blender or a fork, of yogurt, cottage cheese and salsa
12. Cottage cheese blended until smooth, with added finely diced red peppers, ginger and olives
13. Low fat yogurt, ginger, cumin and celery seed, blended
14. Low fat yogurt, minced parsley and small portion of blue cheese, blended
15. Low fat ricotta cheese mixed with capers and Bac' Uns
16. Scrambled egg and tofu mixture topped with salsa
17. Low fat yogurt seasoned with minced garlic, onions, celery and Spicy Mrs. Dash
18. Tuna and low fat yogurt, blended
19. Low fat yogurt and almond butter, blended, with added jalapeno peppers
20. Low fat yogurt mixed with chopped prunes and almonds
21. Low fat yogurt and red caviar
22. Low fat ricotta cheese and sardines blended
23. Soft tofu and Tabasco sauce blended, with added raisins and almonds
24. Broccoli, cauliflower, onions, garlic, low fat yogurt or buttermilk, blended
25. Buttermilk, ricotta cheese, Spicy Mrs. Dash, blended, with added Bac' Uns

26. Leftover chili, vegetable or chicken stew, soups and steamed vegetables
27. Mashed avocado, chopped tomatoes, onions and garlic mixed with low fat yogurt
28. Mashed avocado and salsa mixed with nonfat cottage cheese or low fat ricotta
29. Tempeh, low fat yogurt, salsa, blended
30. Chopped Tempeh, onions, minced garlic, fresh lemon juice, and Tabasco sauce

NOTE: These toppings are designed to be high enough in protein to make the baked (sweet) potato, yam, or grain, a meal. Just add a salad, with a homemade low or nonfat dressing. See *Salad Dressings* chapter, to complete the meal.

BREAKFAST RECIPES

Authentic Muesli

1 cup cold water
1 cup old fashioned oatmeal
Juice of 1 small lemon
1 tbsp wheat germ
2 tbsp pure maple syrup
1 unpeeled apple, finely diced
1 medium banana, sliced

2 tbsp dried fruit, finely chopped
6 almonds, chopped or sliced
2 tbsp sesame seeds
1 cup soy or almond milk or
    plain, low fat yogurt
Cinnamon and Nutmeg, to taste
Nutritional yeast, optional, but
    recommended

1. Combine the water and the oatmeal in a glass bowl. Let stand overnight, covered.
2. Add a little more water if the mixture seems too thick for your preference.
3. Just before serving, stir in rest of ingredients, except soymilk, spices and yeast.
4. Serve in individual bowls and allow each person to add the last 3 items to taste.

Makes 4-6 servings

Berrie Good Kasha

1 cup buckwheat groats
2 cups water
2 tbsp unsulphured raisins
4 chopped dried apricots, unsulphured

1 tbsp pure maple syrup
1 cup fresh berries
6 almonds, chopped
½-1 cup plain, low fat yogurt

1. Bring the water to a boil. Add the groats and return to a boil.
2. Add the dried fruit, and simmer the mixture for 7-10 minutes.
3. When the groats are done, add the maple syrup, berries and almonds, and serve.
4. Top each serving with a generous portion of yogurt.

Makes 3-4 servings

Breakfast Bulgur

1 cup bulgur
3 cups water
2 tbsp dried fruit, unsulphured

1 cup fresh pineapple chunks
1 tbsp pure maple syrup
2 cups soy or almond milk
    or low fat yogurt

1. Bring water to a boil. Add the bulgur and return to a boil.
2. Add the dried fruit and simmer the bulgur mixture for 10 minutes.
3. Remove from the heat and add pineapple chunks and maple syrup.
4. Let sit for 15 minutes and then serve.
5. Top each serving with about ½ cup acidophilus milk or yogurt.

Makes 3-4 servings

Brown Rice Delight

1 cup cooked brown rice
1 cup fresh mango, chopped
2 tbsp sesame tahini

1-2 tsp pure maple syrup or sucanat
½ cup plain, low fat yogurt

Mix together all of the ingredients, and serve.

Variations:
1. Substitute mango with other fresh, ripe fruit.
2. Substitute mango with a combination of pineapple, banana and mango.
3. Substitute tahini with 4-6 chopped almonds, and ¼ tsp almond extract.
4. Substitute mango with 2 tbsp unsulphured dried fruit.

Makes 2 servings

Brown Rice Pudding

A great way to use up leftover cooked brown rice!

1 cup cooked brown rice, chilled	¼ tsp fresh ginger, grated
½ cup plain, low fat yogurt	2 tbsp unsulphured raisins
½ cup vanilla soymilk or almond milk	2 tsp pure maple syrup
½ tsp cinnamon	4 almonds, chopped

1. Mix all of the ingredients together.
2. Can be served heated (not to boiling point) or chilled.

Note: If served chilled, it is best prepared the night before and stored, covered, in the refrigerator. This allows for the flavors to marinate more fully. To maintain the texture of the almonds, add them just prior to serving.

Makes 1-2 servings

Crazy Mixed-Up Grains

ONE:

2 cups mixed leftover grains
4-6 almonds, chopped

3-6 pieces soaked prunes and apricots*
1-2 tbsp pure maple syrup or sucanat

Mix all ingredients together and serve with soy or almond milk or low fat yogurt, and fruit sauce.

* See Prunes and Apricots for Topping on Cereal in **Blended Fruit Toppings** chapter.

Makes 2 servings

TWO:

¼ cup raw millet
¼ cup raw buckwheat groats
¼ cup raw old fashioned oats
¼ cup raw brown rice
½ inch fresh ginger root, peeled
2-2 ½ cups boiling water

1-2 tbsp pure maple syrup or sucanat
4-6 almonds, chopped
3-6 pieces of soaked prunes and
    apricots
Soy or almond milk or plain,
    low fat yogurt

1. Grind each of the grains and ginger root in a coffee mill, or a Vita-Mix machine. In a coffee mill, each will have to be ground separately to preserve the motor, and then mixed together. In a Vita-Mix, they can be ground together at the same time.
2. Add the boiling water to the ground grains and let sit for 30 minutes. Add as much water as necessary to get your desired consistency.
3. Add the maple syrup, fruit and almonds just prior to serving.
4. Top with soy or almond milk or low fat yogurt and fruit sauce, e.g., Apple and Strawberry Sauce, see **Blended Fruit Toppings** chapter.

Makes 2 servings

French Toast

4 thick slices multi-grain bread
2 free-range eggs
½ cup vanilla soy or almond milk
Pure maple syrup (optional)

Olive oil spray
Organic butter
Cinnamon / Sucanat

1. Beat together the eggs and soymilk.
2. Spray a nonstick skillet or griddle with the oil-based spray just to thinly coat it.
3. Heat the skillet at a high heat until a drop of water sizzles when it hits the griddle.
4. Dip the slices of bread in the egg mixture, one at a time, to coat both sides evenly.
5. Cook on each side until the toast is golden brown, crispy on the outside and slightly soft on the inside when pressed with a spatula.
6. Lightly brush on melted butter, cinnamon and sucanat, or a little maple syrup.

Makes 2 servings

Fresh Fruit Salads

Below are some suggestions for combinations of fruit for fruit salads. It is always best to use fruits which are in season. Each combination is approximately 2 servings.

ONE
1 medium banana, sliced
1 cup green seedless grapes
1 medium green apple, chopped

TWO
1 cup fresh pineapple, chopped
1 mango, cubed
1 medium banana, sliced

THREE
1 cup cantaloupe, cubed
1 cup honeydew melon, balled
½ cup watermelon, chopped

FOUR
1 medium banana, sliced
1 medium peach, chopped
1 medium pear, in thin wedges

FIVE
1 papaya, chopped
½ cup fresh pineapple, chopped
½ medium avocado, diced

SIX
1 medium banana, sliced
1 medium nectarine, in thin wedges
1 medium peach, chopped

SEVEN
1 papaya, diced
1 mango, diced
1 cup fresh cherries
1 medium banana, sliced

EIGHT
1 medium pear, diced
1 medium orange, in wedges
1 medium grapefruit, in wedges
½ cup fresh pineapple, cubed

NINE
2 medium bananas, sliced
½ medium avocado, sliced
¼-½ tsp cinnamon

TEN
1 cup fresh strawberries, sliced
½ cup fresh raspberries
½ cup fresh blueberries

Any of the above combinations can be served plain, or with low fat yogurt dressings, or sprinkled with fresh squeezed lemon juice, or with shredded almonds or coconut, or topped with a few sunflower, or pumpkin, or sesame seeds, or any combinations of these ingredients.

Fruity Yogurt

2 cups plain low fat yogurt
½ cup blueberries
1 cup sliced strawberries

1 medium banana sliced
1-1 ½ tbsp pure maple syrup
½-1 tsp cinnamon

1. Blend yogurt, maple syrup and cinnamon together. Fold in all of the fruit.
2. Place in a covered container and let marinate in refrigerator for at least 4 hours, preferably overnight.
3. Serve, as is, in a parfait dish, or sprinkle no added fat granola over the top of the yogurt, for extra fiber.
4. Can use any fruits, in season, in place of above fruits.

Makes 4 servings

The Green Machine Shake

2 scoops Juice Plus+® Complete
1 cup vanilla soymilk or almond milk
1 tbsp wheat germ*
1 tbsp nutritional yeast*

½ cup plain, low fat yogurt
1 medium banana
1 tbsp spirulina powder*
½ cup strawberries,
    or other berries

In a blender or Vita-Mix machine, blend all ingredients together until smooth.

*If you have never used these items before, it is wise to start with about 1 tsp each and gradually, over 3-4 weeks, build up to the recommended amounts in the recipe.

Makes 1 serving

High Protein Breakfast Shake

1 cup vanilla soy milk   1 medium banana
4 large strawberries   1 tsp-1 tbsp spirulina powder
½ cup low fat yogurt, cottage cheese, ricotta cheese, or tofu

1. Blend above ingredients together in blender.
2. If not sweet enough, add 1 tsp pure maple syrup. Drink immediately.

Note: If made in a Vita-mix machine, the texture and blend are much smoother and finer, with greater emulsification.

Makes 1 serving

Hot Oatmeal, Soaked

½ cup old fashioned oats   1 tsp cinnamon
½ inch fresh ginger, ground   2 tbsp unsulphured raisins
Boiling water   1 medium unpeeled apple, chopped
1-2 tbsp wheat germ or bran   2 tsp sucanat or sugar cane crystals (optional)
1 cup vanilla soymilk or plain, low fat yogurt

1. Grind oatmeal and ginger together into a powder, in a coffee mill or Vita-Mix machine.
2. Cover the oatmeal and ginger with boiling water. Let sit for 20 minutes.
3. Mix in the wheat germ, cinnamon, raisins, apple and sucanat.
4. Top with either soymilk, or yogurt, or a combination of the two.

Note: Actually this oatmeal will only be warm by the time you eat it, as prepared above. If you desire hot oatmeal, simply reheat it, just prior to serving. Or sit the covered bowl of oatmeal and ginger over a pot of very hot water during the 20 minute soaking period.

Variations:
1. Substitute any other dried fruit for the raisins.
2. Substitute any fresh ripe fruit for the apple.
3. The oatmeal and ginger can be soaked together in an unground form, and then blended in a blender or Vita-Mix machine, after the soaking period, just prior to the addition of the remaining ingredients.

Makes 2 servings

Low Fat Banana Apricot Loaf

Though this is one item that may require more preparation time than most of the recipes in this book, once prepared you have several quick servings to look forward to. A slice makes an enjoyable breakfast food, a great snack or a special dessert with a flavored low fat yogurt topping. (This was my children's all time favorite baked goodie. And it's healthy too!)

Dry ingredients:
1 ½ cups whole-wheat flour
½ cup old fashioned oats
⅛ cup wheat germ
1 ½ tsp non-aluminum
    based baking powder
½ tsp baking soda
1 tsp ground cinnamon
¼ tsp ground nutmeg
⅛ tsp ground cloves
¼ cup dried apricots, finely chopped

Moist ingredients:
2 free-range eggs
½ cup buttermilk
3 large or 4 medium bananas
½ cup dried prune puree*
    or applesauce
⅛ to ¼ cup pure maple syrup
Olive oil Spray

1. Spray a nonstick or Pyrex loaf pan with an olive oil spray.
2. In a large glass bowl, mix all of the dry ingredients, adding the apricots last.
3. In a blender, whip all of the moist ingredients until very well blended.
4. Fold the moist ingredients into the dry ingredients until just blended. Do not over mix, or tunnels will form in the finished baked product.
5. Bake in a preheated 325°-350° oven, for approximately one hour. Use a knitting needle or fork to test the middle of the loaf for doneness.

* Prune Puree: To prepare 1 cup of prune puree, combine 8 ounces (1 ⅓ cups) of pitted prunes with 6-8 tbsp of hot water in a Vita-Mix machine or food processor.

An alternative to preparing your own puree is to buy a commercial product called **Dried Plum Puree.** See the *Food Products* chapter for information on where to find this product.

Millet Fantasy

½ cup millet, uncooked
Boiling water
½ cup vanilla soy or almond milk
½ tsp cinnamon
1 medium peach or banana, chopped

1 tbsp unsulphured dates, chopped
3 almonds, chopped
1-2 tsp pure maple syrup
½ cup low fat plain yogurt

1. Grind the millet to a powder in either a coffee mill or a Vita-Mix machine.
2. Cover the millet with boiling water. Let sit for 20 minutes. *A great opportunity to get ready for the day ahead!*
3. Mix the maple syrup and yogurt together. Let sit while you prepare the rest.
4. Mix the soymilk and cinnamon into the soaked millet.
5. Add the chopped fruit, dates and almonds.
6. Top with low fat yogurt.

Makes 1-2 servings

Oatmeal Pancakes

½ cup whole wheat flour
¼ cup rolled oats
1 tsp baking soda
1 free-range egg
¾ cup buttermilk

¼ cup applesauce
½ tsp cinnamon
Olive oil spray
Fruit preserves
Applesauce

1. Combine all of the dry ingredients, including the cinnamon, in a glass bowl.
2. Whip together all of the liquid ingredients in a blender.
3. Fold the liquid ingredients into the dry just until blended. Let sit for a few minutes.
4. Pour the pancake batter onto a hot, lightly sprayed, griddle or skillet.
5. When tiny bubbles which form on the pancakes begin to burst, turn the pancakes. This takes about 1-1 ½ minutes on each side.
6. Serve pancakes hot with fruit preserves or applesauce.

Makes 6-8 pancakes or 3-4 servings

Potato and Egg Scramble

½ medium onion, chopped
2 cloves of garlic, chopped
2 free-range eggs, lightly beaten
4 ounces firm tofu, crumbled
Organic butter to taste, optional

2 leftover baked potatoes, diced
Mrs. Dash or Spicy Mr. Dash, to taste
Hot pepper sauce, to taste
Olive oil spray

1. Spray a medium skillet lightly with an olive oil spray.
2. Briefly sauté the garlic and onion, for about 1 minute, at medium to high heat.
3. Add diced potato and briefly sauté for about 1 minute more.
4. Add crumbled tofu and beaten eggs.
5. Scramble until firm, adding seasoning and butter just prior to completion of cooking.

Makes 2 servings

Raspberry Delight: Healthy Shake

2 cups vanilla soymilk, chilled
1 cup fresh raspberries, chilled
1 medium banana
1-2 tbsp untoasted wheat germ

¼ tsp almond extract
2 tsp spirulina powder
1-2 tsp pure maple syrup (optional)

1. Blend all ingredients together in a blender or a Vita-Mix machine.
2. If not sweet enough, add 1-2 tsp pure maple syrup.

Note: If made in a Vita-Mix machine, the texture and blend are much smoother and finer. However blend for only a few seconds to avoid heating the product, as the power of the motor generates heat while it blends. To counteract this heating action, simply add 3 or 4 ice cubes with the other ingredients, during the blending process.

Makes 2 servings

Scrambled Eggs and Tofu

Olive oil spray
4-6 ounces firm tofu
2 large free-range eggs, lightly beaten
2 tbsp low fat grated cheddar cheese or cheddar tofu cheese

¼ cup scallions, chopped
Mrs. Dash or Spicy Mrs. Dash
⅛-¼ tsp paprika

1. Spray a 10-inch nonstick skillet with enough spray to evenly coat it.
2. Heat the pan on a medium temperature, while crumbling the tofu into the pan.
3. As the tofu is cooking it dries slightly; then add the scallions and cook for about 3 minutes.
4. Add the lightly beaten eggs to this mixture and scramble until firm, adding the grated cheddar just before removing the pan from the heat.
5. Season to taste.

Makes 2 servings

Scrambled Tofu and Tomatoes

Olive oil Spray
½ medium onion, chopped
2 cloves fresh garlic, chopped
6 ounces of firm tofu

½ large green pepper, sliced
2 medium fresh tomatoes
Mrs. Dash or Spicy Mrs. Dash,
    to taste
Cayenne pepper, to taste

1. Lightly spray a medium skillet with an olive oil spray.
2. Briefly sauté the garlic and onions, for about 1 minute, at medium to high heat.
3. Crumble the tofu into the skillet. Add the green peppers and tomatoes.
4. Sauté the mixture, at medium heat, for about 2-3 minutes.
5. Add seasoning to taste and serve.

Makes 2 servings

Tropical Fruit Salad

1 papaya, diced
1 mango, diced
1 medium banana, sliced

1 cup pineapple, cubed
1 kiwi, sliced

1 medium orange, in sections
Juice of 1 lime
2 tbsp unsweetened shredded
    coconut
2 tbsp chopped dates or figs
Juice from prepared fresh fruit

Mix all ingredients together and serve immediately in your most elegant dishes.

Makes 4 servings

Vibrant Fruit Salad

1 medium peach, chopped
1 medium orange, in sections
¼ of a fresh pineapple, chopped
6 strawberries, sliced
1 medium banana, sliced

½ cup plain, low fat yogurt
½ tsp raspberry extract
2 tsp pure maple syrup
2 tbsp unsweetened shredded
    coconut

1. Blend the yogurt, maple syrup and extract together.
2. Fold in all of the prepared fruit, including any juice from the pineapple.
3. Serve in your most elegant glass dessert dishes.
4. You may top with additional plain, low fat yogurt.
5. Sprinkle shredded coconut on the top of each serving.

Variation: Can substitute any in-season fruit.

Makes 2 servings

FESTIVE BEVERAGES FOR HEALTH AND VITALITY

Ginger Tea

1 ½ inches fresh ginger root, peeled
4 cups water
1 cup skimmed/lite evaporated milk, or unsweetened vanilla soymilk
1-2 tsp pure maple syrup

1. Bring water to a rolling boil. Add peeled ginger root.
2. Simmer ginger root in water for about 20-25 minutes.
3. Remove pot with ginger and water from heat.
4. Add evaporated milk or soymilk, and maple syrup.

Makes 3-4 servings. Can be served hot or iced.

Immune Enhancing Green Tea Chai

2 liters water
15 whole cardamom pods
  (crush slightly)
3 sticks of cinnamon
12 whole cloves

12 whole black peppercorns
8 slices fresh ginger (¼" thick)
Pure maple syrup or organic
  Sucanat, to taste
2 cups organic vanilla soymilk

1. Bring the 2 liters of water to a boil.
2. Add the spices and ginger and simmer for 30-40 minutes.
3. Add more water as it simmers, so that you end up with about 2 liters.
4. Remove from heat and let the spices sit in the water for several
5. hours or overnight.
6. Before serving, bring to a boil again and remove from heat.
7. Add 2-3 tsp loose green tea leaves. Let steep for 5 minutes.

Option: Can strain mixture.

8. Add soymilk and sweetener. Can be served hot or cold.

Variations: 1. Substitute chocolate soymilk for the vanilla.
              2. Experiment with the spices to determine your favorite
                 blend.

Real Lemons Lemonade!

4 Lemons, large, organic
½ cup pure maple syrup, or organic sucanat
4 cups Boiling water

Makes about 4 cups — Can be served hot or cold

1. Scrub lemons, halve, then squeeze out the juice.
2. Place juice and pulp of the 4 lemons in a large jug or bowl with syrup or sucanat.
3. Pour 1 ½ cups boiling water over. Stir until sugar dissolves.
4. Add lemon halves, each cut into ¼'s, and another 2 ½ cups boiling water.
5. Stir well, then cover to steep, and let cool.
6. Strain, squeezing out any remaining juice from lemon sections, and serve.
7. For cold lemonade, fill 4 large glasses with ice and divide the lemon (-ginger) mixture among them.
8. Garnish each glass (or mug, if hot lemonade) with mint sprigs and lemon wedges.

Variations:
1. Top off each serving (just prior to step #8) with ¼ cup sparkling water for some fizz!
2. Add slices of fresh ginger in step #4, for a unique gingery accent.
3. Slices of lime add a delicious twist to either the hot lemonade (added in Step 4) or the cold.

Spiced Apple Cider

7 cups organic apple cider
3 cups orange juice, fresh squeezed
4-6 cinnamon sticks
¼ tsp nutmeg
4-6 whole cloves
1 large unpeeled orange, thinly sliced

1. Combine all ingredients in a Dutch oven or stock pot.
2. Heat just to boiling. Cover and keep hot on very low heat.
3. Ladle servings as desired. Include a slice of orange on the surface of each.

FRUIT SMOOTHIES

Each recipe makes 2 servings

1: Berrie Good

1 cup fresh berries
1 medium banana

1 cup pure organic apple cider
1 tbsp spirulina powder

In a blender or Vita-Mix machine, blend all ingredients together until smooth.

2: High Energy

1 cup plain, low fat yogurt
1-2 tsp pure maple syrup or sucanat
1 tbsp sesame seeds
1 fresh papaya
1 medium banana

(Build up to These)* ☺
1 tbsp nutritional yeast * ☺
1 tbsp spirulina powder * ☺
1 tbsp wheat germ * ☺

In a blender or Vita-Mix machine, blend all ingredients together until smooth.

Variations: Add or substitute strawberries, blueberries, raspberries, mango, peaches, apricots, pineapple, pear, or other fresh, ripe fruit.

* If you have never used these products before (i.e., wheat germ, nutritional yeast, and spirulina powder), it is wise to start with about 1 tsp each and gradually, over 3-4 weeks, build up to the recommended amounts in this recipe.

☺ Any of these items can be added to any blended drink included in this book, as well as to sandwich fillings, or sprinkled on the top of salads, or mixed into loaves, burgers, or soups. They are so packed full of valuable nutrients, that it would be a shame to miss such easy opportunities to include them in your diet.

3: Melon Ice

1 medium cantaloupe
l-2 tbsp spirulina powder

4-6 ice cubes

In a blender or Vita-Mix machine, blend all ingredients together until smooth.

4: <u>Ginger Snap</u>

1 cup raspberries   1 cup fresh pineapple
4 fresh or dried, soaked apricots   ½ inch fresh ginger root

In a blender or Vita-Mix machine, blend all ingredients together until smooth.

Variations: 1.   Substitute the fruits in **Ginger Snap** recipe with 1 papaya and 1 banana.
              2.   Substitute the fruits in recipe **Ginger Snap** with 1 cup any berries, 1 banana, and 1 cup organic apple cider.
              3.   **Plain, Low fat Yogurt Fruit Smoothies**: add 1 cup of plain, low fat yogurt to any of the Smoothies listed above, except the **High Energy recipe.** If the taste is too tart or too tangy, add 1-2 tsp pure maple syrup or sucanat. Gradually reduce the sweetener each time you prepare the smoothie, until you no longer need it.

These recipes are healthy, delicious, easy to make, and enticing. Anyone can blend these together in a minute or two, for an on-the-run breakfast, snack, after-workout pick-me-up, or meal replacement.

However, I am asked continuously, at every seminar or event I facilitate, what I recommend for a person who has a compromised immune system, or is experiencing a challenging illness. Well, years ago I developed a delicious, yet extremely wholesome smoothie recipe, which can be used by anyone, anytime. However, it was primarily formulated with my patients in mind. You can find the recipe for the **SUMPTUOUS IMMUNE BALANCING SMOOTHIE** in the chapter, *Dr Joyce Recommends* . . .

Enjoy!

FRUIT FRAPPES

Make frappes in a blender or Vita-Mix machine, blending suggested fruits with 4-6 ice cubes. Try mixing your own blends of fruits. Serve immediately. Each combination makes 2 servings.

Variations:

1. **Apple and Strawberry Frappe**: 1 cup pure organic apple cider and 1 cup fresh strawberries plus ice. Can substitute strawberries with pineapple, grapes, peach, papaya, banana, or pear.

2. **Banana and Papaya Frappe**: 1 ripe banana and 1 ripe papaya plus ice.

3. **Cantaloupe Frappe**: Pulp of 1 small cantaloupe plus ice.

4. **Mango and Papaya Frappe**: 1 ripe mango and 1 ripe papaya plus ice.

5. **Peach and Banana Frappe**: 1 ripe peach with skin and 1 ripe banana plus ice.

6. **Pineapple and Mango Frappe**: 1 fresh ripe mango and 1 cup fresh pineapple plus ice.

7. **Raspberry and Banana Frappe**: 1 cup fresh or frozen raspberries and 1 ripe banana plus ice. Can use strawberries or blueberries instead.

8. **Yogurt Frappe**: Plain, **low fat yogurt** can be added to any of the above combinations.

Note: If a sweeter taste is preferred, add 1-2 tsp pure maple syrup or sucanat or stevia. However, the goal is to reduce your desire for sweets, so gradually reduce the amount of sweetener added each time you prepare the frappes.

FRUIT AND YOGURT WHIPS AND PUDDINGS

The following recipes can be prepared in a blender or a Vita-Mix machine. The Vita-Mix machine produces a much finer and smoother consistency.

Chill each blend in the freezer for at least 1 hour before serving.

Each recipe makes 2 servings

Berry-Ricotta Surprise

In a blender or Vita-mix machine, blend 1 cup low fat ricotta cheese with 1 cup of berries, (any one of, or a combination of, strawberries, raspberries, blueberries, blackberries), ¼-½ tsp brandy extract, ½ tsp cinnamon, and 1 tbsp pure maple syrup or sucanat. Chill in the freezer for at least 1 hour before serving.

Variations: 1. **Fruit-Ricotta Surprise**, substitute any fresh fruit in season for the berries. Peaches are particularly good. Use 2 medium peaches, unpeeled.
2. **Tropical Fruit-Ricotta Surprise**, substitute tropical fruits, e.g. pineapple, kiwi, mango, papaya, or banana, or a combination of these. Add ½ tsp dried ginger, or ½ inch fresh ginger, grated, to this blend.

Fresh Low Fat Banana Yogurt

Blend 1 cup plain low fat yogurt, 1 ripe banana and 2 tsp pure maple syrup together. Add a drop of almond extract or a ½ tsp of cinnamon or ginger for variety.

Variations: **Tropical Fruit Yogurt**, substitute 1 cup of tropical fruits, e.g. pineapple, mango, papaya, kiwi, banana, or avocado. It can be one of these or a combination.

Two methods: a) Blend ingredients together; or b) Mix chunks of fruit into plain, low fat yogurt. For both methods, chill overnight to blend flavors.

Home-Blended Low Fat Vanilla Yogurt

Blend 1 cup plain, low fat yogurt, 2 tsp pure maple syrup, ¼-½ tsp pure vanilla extract. This combination can be the base for a variety of fruit and yogurt combinations.

Variations:
1. **Whipped Vanilla and Strawberry Yogurt**, add 1 cup fresh strawberries to the above ingredients and whip.
2. **Sweet Potato and Raisin Yogurt Whip**, add 1 medium unpeeled baked sweet potato, and 2 tbsp unsulphured raisins to the above basic combination and whip.

Whipped Prunes and Almond Yogurt

Whip together 1 cup plain, low fat yogurt, ¼-½ tsp almond extract, and ½ cup soaked unsulphured pitted prunes (drained).

Variations:
1. **Apricot Dream**, substitute ½ cup soaked unsulphured apricots (drained) for the prunes, and add 4-5 raw almonds.

2. **Date and Almond Whip**, substitute ½ cup of soaked unsulphured dates (undrained) for the prunes, and add 6 raw almonds.

3. **Pineapple Almond Whip**, substitute 1 cup fresh pineapple for the prunes, and 1 tsp sucanat, if necessary.

4. **Tofu-Yogurt Almond Pudding with Raspberry Puree**, add ½ cup soft tofu, 5 raw almonds and 2 tsp sucanat. Top with Raspberry Puree, see *Blended Fruit Toppings* chapter

5. **Sweet Potato and Raisin Yogurt Almond Whip**, substitute 1 medium unpeeled baked sweet potato, and 2 tbsp unsulphured raisins for the prunes.

6. **Whipped Peaches and Almond Yogurt**, substitute 1 large ripe peach for the prunes, and add 1 tsp sucanat.

BLENDED FRUIT TOPPINGS

All of these blends can be used as either a sauce or a topping.

Apple and Strawberry Sauce

1 fresh sweet unpeeled apple, cored   ¼ cup low fat, plain yogurt
1 cup fresh strawberries   ¼ tsp brandy extract

In a blender, or Vita-Mix machine, blend all ingredients until smooth. The consistency is much smoother when blended in a Vita-Mix machine.

Variations:

1. **Apricot Sauce**: substitute 1 cup soaked unsulphured (drained) apricots for the apple and strawberries. Or substitute ½ cup apricots for only one of the fruits, creating **Apricot-Apple Sauce** or **Strawberry-Apricot Sauce.**

2. **Banana and Pineapple Fruit Sauce:** substitute 1 ripe banana and 1 cup of fresh pineapple for the apple and strawberries.

3. **Blueberry Sauce:** substitute 2 cups of blueberries for the fruit.

4. **Non-Creamy Blended Fruit Topping**: prepare as above, but eliminate the yogurt.

5. **Raspberry Puree**: substitute 2 cups of fresh raspberries for the apple and strawberries. You can eliminate the yogurt for a rich berry flavor.

6. **Tropical Fruit Sauce:** substitute 1 mango, 1 papaya and 1 cup fresh pineapple, for apple and strawberries.

7. Substitute the brandy extract with almond, vanilla, lemon, orange, etc.

8. Substitute the apple with any other fruits in season.

9. Substitute the strawberries with any other berries in season.

10. Add 1-2 tsp pure maple syrup or sucanat, if a sweeter taste is desired. The riper the fruit, the sweeter the sauce is naturally, without added sweetener.

11. Substitute the fresh fruit with soaked unsulphured dried fruits such as cranberries, raisins, bananas, prunes, apples, or apricots, and some of the soaking liquid.

12. Add chopped walnuts, almonds, or pecans, or pumpkin, sesame, or sunflower seeds or any combination of these. Sprinkle over, or mix into, the blended fruit.

Note: For information on how to soak dried fruits, see the recipe for **Prunes and Apricots for Toppings on Cereal.**

Fresh Homemade Applesauce

1 apple, unpeeled, cored   1-2 tsp pure maple syrup
½ tsp cinnamon   1-2 tbsp pure apple cider (optional)

1. Process in blender for about 30 seconds or Vita-Mix machine for about 10 seconds.
2. Can add a little pure apple cider, to thin it down or for added flavor.

Makes 1-2 servings

Prunes and Apricots for Topping on Cereal

½ cup of dried prunes, unsulphured
½ cup of dried apricots, unsulphured

Boiling water

1. Just cover with boiling water, in the same bowl, the dried prunes and dried apricots.
2. Cover the bowl with a thick tea towel. Let it sit overnight.
3. Serve 3-4 pieces of fruit, and some of the soaking liquid, per person, on the cereal.
4. Refrigerate the undrained fruit, in a covered container, for future use. Use all of the fruit topping within 1 week.

FROZEN FRUITS

Variations:
1. **Blended Frozen Bananas with Raisins**: blend 1 frozen banana and 2 tbsp. unsulphured raisins together. Can also add ¼ tsp almond extract to the blend.

2. **Frozen Bananas**: use only ripe bananas with brown spots on the skin. Peel bananas and freeze in zipper freezer bags. Slice and eat, or run them through the blender for a creamier consistency.

3. **Frozen Banana and Date Delight**: blend 1 frozen banana and ¼-½ cup soaked unsulphured dates (drained) together. Refreeze before eating. For a creamier consistency, run through the blender again just before serving. Makes 2 servings.

4. **Frozen Grapes**: remove seedless grapes from vines, wash thoroughly and dry. Put grapes into zipper freezer bags, removing any air. Freeze grapes and eat as desired.

5. Freeze other fruits, e.g. blueberries, peaches, pineapple, cantaloupe, mango, etc. Eat either as they are, or run them through the blender.

Note: When blending any of the above frozen fruit combinations, use "whip" speed on blender, or "high" speed on Vita-Mix machine. Refreeze after whipping and then serve. For a creamier blend, whip again very briefly, and serve.

DIPS, SPREADS, CRUDITIES

Beans as Dips, Spreads or Dressings

1. To make **Salad Dressings, Sauces or Sandwich Spreads,** simply adjust the amount of liquid in the recipe. Adding more liquid creates a thinner more dressing-like consistency. Eliminating some of the liquid creates a thicker consistency, which is more appropriate for a spread.
2. For most dips, dressings and spreads which use beans as a base, experiment with flavors, substituting one type of bean for another in the recipe. For example, substitute black beans for chickpeas, or vice versa. Or substitute pinto beans or black-eyed peas for chickpeas or black beans. *The sky is the limit when you become adventurous with your taste sensations!*

Cottage Cheese and Applesauce Spread

½ cup low fat cottage cheese   ½ tsp cinnamon
½ cup applesauce, commercial   ¼ tsp nutmeg or homemade*

1. Either mix all of the ingredients together for a more lumpy consistency, or blend together for a smoother consistency. (My preference is smooth, because it spreads more easily.)
2. After blending the mixture, let it sit for 30-60 minutes to blend the flavors.

Variation: Ricotta cheese can be substituted for the cottage cheese.

* See the recipe for Homemade Applesauce in the *Blended Fruit Toppings* chapter.

Makes 2 servings

EVENING WITH FRIENDS:

Raw Vegetable Platter

Bell peppers, tomatoes, mushrooms, broccoli, cauliflower, zucchini, carrots, celery, etc.

Baked Tortilla Chips, Pita Chips, Rice Chips, Rye Crackers, Flax Crackers

DIP 1:   **Salsa Chunky Dip**

½ cup medium salsa
½ cup plain, low fat yogurt
½ cup nonfat cottage cheese
1 tsp minced garlic

Put all ingredients together in a bowl. Mix well and let marinate in refrigerator for at least 2 hours.

DIP 2:   **Salsa Smooth Blend**

Above ingredients (Dip #1) + extra ¼ cup nonfat cottage cheese
Juice of 1 small fresh lemon
½ small onion, chopped
¼ cup fresh parsley, chopped
¼ tsp dry mustard powder
¼ tsp black pepper

Blend all of ingredients together in a blender. Let marinate in a covered container in refrigerator for at least 2 hours.

DIP 3:   **Spicy Tuna Dip**

1 can (6 ounces) water-pack tuna, drained and rinsed
Juice of 1 small fresh lemon
1 tsp minced garlic
½ medium onion, chopped
Few drops hot pepper sauce
½-1 tsp curry powder
¼ cup fresh parsley, chopped

Blend all ingredients together in blender, until almost smooth. Let marinate in refrigerator overnight.

DIP 4: **Veggie Bean Dip**

1-16 oz. can vegetarian baked beans
½ medium onion, chopped
Juice of 1 fresh lemon
1 tsp minced garlic
1 tsp dry mustard powder
½ tsp hot pepper sauce
¼-½ tsp Worcestershire sauce
¼ tsp black pepper
½ tsp Mrs. Dash

Blend all of ingredients together in blender. Let marinate in refrigerator for at least 2 hours.

Note: 1. To thicken any of above dips, use coffee grinder to grind raw oatmeal to a powder. Then add powder to mixture prior to marinating period.
2. All of the above dips make an excellent topping over baked potatoes, which have already been topped with steamed vegetables and all natural butter sprinkles.
3. **Bonus:** Adding ground oatmeal to a dip or spread increases the fiber content, as well.
4. If using a *Vita-Mix* to prepare these dips, a wonderful benefit is that only ½ of a whole lemon, skin, seeds, and all (only if organic) is required to replace the juice of 1 whole lemon. In fact, all of that labor-intensive mincing, chopping and squeezing of ingredients can be virtually eliminated!

Garlic Cheese Dip

1 cup nonfat cottage cheese
2 medium cloves of garlic
1 tbsp all natural butter sprinkles

1 tsp dried chives
⅛-¼ tsp fresh ground pepper

In a blender or Vita-Mix machine, blend all ingredients until smooth. Cover and refrigerate for at least 4 hours prior to serving.

Guacamole Dip

1 medium onion, chopped	1 tbsp Bragg Liquid Aminos
2 large cloves of garlic	⅛-¼ tsp hot pepper sauce
2 avocados	Juice of ½ fresh lemon
¼ cup plain, low fat yogurt	2 medium tomatoes. diced

In a blender or Vita-Mix machine, blend all ingredients, except the tomatoes, until smooth. In a bowl, mix the tomatoes into the blended mixture. Chill for at least 1 hour prior to serving. Garnish with chopped scallions and tomatoes.

Variation: For **Chickpea Guacamole Dip and Spread**, add 1 can (16 ounces) of chickpeas and an additional ½ cup of plain, low fat yogurt to the mixture, prior to blending all of the ingredients, except the tomatoes. For a chunkier consistency reduce the blending time. As above, *mix* the tomatoes in last.

Note: Chickpeas and **Garbanzo Beans** are the same thing!

Hummus: Chickpea Dip / Chickpea Spread

1 can (16 ounces) chickpeas, drained	2 tbsp tamari
2-3 medium cloves garlic	3 tbsp fresh parsley, chopped
2 tbsp tahini	¼ tsp cumin
Juice of 1 fresh lemon	⅛-¼ tsp hot pepper sauce

In a blender or Vita-Mix machine, blend all ingredients until smooth. It should be thick. Cover and refrigerate for at least 4 hours to meld the flavors.

Variation: For **Curried Chickpea Dip and Spread**, eliminate the tamari and cumin, and add 1-2 tsp curry powder, 1 tsp Spicy Mrs. Dash and 1 large tomato, diced. Blend all of the ingredients, except the tomatoes. Stir in tomatoes and chill as above.

Nippy Dippy

1 can (16 ounces) black beans, drained and rinsed
2 medium cloves of garlic
½ medium onion, chopped

½ tsp cumin
⅛-¼ tsp hot pepper sauce
Juice of 1 fresh lemon
Water, as needed

In a blender or Vita-Mix machine, blend all of the ingredients until smooth, about 1 minute. Only add water if necessary.

Ricotta Cheese and Fruit Spread

½ cup ricotta cheese
1 tbsp unsulphured raisins or dates

½ medium banana

In a blender or Vita-Mix machine, blend all ingredients together until smooth.

Variations:
1. Add 1 mango to the existing recipe.
2. Substitute 1 mango for the banana in the recipe.
3. Substitute with any fresh ripe fruit in season.
4. Substitute the dried fruit with ½ of a fresh, ripe avocado.
5. Substitute the ricotta cheese with nonfat cottage cheese.
6. Substitute the dried fruit in the recipe with dried apricots.
7. Eliminate the dried fruit in the recipe.

Makes 2 servings

Seafood Dip / Seafood Spread

½ lb. crabmeat, flaked
4 ounces low fat cream cheese
½ cup plain, low fat yogurt
½ medium onion, diced

1-2 tsp Bragg Liquid Aminos
⅛-¼ tsp hot pepper sauce
1 tbsp prepared horseradish
Paprika

1. In a blender, blend the cream cheese and yogurt together.
2. In a bowl, thoroughly combine all of the ingredients, including the blended mixture.
3. Cover and refrigerate for at least 30 minutes. Sprinkle with paprika.

Note: Tuna, Salmon, Shrimp, can be substituted for the crabmeat.

Tangy Chili Dip

1 can (16 ounces) pinto beans
1 cup plain, low fat yogurt
½ cup canned green chilis
½ medium onion, chopped

¼ tsp cumin
2 tbsp Parmesan cheese
2 tsp chili powder

In a blender or Vita-Mix machine, blend all ingredients until smooth. Cover and refrigerate for several hours prior to serving.

SOUPS

Curried Lentil Soup

1 lb. lentils
10 cups of water
1 large onion, chopped
3 medium cloves of garlic, minced
2 large carrots, sliced
1 large stalk of celery, chopped
3 large unpeeled potatoes, chopped

2-3 tsp curry powder
¼ cup fresh parsley, chopped
½ inch fresh ginger root, grated
1-2 tsp Spicy Mrs. Dash
¼ tsp fresh ground pepper
Plain, low fat yogurt

1. Put all of the ingredients, except the yogurt, into a Dutch oven. Bring to a boil.
2. Cover and simmer for 1 hour, until lentils are tender.
3. Top each serving with a dollop of yogurt.

Makes 8-10 servings

Instant Miso Soup

Boil 1 cup of water. Pour a small amount of the water into a cup. Cream 1 tbsp of red or barley miso in this water, and then pour the rest of the water into the cup. Mix and then top with tiny tofu pieces and finely chopped scallions. *A healthy mid-afternoon pickup!*

Lentil Vegetable Soup

1 lb. lentils
10 cups water
1 large onion, chopped
2 large cloves of garlic, minced
2 large carrots, sliced
2 large stalks celery, chopped
1 small green pepper, chopped
1 carton (26 ounces) Pomi tomatoes
1 lb. fresh spinach, chopped

¼ cup fresh parsley, chopped
½ tsp dried oregano
½ tsp ground cumin
1 bay leaf
½ tsp dried red pepper
¼ tsp fresh ground pepper
1 tsp Mrs. Dash
Juice of one lemon

1. Put all of the ingredients, except lemon juice, into a Dutch oven, and bring to a boil.
2. Cover and simmer for about 1 hour, until the lentils are tender, stirring occasionally.
3. Add lemon juice when cooking is complete, and let the pot sit off the heat, covered, for 15 minutes, before serving.

Variations:
1. **Potato Lentil Soup-1**: add 4 unpeeled, chopped potatoes to the Dutch oven, with the rest of the ingredients, and cook for 1 hour as above. Add lemon juice at end of cooking and let sit before serving.
2. **Potato Lentil Soup-2**: eliminate the carton of tomatoes and the spinach, and add 6 unpeeled, chopped potatoes. The lemon juice is optional with this variation.

Note: This soup tastes even better the next day. But don't boil it the next day when you are reheating it, as this can result in a bitter aftertaste.

Makes 8-10 servings

Minestrone Soup

4 cups hot water
2 large cloves of garlic, minced
1 medium onion, chopped
2 large carrots, chopped
1 large stalk of celery, chopped
1 carton (26 ounces) Pomi tomatoes
¼ cup fresh parsley, chopped
3 medium unpeeled potatoes, chopped
1 tsp dried basil
1 tbsp Spicy Mrs. Dash

½ cup whole grain macaroni
2 small zucchini, chopped
1 cup kale, chopped
1 cup spinach, chopped
½ cup green cabbage, shredded
1 can (16 ounces) kidney beans,
    drained and rinsed
¼-½ tsp hot pepper sauce (optional)
Parmesan or Romano cheese

1. In a Dutch oven, bring the 4 cups of water to a boil. Add all of the ingredients in the first column and return to a boil.
2. Cover and simmer for about 20 minutes.
3. Add the rest of the ingredients, except the hot pepper sauce, and simmer for another 25 minutes. More water can be added as necessary, if the soup becomes too thick.
4. Add hot pepper sauce when cooking is complete, and let marinate for about 10 minutes before serving.
5. Top each serving with a sprinkling of Parmesan or Romano cheese.

Makes 6-8 servings

Miso Soup with Tofu Cubes

4 cups of water
4 pieces, 1 inch each, of wakame
   seaweed, dried
½ cup of water
½ cup carrots, thinly sliced

½ cup daikon radish, thinly sliced
4 mushrooms, quartered
4 ounces firm tofu, cubed
4 tbsp red or barley miso
2 scallions, finely sliced

1. Reconstitute the wakame in ½ cup of water.
2. Bring 4 cups water to a boil. Add carrot and daikon and cook for 2 minutes.
3. Add mushrooms and cook for another 3 minutes.
4. Reduce to medium heat and add tofu cubes. Water should not boil after tofu is added. (Tofu will become hard if it is boiled.)
5. Add wakame and soaking water, when tofu floats to the surface. Do not boil water!
6. Remove ⅓-½ cup of water from the pot and use to cream the miso. Only when the paste has been fully dissolved, is it returned to the pot. Do not boil the soup!
7. After soup is removed from the heat, sprinkle with scallions and serve.

Makes 4 servings

Split Pea Soup

1 lb. dried green split peas	½ tsp Real Salt
8 cups hot water	1 tsp Spicy Mrs. Dash
4 large carrots, chopped	¼ tsp fresh ground pepper
4 large stalks celery, chopped	½ tsp dried basil
1 medium onion, chopped	¼ tsp ground cumin
2 large cloves of garlic, minced	½ tsp dried marjoram
1 tbsp pure virgin olive oil (optional)	Juice of 1 fresh lemon
Hot pepper sauce, to taste	

1. Sort and wash peas. Place in a Dutch oven with the hot water.
2. Add the remaining ingredients, except the lemon juice and hot pepper sauce.
3. Bring to a boil, and then simmer for about 1 ½ hours, until the peas are soft and the vegetables are tender.
4. When the soup is finished cooking, add the juice of the lemon, and the hot pepper sauce. Let the soup sit for about 15 minutes before serving to allow the flavors to develop.

Variation: **Mediterranean Lentil Soup**: add 1 carton (26 ounces) of Pomi tomatoes, 1 medium green pepper, chopped, and ½ inch fresh ginger, grated, with the rest of the ingredients, at the start of cooking. Then add 3 medium zucchini, sliced, 10 minutes before cooking is complete. As in Step #4 above, add lemon juice and hot pepper sauce, and let sit 15 minutes before serving.

Note: This soup tastes even better the next day. But don't bring it to a boil again after the lemon juice and hot pepper sauce have been added! It will develop a slightly bitter after taste.

Makes 6-8 servings

SANDWICHES

Almond Butter, Tomato and Sprouts on Multigrain Bread

Though a bit high in fat, this sandwich is packed full of nutrition!

Go easy on the almond butter; no more than 2 tbsp. The rest is self-explanatory. Other veggies that go well with almond butter include cucumber slices, green pepper rings, onions, avocado (Cut the almond butter down to 1 tbsp if you use ¼ of an avocado.), fruit preserves, dried fruits, chunky salsa and radish slices.

Note: Always buy fresh ground, natural almond butter out of a refrigerated case instead of taking it from a shelf, as it tends to go rancid quickly in warmer temperatures. And due to being ground, there is more surface area of the product exposed to the oxygen in the air, which is the reason for rancidity occurring in the first place.

Variations: Any of the wide variety of delicious beans available today can be substituted for the pinto beans. See the long list of beans to choose from in the chapter on *Scoop on Beans and Lentils*.

Select vegetables in season, and experiment with various combinations. You can also use any raw or cooked vegetables you have leftover from dinner.

Bean Burritos with Diced Vegetables

1 can (16 oz) Pinto Beans, organic
1 cup fresh vegetables, diced

4 oz nonfat grated cheese
4 sprouted corn or whole wheat
   tortillas

1. Put beans and vegetables into a medium-sized saucepan and heat on low until just warm. If it begins to simmer, you have over-heated the mixture. Remove it immediately.
2. Spoon ¼ of the heated beans and vegetables, slightly off center, onto a sprouted corn or sprouted wheat tortilla.
3. Sprinkle 1 oz of nonfat grated cheese onto each of the burritos prior to folding.
4. Fold the short sides of the tortilla over the filling. Then fold over the long sides, placing the seam side down on the plate.

Chicken Pita Sandwich

1 ½ cups skinless chicken breast
   cooked and diced
1 stalk of celery, diced
½ green pepper, diced
½ cup unwaxed cucumber, diced
4 scallions, diced
Juice of ½ fresh lemon

2 tbsp Nayonnaise
¼ cup plain, low fat yogurt
1 tbsp Dijon mustard
⅛ tsp Tabasco sauce
2 large pitas, whole grain, in halves
Alfalfa sprouts

Mix all of the ingredients together except the pitas and the sprouts. Fill each of 4 pockets with the filling and top each with alfalfa sprouts.

Variations:
1. Substitute the Dijon mustard with 1-2 tsp curry powder.
2. **Tuna Salad Sandwiches**: substitute the chicken with 1 can (6.5 ounces) water-packed, drained and rinsed tuna. Use 8 slices of whole grain bread, or 4 large whole grain rolls.
3. Fresh green leaf lettuce and slices of tomato can be used on each sandwich, or stuffed into the pita pockets.

Eggless "Egg" Salad Sandwich

½ lb. firm tofu
1 medium carrot, shredded
2 scallions, finely chopped
¼ cup fresh parsley, chopped

1 tbsp tahini
1 tbsp Dijon mustard
1 tsp Spicy Mrs. Dash
¼ tsp fresh ground pepper

1. Mash the drained tofu with a fork to form very loose curds.
2. Combine thoroughly with the rest of the ingredients.
3. Spread on wholegrain bread, toast or crackers. Also great with low fat tortilla chips, or with vegetables, as a **Tofu Vegetable Dip.**

Note: This product is best used immediately. It does not store well.

Marinated Tofu and Sprout Sandwich

1. Slice an 8 ounce block of extra firm tofu into ¼ to ½ inch thick slices.
2. Place the slices side by side in a shallow oven proof glass baking dish.
3. Cover the slices with a marinade of your choice (see **Marinades** chapter). Be adventurous and try a different one each time you do it.
4. Then cover the dish and refrigerate for at least 4 hours, preferably overnight.
5. When ready to serve, simply place several slices of marinated tofu on a slice of whole grain bread, add some fresh tomato slices and a generous portion of alfalfa sprouts.

So you're in a hurry? You have no time to marinate tofu, but that's what you want to eat. Place a few slices of tofu on a flat plate and pour some Bragg Liquid Aminos over them, followed by some fresh squeezed lemon or lime juice. Wait about 5 minutes, and there you have it! Marinated tofu in a flash!

Variations:
1. **Marinated Tempeh Sandwich:** substitute the tofu slices with any of the many varieties and flavors of tempeh.
2. A **Tempeh Sandwich** does not have to start with marinated tempeh. Tempeh comes in many flavors which are very tasty as they are. Dress this sandwich as suggested for the marinated tofu sandwich. You could also add a touch of Dijon mustard or Nayonnaise.

Nonfat Cheese and Avocado Pita Pocket with Sprouts

1. Into a whole wheat pita pocket, put strips of fresh, ripe avocado; about ¼ of a medium avocado.
2. Sprinkle 1 ounce of grated nonfat cheese over the avocado.
3. Stuff the pocket with chunky salsa and clover or alfalfa sprouts.
4. Pour **Tahini and Buttermilk Dressing,** see *Salad Dressings* chapter, over the filling in the pocket.

Salmon Dill Sandwich on Sprouted Bread

½ cup plain, low fat yogurt
2 tbsp Vegenaise
2 scallions, finely chopped
1 tsp dried dill weed
1 clove of garlic, minced

⅛-¼ tsp hot pepper sauce
Mrs. Dash, to taste
1 stalk of celery, diced
1 can (7.5 ounces) water-packed
    salmon, drained and rinsed

1. Blend all of the seasoning ingredients together well.
2. Add the salmon and celery, and combine thoroughly with the blended seasoning sauce.
3. Cover and refrigerate for at least 1 hour.
4. Prepare sandwiches on sprouted wholegrain bread. Delicious with alfalfa sprouts, tomato slices, and green or red leafy lettuces.

Turkey Burger, American Style

1 lb. ground turkey breast
½ medium onion, diced
1 stalk of celery, diced
½ medium red or green pepper, diced
2 cloves of garlic, minced

1 tsp paprika
¼ tsp fresh ground pepper
1 tbsp Bragg Liquid Aminos
4 whole wheat burger buns
Dijon mustard, lettuce,
    tomatoes

1. Combine the ground turkey and the seasonings.
2. Shape the mixture into 4 patties.
3. Grill, or pan fry in a nonstick skillet until cooked throughout, about 5 minutes per side.

Variations: Dress your burger with a variety of toppings such as:

cucumber slices
alfalfa or clover sprouts
nonfat chili beans
Nayonnaise
grated nonfat cheese

radishes
chutneys
onion slices
Dijon mustard
Gourmet mustards

sliced mushrooms
chunky salsa
tomato slices
shredded lettuce
grilled asparagus

Turkey Burger, Asian Style

1 lb. ground turkey breast
½ medium onion, diced
1 tbsp soy sauce, reduced sodium
2 cloves of garlic, minced

½ inch fresh ginger root, grated
1 ½ tsp cold pressed sesame oil
¼ tsp dry mustard powder

1.   Thoroughly combine all of the ingredients.
2.   Shape the mixture into 4 patties.
3.   Grill, or pan fry in a nonstick skillet until cooked throughout, about 5 minutes each side.
4.   See Variations above for ways to dress your burger.

Turkey Loaf on Whole Grain Kaiser Roll

See recipe in *Main Entrees* chapter for Turkey Loaf.
Spread Dijon mustard or Nayonnaise, or a combination of both on the Roll.
Slices of each of, a red onion, and a ripe tomato, add a flavorful accent.

Turkey and Tomato on Rye

1.   On 100% rye bread, spread a combination of 1 tsp Nayonnaise and 1 tsp Dijon or grain mustard.
2.   Place 2 ounces of thinly sliced turkey breast on the spread.
3.   Dress with green leaf lettuce, and cucumber and tomato slices.
4.   Top with another slice of wholesome rye bread.

Whole Wheat English Muffin Pizzas

1.   Spread some bottled nonfat natural marinara sauce onto 2 halves of an English muffin.
2.   Sprinkle a little bottled minced garlic and some diced scallions over the sauce.
3.   Arrange slices of fresh mushrooms, and some grated nonfat or low fat cheddar or mozzarella cheese on top.
4.   Sprinkle with Parmesan cheese and fresh ground pepper.
5.   Bake, on a lightly sprayed cookie sheet, at 450°, until cheeses are melted.

SALADS

Broccoli-Cauliflower Salad

¼ cup buttermilk
¼ cup Nayonnaise
2 tbsp plain, low fat yogurt
1 tbsp sucanat
¼ tsp fresh ground pepper
Juice of 1 fresh lemon or lime

2 cups broccoli florets, small
2 cups cauliflower florets, small
2 scallions, chopped
½ large red pepper, chopped
½ small red onion, chopped
Hot pepper sauce (optional)

1. Blend all of the ingredients together in the first column.
2. In a large bowl, combine all of the vegetables in the second column.
3. Pour the dressing over the vegetables and toss lightly. Store in the refrigerator.

Note: For added flavor and nutrition, a handful of seeds, such as sesame, pumpkin or sunflower, can be sprinkled on top just prior to serving.

Makes 4-6 servings

Caesar Salad

Tear the leaves of 1 large head of romaine lettuce into large bite-size pieces. Toss gently, but thoroughly, with the Caesar Dressing in the Dressings section. Top with nonfat seasoned croutons, available at most health food stores.

Variations:
1. **Chicken Caesar** or a **Fish Caesar**, top the salad with pieces of grilled chicken or fish, or canned tuna.
2. **Seafood Caesar** by topping with a mixture of grilled shrimp, scallops, crabmeat, lobster and whitefish.
3. Sprinkle 2 tbsp of grated low or nonfat cheese and a few sesame seeds on top.

Citrus Rice and Bean Salad

2 cups brown rice, cooked
3 scallions, finely chopped
1 can (16 ounces) black beans,
  drained and rinsed
1 can (6 ounces) water-packed tuna
  or salmon, drained and rinsed
1 large orange, seedless, peeled
  and chopped

½ cup orange juice, fresh
  squeezed
2 tbsp fresh cilantro, chopped
1 tbsp pure virgin olive oil
¼ cup low fat, plain yogurt
2 tbsp coarse grain mustard or
  Dijon mustard

1. In a Vita-Mix machine or blender combine all of the ingredients in the second column. Refrigerate until ready to use. Can be made ahead
2. In a large bowl, combine all of the ingredients in the first column.
3. Pour the prepared dressing over the rice combination, and toss until well mixed.
4. Refrigerate until ready to serve.

Variations:
1. Substitute the tuna or salmon with 6-8 ounces (about 1 cup) of diced skinless chicken or turkey breast.
2. Substitute the tuna or salmon with **Marinated Tofu or Tempeh.** (See recipe under **Sandwich Fillings** or under **Lively Chef's Salad.**)
3. For a unique flavor, substitute the fresh squeezed orange juice in the dressing, with the juice of 1-2 fresh limes.

Makes 6 servings

Crabmeat Salad

1 lb. crabmeat, chopped
1 tbsp pure virgin olive oil
2 medium cloves of garlic, minced
Juice of 2-3 fresh limes (½ cup juice)
1 tsp Mrs. Dash or Spicy Mrs. Dash
½ tsp red pepper flakes
1 small red onion, diced

2 large tomatoes, chopped
1 medium red pepper, chopped
1 medium green pepper, diced
2 tbsp fresh cilantro, chopped
⅛-¼ tsp hot pepper sauce

1. Combine all of the seasonings. Let sit while you chop the vegetables and meat.
2. Add the chopped vegetables, cilantro and crabmeat to the sauce.
3. Cover and refrigerate for at least 1 hour prior to serving. Keeps up to 3 days in the refrigerator.

Variations:
1. Instead of crabmeat, any variety of cooked white fish or seafood can be used.
2. **Bay Scallop Salad:** just substitute 1 lb. of bay scallops for the crabmeat. Scallops are especially good prepared with this recipe.
3. **Creamy Crabmeat Salad:** to serve over a baked potato or grains, reduce the amount of lime juice to that of 1 fresh lime and add ½ cup plain, low fat yogurt. Refrigerate for at least 1 hour.

Makes 4 servings

Creamy Potato Salad

¾ cup plain, low fat yogurt
¼ cup Nayonnaise
¼ cup organic cider vinegar
2 medium cloves of garlic, minced
1 tsp Mrs. Dash or Spicy Mrs. Dash
1 tsp curry powder
½-1 tsp dry mustard powder
½ tsp fresh ground pepper
Hot pepper sauce, to taste (optional)

8 medium potatoes, baked with skin
½ large red onion, chopped
2 large celery stalks, chopped
5 radishes, sliced
2 free-range hard-boiled eggs, sliced (optional)

1. In a large bowl, thoroughly combine all of the ingredients in the first column.
2. Chop the unpeeled potatoes into small bite-size pieces, and add to the bowl.
3. Add the remaining ingredients in the second column, except eggs, and toss gently.
4. Top the salad with the egg slices.
5. Cover and refrigerate for at least 30 to 60 minutes.

Makes 8 servings

Cucumber and Tomato Raita

2 cups plain, low fat yogurt
2-3 large cloves of garlic, minced
2 tbsp fresh mint, chopped
1-2 tsp Spicy Mrs. Dash

1 medium onion, thinly sliced
1 large fresh, unwaxed cucumber
2 large fresh tomatoes
⅛-¼ tsp hot pepper sauce
(optional)

1. Blend the yogurt, garlic and seasonings together. Set aside.
2. Dice the unpeeled cucumber and let it drain on paper towels.
3. Dice the tomatoes, and prepare the onions. Then combine the cucumbers, onions and tomatoes with the yogurt mixture.
4. Chill thoroughly, allowing at least 1-2 hours for the flavors to marinate and blend.

Variations: **Zucchini Salad**: substitute the cucumber with 3 medium zucchini. For another version of **Zucchini Salad**, substitute the cucumber with the zucchini, eliminate the yogurt mixture, and top with the **Spicy Dressing**.

Note: This is a delicious side dish with spicy entrees, and with East Indian and Middle Eastern menus.

Makes 4-6 servings

Curried Brown Rice Salad

6 cups cooked brown rice
4 cups cooked chicken or turkey
   breast, diced
2 large stalks of celery, chopped
1 small green pepper, chopped
1 small red pepper, chopped
1 can (16 ounces) chickpeas, drained
   and rinsed
1 cup fresh pineapple chunks
1 small red onion, diced

1 cup plain, low fat yogurt
⅓ cup balsamic vinegar
3 medium cloves of garlic, minced
2 tsp sesame oil
1 tbsp Bragg Liquid Aminos
2 tbsp sucanat
2 tsp curry powder
1 tsp dry mustard powder
1 tsp Mrs. Dash
¼ tsp fresh ground pepper

1. In a blender, thoroughly mix all of the dressing ingredients in the second column. Cover and refrigerate until ready to use.
2. In a large bowl, combine all of the salad ingredients in the first column.
3. Pour chilled dressing over the salad combination. Toss gently.
4. Cover and refrigerate for at least 30 minutes to blend the flavors.

Variations:
1. Substitute the chicken or turkey with equal portions of chopped fish, or shellfish, or crabmeat, or a combination of scallops, shrimp, and whitefish.
2. Eliminate chicken or turkey, and add 1 cup of fresh green peas.
3. Substitute the poultry with marinated tofu or tempeh slices or cubes. Double the dressing recipe above and marinate the tofu or tempeh slices in this mixture, overnight, prior to use.
4. **Curried Brown Rice, Salmon and Vegetable Salad**: substitute the chicken or turkey with 1 can (15 ounces) water-packed salmon, drained and rinsed, or 3 cups diced fresh baked salmon. Substitute the chickpeas with 1 can (16 ounces) of black-eyed peas. And add 1 cup of finely chopped raw broccoli and/or raw cauliflower.

Makes 8-10 servings

Fresh Organic Salad Mix

Available, as is, ready to use, from various sources: farms which produce organic produce for wholesale and for mail order, see *References & Resources* chapter, health food stores, farmers' markets, and more recently, produce sections of many grocery stores.

Greens and Tomatoes

Mix about 3 different green (or red) leafy vegetables together and top with your favorite, in-season tomatoes, in chunks or slices, and your favorite dressing.

Kitchen Sink Salad

This is basically what it sounds like! Anything you need to use up is perfect for this salad. As long as it is fresh, natural and organic, throw it in. Include some leafy greens, a few other veggies, a little protein (tofu, legumes, fish or chicken), and top it off with some colorful fresh tomatoes. Select one of your favorite low fat or nonfat dressings and *enjoy to your heart's content, your body's content, and your mind's content!!*

Lively Chef's Salad

1 head dark green or red lettuce	6 cherry tomatoes, in halves
6 mushrooms, sliced	½ cup chickpeas
½ large green pepper, in thin strips	½ cup kidney beans
3 scallions, chopped	Marinated cubes of tempeh or tofu
2 medium cloves of garlic, minced	Parmesan or Romano cheese

Dressing of your choice. See *Salad Dressings* chapter.

1. In a large bowl, combine all of the ingredients in the first column, and toss lightly.
2. Add the cherry tomatoes and toss very gently, just to distribute them.
3. Top each serving of salad with a spoonful of each of the beans, and a few cubes of tempeh or tofu. Sprinkle about 1 tbsp of cheese onto each serving as well.

Variations:
1. Leftover pieces of chicken or fish can be used instead of the beans.
2. Grated low or nonfat cheese can be used in place of Parmesan or Romano.
3. The basic salad, without the beans and tempeh, can be used as a side salad for another meal.

Note: To make **Marinated Tempeh**, or **Marinated Tofu**, simply slice the tempeh or the extra firm tofu into ¼-½ inch thick slices, and place these slices side by side in a shallow glass dish. Cover the slices with a marinade of your choice, see *Marinades* chapter. Then cover the dish and refrigerate for at least 4 hours, preferably overnight, if possible. When ready to serve, cut the slices into the size of cubes you desire. Whatever you do not use can be kept, covered, in the refrigerator, for up to 5 days, and used as desired.
Makes 4 servings

Low Fat Creamy Coleslaw

1 large head of green cabbage, sliced
1 medium onion, chopped
2 large carrots, shredded
3 tbsp Nayonnaise
½ cup plain, low fat yogurt

¼ cup balsamic vinegar
Juice of 1 fresh lemon
1 tbsp Bragg Liquid Aminos
½ tsp fresh ground pepper
1 tbsp pure maple syrup

1. Blend everything, but the vegetables together. Let sit.
2. In a large bowl, toss the vegetables together.
3. Pour the dressing over the vegetables and toss well to combine. Chill thoroughly.

Variation: **Nippy Dijon Coleslaw**: eliminate the lemon juice and maple syrup. Reduce the Bragg liquid Aminos to 1 tsp and add 2 tbsp Dijon mustard, ¼ to ½ tsp dry mustard powder, ⅛ tsp celery seeds and 1 tbsp tahini.

Makes 6-8 servings

Marinated Tomato, Onion and Cucumber Slices

Marinate the vegetables in a vinaigrette or herb dressing for 30-60 minutes. See *Salad Dressings* chapter. Cover and refrigerate while marinating.

Mediterranean Potato Salad

1 tbsp pure virgin olive oil
Juice of 1 fresh lemon
¼ cup balsamic vinegar
½ medium ripe avocado
½ cup plain, low fat yogurt
2 medium cloves of garlic, minced
1 tsp dried tarragon
¼ tsp fresh ground pepper
1 tsp Spicy Mrs. Dash

6 medium potatoes, baked
1 large stalk celery, chopped
4 scallions, chopped
½ large green pepper, chopped
1 large tomato, chopped
10-15 black olives, chopped

1. In a large bowl, blend all of the ingredients in the first column thoroughly.
2. Chop the unpeeled potatoes into small bite-size pieces, and add to the bowl.
3. Add the remaining ingredients in the second column, and toss gently.
4. Cover and refrigerate for at least 30 to 60 minutes before serving.

Makes 6-8 servings

Red and Green Cabbage Slaw / Creamy Cabbage Slaw

1 medium head of red cabbage
1 medium head of green cabbage
2 large carrots, shredded
1 medium onion, chopped
1 large yellow pepper, in thin strips
⅓ cup Nayonnaise

⅓ cup plain, low fat yogurt
¼ cup organic cider vinegar
1 tbsp pure maple syrup
¼ tsp celery seeds
¼ to ½ tsp hot pepper sauce

1. Blend the Nayonnaise, yogurt, vinegar, syrup, seeds and hot pepper sauce together.
2. Thinly slice the red and green cabbages.
3. Toss all of the vegetables together in a large bowl.
4. Pour the dressing over the vegetables and toss well to combine. Chill thoroughly.

Makes 8-10 servings

Romaine, Watercress and Tomato Salad

1 head of romaine lettuce
2 cups watercress leaves
2 scallions, finely chopped

3-5 radishes, sliced
1 large tomato, in chunks

1. Tear the romaine leaves into bite-size pieces.
2. Snip the watercress leaves into manageable pieces, with kitchen shears.
3. Toss all of the ingredients together and drizzle your favorite dressing over the salad.

Variation: **Romaine and Tomato Salad**: eliminate the watercress. Then give this salad a real kick with a watercress dressing. See *Salad Dressings* chapter

Makes 4 servings

So What's in a Salad Bar?

The following is a set of lists to help you develop your own repertoire of salad bar ingredients! Be creative. Select different items from time to time, for interest and variety. Widen your scope of experience with respect to flavor and color combinations.

Start with the Greens: *Each week select a few of these to include in your own potential salad bar.*

Alfalfa sprouts
Amaranth
Arugula
Beet greens (tops)
Bibb lettuce
Cabbage, red and green
Celery tops
Chicory
Chinese cabbage
Cilantro
Clover sprouts
Collard greens
Corn salad (Lambs lettuce)
Dandelion greens

Then add Some Variety in Colors and Textures *with more dense salad items. Use in smaller quantities.*

Artichoke hearts, in water
Asparagus
Beets, raw, grated, or cooked
Bell peppers, red, green & yellow
Broccoli, raw or lightly steamed
Broccolini, raw or lightly steamed
Carrots, shredded, sliced, steamed
Cauliflower, raw or lightly steamed
Celery
Chives
Corn
Cucumbers
Green & yellow beans
Jicama

Endive
Escarole
Green Cabbage
Ithaca Head Lettuce
Kale
Kolrabi
Lambsquarter
Mint
Mustard greens
Parsley
Red Cabbage
Red or Green leaf lettuce
Rocket
Romaine lettuce
Savoy Cabbage
Spinach
Swiss Chard
Watercress

Legumes: chickpeas, black-eyed peas
black beans, edamame, kidney
    beans northern beans
Mushrooms, brown and white
Okra
Onions, red and white, Bermuda
Parsnips
Pickles, low sodium
Pickled peppers, low sodium
Potatoes, cooked
Radishes, red and daikon
Scallions
Sea vegetables
Snow peas
Sweet peas
Sweet potatoes
Sprouts, any variety
Squash, winter & summer
Tomatoes, any variety
Zucchini

And Then Complete the Makings of a Great Salad, before you dress it!

Avocados, fresh and ripe (Go easy!)
Bamboo shoots
Bread, wholegrain varieties
Brown rice, cooked
Buckwheat groats, cooked
Bulgur wheat, cooked
Cheese, nonfat or low fat
Chili Peppers
Chicken, skinless breast, cooked
Crackers, wholegrain, nonfat
Croutons, wholegrain, nonfat
Eggs, free-range, hard boiled
Fish, cooked
Ginger Root
Herbs and Spices
Kasha, cooked
Marinated beans, nonfat or low fat

Millet, cooked
Nuts, esp. almonds (Go very easy!)
Olives, black or green (Go easy!)
Pasta, wholegrain or vegetable, cooked
Poppy seeds
Pumpkin seeds
Quinoa, cooked
Raisins
Salmon, canned, water-packed
Salsa
Sesame seeds and Tahini (Go Easy!)
Sunflower seeds
Shellfish, cooked, sparingly
Tempeh, as is, or marinated
Tofu, as is, or marinated
Tuna, canned, water-packed
Turkey, skinless breast, cooked

The Grand Finale for Any Salad Bar is, of course, a variety of delicious salad dressings and flavorful dips, for nonfat tortilla chips, nonfat crackers, and vegetable sticks. (See *Dips, Spreads & Crudities; and Salad Dressings.*)

Spinach and Mushroom Salad / Spinach and Tomato Salad

Mix any variety of spinach (some examples are leaf or spring spinach, Malabar spinach, and New Zealand spinach) with sliced brown or white mushrooms and/or tomatoes. Dressings with a lemon, lime or mustard base make a tasty accent.

Three-Bean Salad

¼ cup red wine vinegar
2 tbsp organic cider vinegar
1 tbsp pure virgin olive oil
2 medium cloves of garlic, minced
¼-½ tsp cayenne pepper
1 tbsp pure maple syrup
½ tsp dry mustard powder

½ medium red onion, sliced
2 large stalks of celery, chopped
2 cans (16 ounces each) red kidney beans, drained and rinsed
1 can (16 ounces) chickpeas, drained and rinsed
1 lb. fresh green beans, lightly cooked

1. Combine all of the ingredients in the first column, in a large bowl.
2. Add the onions, celery and beans, and toss gently. Cover and refrigerate.

Note: Make this salad the day before to allow the flavors to blend. Though it must be kept refrigerated when made ahead, this salad is best served at room temperature for fullest flavor.

Makes 8-10 servings

Tossed Green Salad / Mixed Green Salad

You can use the organic salad mix, or mix your own variety of green, leafy vegetables. Look for the darkest green leaves, or the brightest red leaves. *Iceberg lettuce is not, by itself, a tossed green salad, as most restaurants would have you believe.* Some greens for you to explore, include:

arugula	Chinese cabbage	dandelion greens
beet greens	cilantro	endive
bibb lettuce	collard greens	escarole
chicory	corn salad (lamb's lettuce)	green cabbage
head lettuce (Ithaca)	parsley	Savoy cabbage
kale	red cabbage	spinach
leaflettuce (Buttercrunch)	rocket	Swiss chard
mustard greens	romaine	watercress

Tri-Color Pasta and Vegetable Salad

1 package (16 ounces) fresh vegetable
    pasta: 3 colors in one package
1 can (16 ounces) black beans,
    drained and rinsed
2 medium zucchini, thickly sliced
½ lb. fresh broccoli, cauliflower or
    baby carrots, chopped
1 red and 1 green pepper, chopped
3 scallions, chopped
¼ cup fresh cilantro, chopped

1 cup plain, low fat yogurt
1 cup chunky fresh salsa, medium
3 medium cloves of garlic, minced
½ tsp ground cumin
½ tsp fresh ground pepper
Juice of 1 fresh lime
Parmesan or Romano cheese, for
    topping as desired

1. Combine all of the ingredients in the second column, except the cheese.
2. Cook the pasta according to the directions on the package.
3. Combine the cooked pasta, vegetables and dressing. Bake at 325 degrees for 30 minutes in a lightly sprayed casserole dish. *(The vegetables should not be soft.)*

Variations:

1. Instead of heating this salad, serve it as a cold salad. As above, combine the cooked pasta, raw vegetables, and dressing. Chill thoroughly before serving. Sprinkle with Parmesan or Romano.

2. Substitute any vegetables in season you desire for the carrots, broccoli or cauliflower, or use a combination of fresh vegetables.

3. Grated low or nonfat cheddar or mozzarella cheese can be used instead of Parmesan or Romano.

4. To make a **Tuna, Salmon or Crab Pasta Salad**, simply replace the beans in the recipe with a 6 ounce can of tuna or salmon, or 6-8 ounces of flaked crabmeat. Serve hot or cold.

5. **Pasta Salad**: see the above variations listed. Instead of using the tri-color variety of pasta, experiment with any wholegrain, rice pasta or vegetable pasta that appeals to you. Eat it cold or hot. The choice is yours!

6. A quick and easy **Pasta and Vegetable Salad**: Great for those sudden potluck invitations or a very hurried dinner. Make it by cooking a batch of pasta, and a batch of frozen vegetables (the Mediterranean variety is delicious!). And then toss them together with any salad dressing of your choice. See *Salad Dressings* chapter. Or just use the dressing from the above recipe.

Makes 6-8 servings

SALAD DRESSINGS

General Guidelines for Making and Using Dressings

1. The easiest and fastest way to prepare salad dressings is by using a Vita-Mix machine. This eliminates the chopping and mincing steps. The ingredients can simply be thrown into the machine and it does the chopping, mincing, blending and emulsifying.
2. Dressings are best prepared at least 30 minutes prior to being served. The flavors need time to marinate. Overnight is even better.
3. Dressings will usually keep well for up to 1 week, if refrigerated and stored in a tightly covered bottle or container.
4. Shake the bottle well just before each use, as ingredients tend to separate when dressing is sitting for any length of time.
5. If you have just a little of two different dressings left, don't throw them out! Try mixing them for a new taste.
6. The following dressings are not limited to use on salads. Be adventurous and try various dressings on steamed vegetables, as well as baked, grilled or broiled fish, poultry and wild game meats.

Balsamic Garlic Dressing

2 tbsp pure virgin olive oil
¾ cup balsamic vinegar
5 medium cloves of garlic, minced

½ cup fresh parsley, chopped
1 tsp Spicy Mrs. Dash

Either mix in a bottle or blend in a blender. Let sit in a covered glass bottle or jar, on a shelf that gets direct sunlight for at least half a day, to marinate the flavors.

Variation: **Balsamic Dressing:** (basic), reduce the garlic to 2 cloves and add ¼-½ tsp fresh ground pepper. Use the same procedure for preparation.

Caesar Salad Dressing

This is best done in a Vita-Mix machine. Failing that, use a blender.

Because of the potential for salmonella poisoning from raw eggs, I have resorted to an egg substitute in this recipe. Since everything else in the recipe is fresh and natural, this is still a much more wholesome alternative than the many commercial varieties! And though there is some fat in this recipe, when divided into 6 servings, it is not enough to do any harm. And it's certainly a more healthy variety of oil than the hydrogenated oils used in the bottles of dressings found on the grocery store shelves! So go ahead and enjoy a treat!

2 tbsp pure virgin olive oil
⅓ cup red wine vinegar
¼ cup egg substitute
2 medium cloves of garlic, minced
1 tbsp Dijon mustard

½-1 tsp Spicy Mrs. Dash
¼-½ tsp fresh ground pepper
3 tbsp Parmesan or Romano cheese
¼-½ tsp hot pepper sauce
2 tsp anchovy paste

In a Vita-Mix machine, or blender, blend all of the ingredients together until very smooth. Cover and chill thoroughly before serving.

Variation: **Nonfat Caesar Dressing:** eliminate the oil and anchovy paste, and use nonfat Parmesan cheese. See **Dairy** in the *Food Products* chapter

Cheesy Ginger Dressing

1 cup ricotta cheese
¼ cup buttermilk
Juice of 1 fresh lemon
2 medium cloves of garlic (optional)

½ medium onion, chopped
½ inch fresh ginger root, grated
2 tbsp pure maple syrup

In a blender, or Vita-Mix machine, blend all of the ingredients together until smooth and creamy. Chill thoroughly prior to serving.

Cheesy Herb Dressing, Low Fat

1 cup plain, low fat yogurt
1 cup nonfat cottage cheese
4 tbsp Parmesan or Romano cheese
2 scallions, chopped
2 medium cloves of garlic, minced

Juice of ½ fresh lemon
1 tbsp pure maple syrup
1 tbsp Dijon mustard
1 tsp dried basil
⅛-¼ tsp hot pepper sauce

Either combine all of the ingredients in a blender, or use a Vita-Mix machine to save a lot of work and to provide a much smoother consistency. Chill thoroughly before use.

Creamy Basil or Coriander Dressing

12 oz soft or firm tofu
1 medium sized onion
3 large cloves of garlic
¼ cup Bragg Liquid Aminos

1 fresh lime
½ cup fresh basil, chopped
¼ organic cider vinegar
¼ cup purified water

Variation: **Coriander (Cilantro) Dressing**: substitute fresh coriander for fresh basil

Creamy Mustard-Yogurt Dressing, Low Fat

¾ cup plain, low fat yogurt
2 tbsp dry mustard powder
Juice of ½ lemon

Mrs. Dash, to taste
Fresh ground pepper, to taste

In a blender, blend all of the ingredients together. Chill thoroughly before serving. Keeps about 2-3 days in refrigerator.

French Dressing

1 tbsp pure virgin olive oil
2 tbsp fresh parsley, chopped
Juice of 3 fresh lemons
2 scallions, finely chopped
2 medium cloves of garlic, minced

¼ tsp dried rosemary
¼ tsp dried thyme
½ tsp dried oregano
½ tsp dried basil
⅛ tsp paprika

Either combine all of the ingredients by hand, or use a Vita-Mix machine to save yourself some work. Chill thoroughly before serving.

Green Goddess Buttermilk Dressing

½ cup buttermilk
½ cup Nayonnaise
Juice of ½ fresh lemon
2 tbsp white wine vinegar

2 medium cloves of garlic, minced
¼ cup fresh parsley, chopped
¼ tsp dried tarragon
¼ tsp fresh ground pepper

In a blender, blend all of the ingredients together until smooth. Chill thoroughly before use.

Herb Dressing, Nonfat

½ cup organic apple cider
¼ cup white wine vinegar
3 medium cloves of garlic, minced
1 tsp Spicy Mrs. Dash
2 scallions, finely chopped

½ tsp dried basil
½ tsp dried oregano
½ tsp dried rosemary
1 tsp Dijon mustard

Combine all of the ingredients and let sit, refrigerated, for about 30 minutes before use.

High Omega-3 GLA Dressing

1 tbsp cold pressed flaxseed oil
1 tsp cold pressed sesame oil
Juice of 2 fresh lemons
Rind of 1 lemon, grated
⅛ tsp hot pepper sauce

2 medium cloves of garlic, minced
½ inch fresh ginger root, grated
1 tbsp Bragg Liquid Aminos
1 tsp Mrs. Dash

In a blender, blend all of the ingredients together thoroughly. Let flavors marinate prior to serving.

Note: Flaxseed Oil and Udo's Oil *can be substituted for any of the oils used in the various dressing recipes.* However, be aware of the fact that they do have a particular flavor that is not as readily accepted as that of other oils. The good news is that with continued use, a taste for these oils can be acquired. After a few years of regular use and a lot of experimentation with recipes, I really enjoy the flavor now. Of course the fact that these oils are so beneficial to my body's health makes it all the more enjoyable to me!

REMEMBER! Never ever cook Flaxseed Oil or Udo's Oil **AND** always keep refrigerated!

Honey-Mustard Dressing

½ cup Nayonnaise
½ cup plain, low fat yogurt
Juice of ½ fresh lemon

2 tbsp Dijon mustard
1 tbsp natural honey
¼ tsp fresh ground pepper

In a blender, blend all of the ingredients together. Chill for at least 30 minutes.

Variations: **Honey-Lemon Dressing**: eliminate the mustard, and add the grated lemon rind from ½ lemon.
Lemon Dressing: eliminate the honey or reduce to 1 tsp, use the juice of 1 whole lemon, and include the grated lemon rind from ½ lemon.

Miso Dressing

1 cup of soft tofu
2 tbsp red miso paste
1 tbsp pure virgin olive oil
Juice of 1 fresh lemon

2 medium cloves of garlic, minced
1 tbsp pure maple syrup
½ tsp paprika

In a blender, blend all of the ingredients until smooth. Chill prior to serving.

Variations: **Miso Spread**: substitute the soft tofu with very firm tofu, and the maple syrup with sucanat.
Sesame Miso Dressing: substitute cold pressed sesame oil for pure virgin olive oil

Mock Sour Cream Dressing

8 ounces soft tofu
2 tbsp pure virgin olive oil
Juice of ½ fresh lemon

2 tsp pure maple syrup
1 tsp Mrs. Dash

In a blender, blend all of the ingredients together until smooth. Use in recipes which call for sour cream, or use as is, as a topping or dressing.

Mustard Vinaigrette Dressing, Nonfat

¼ cup apple cider vinegar
¼ cup white wine vinegar
1 scallion, finely chopped
2 medium cloves of garlic, minced

1 tsp black mustard seeds, ground
¼ inch fresh ginger, grated
1 tsp Dijon mustard
Mrs. Dash, to taste

Combine all of the ingredients by hand, or save yourself some work and blend them together in a Vita-Mix machine.

Mustard Yogurt Dressing

½ cup plain, low fat yogurt
¼ cup Nayonnaise

½ small onion, finely chopped
1 ½-2 tbsp Dijon mustard

Mix the ingredients together thoroughly. Cover and refrigerate.

Variation: **Dill Yogurt Dressing**: substitute the Dijon mustard with 1 tsp dried dill weed. Cover and refrigerate.

Salsa-Yogurt Dressing

½ cup plain, low fat yogurt
½ cup fresh, medium salsa
2 medium cloves of garlic, chopped

Juice of 1 fresh lime
3 scallions, finely chopped

Mix all of the ingredients together. Chill thoroughly prior to use.

Note: Many grocery stores and health food stores carry fresh salsa, made daily, in their deli sections. These are the only ones I buy! Avoid those almost dead brands which sit on the shelves forever without needing refrigeration! Remember, fresh is best!

Seasoned Yogurt and Tofu Topping

1 cup (8 ounces) soft tofu
½ cup plain, low fat yogurt
2 medium cloves of garlic, minced
Juice of 1 fresh lemon

1 tbsp pure maple syrup
1 tbsp Bragg Liquid Aminos
⅛ to ¼ tsp hot pepper sauce
¼ cup fresh parsley, chopped

In a blender or a Vita-Mix machine, blend all of the ingredients until smooth. Chill thoroughly prior to use.

Variation: **Tuna and Seasoned Yogurt Topping**: substitute the tofu with 6 ounces of water-packed canned tuna, well drained and rinsed. And eliminate the maple syrup. *This a high protein, high omega-3, EPA topping for baked potatoes, as well as a great dip or dressing for other vegetables.*

Spicy Dressing

1 tbsp pure virgin olive oil
½ cup low sodium tomato juice
Juice of ½ fresh lemon
2 tbsp organic cider vinegar
¼ of large red onion, chopped
½ tsp dry mustard powder

2 medium cloves of garlic, chopped
½-1 tsp uncreamed horseradish
⅛-¼ tsp cayenne pepper
½ tsp dried oregano
1 tbsp pure maple syrup

In a blender, blend all of the ingredients together until smooth. Let sit for at least 1 hour before serving to enhance the blend of flavors.

Spicy Ginger Dressing

1 tbsp pure virgin olive oil
1 tsp sesame oil
Juice of 2 fresh limes
Rind of 1 lime, grated
¾-1 inch fresh ginger root, grated

2 medium cloves garlic, minced
⅛-¼ tsp hot pepper sauce
1 tbsp tamari sauce
1 tbsp pure maple syrup

Either blend in a blender, or, for ease of preparation, use a Vita-Mix machine. Let sit for at least 1 hour before serving to enhance the blend of flavors.

Variation: **Lemon-Ginger Dressing**: substitute the lime juice with the juice of 2 fresh lemons, and substitute the lime rind with the grated rind of 1 lemon.

Tahini and Buttermilk Dressing

½ cup buttermilk
¼ cup sesame tahini
2 medium cloves of garlic, minced
Juice of ½ fresh lemon

1 tsp Spicy Mrs. Dash
½ tsp fresh ground pepper
¼ tsp dry mustard powder

In a blender, blend all of the ingredients together thoroughly. Chill prior to serving.

Tangy Herb Dressing

½ cup cider vinegar
3 medium cloves of garlic
2 tbsp Sucanat
¼ cup Bragg Liquid Aminos
½ medium onion
¼ cup purified water

1 tsp Dijon mustard
½ tsp dried basil
½ tsp dried oregano
½ tsp dried rosemary
2 tsp pure virgin olive oil

Blend all ingredients in a blender. Blend thoroughly. Pour into a salad dressing shaker bottle. Refrigerate for at least 4 hours before serving. Shake bottle just before each use.

Tofu Curry Dressing

8 ounces soft tofu
1 tsp cold pressed sesame oil
Juice of 1 fresh lemon
1 tbsp natural honey
2 medium cloves of garlic, minced

1 tsp curry powder
½ inch fresh ginger root, grated
1 tsp Spicy Mrs. Dash
⅛-¼ tsp hot pepper sauce
   (optional)

Either in a blender or a Vita-Mix machine, blend all of the ingredients together until very smooth. Chill thoroughly prior to serving.

Tomato-Basil Dressing, Nonfat

½ cup low sodium tomato juice   2 medium cloves of garlic, minced
Juice of ½ fresh lemon   2 tsp fresh basil, chopped
1 tsp pure maple syrup   1 tsp Spicy Mrs. Dash

Combine all of the ingredients and let sit, refrigerated, for at least 30 minutes, to marinate the flavors.

Vinaigrette Dressing

½ cup balsamic vinegar   2 tsp Dijon mustard
1 tbsp pure virgin olive oil   ¼-½ tsp fresh ground pepper
2 medium cloves of garlic, minced

In a blender, blend all of the ingredients together. Chill thoroughly before serving.

Watercress Buttermilk Dressing

½ cup buttermilk   ¼ tsp fresh ground pepper
¼ cup seasoned rice wine vinegar   ½ tsp dried tarragon
2 scallions, chopped   1 tsp pure maple syrup
2 medium cloves of garlic, chopped   ½ tsp Spicy Mrs. Dash
½ cup watercress leaves, packed   Rind of 1 lime (optional)

Either in a blender, or in a Vita-Mix machine (which will save you the work of chopping vegetables), blend all of the ingredients until smooth. Chill thoroughly before use.

Variation: **Honey Dijon Watercress Dressing**: substitute the maple syrup with 1 tbsp natural honey, eliminate the tarragon and the rind of a lime, and add 1-2 tbsp of Dijon mustard.

MARINADES

General Guidelines For Using Marinades

1. Marinades can be used for enhancing the flavor of firm to very firm tofu, fish, poultry and vegetables.
2. Generally the longer the marinating time, the better the flavor of the finished product.
3. Marinate tofu and fish for a minimum of 2-4 hours, preferably overnight.
4. Marinate chicken and turkey, and most game meats for a minimum of 4-6 hours, preferably overnight.
5. Marinate most vegetables for about 1-4 hours before eating as they are, or cooking them. Vegetables with lower water content are the best for marinating.
6. Vegetable sticks can be placed in a zipper baggie or a tightly sealed container, with some marinade, and carried to the office or on a hiking trip, for a flavorful addition to a meal or as a snack.
7. Most marinades keep well, in the refrigerator, for up to 1 week, in a tightly sealed jar or container.
8. Marinades with a yogurt or buttermilk base, are best used within 2-3 days.

The Drunken Limey Marinade

Juice of 2 fresh limes
Rind of 1 lime, grated
½ cup dry white wine
3 medium cloves of garlic, minced
1 tbsp pure maple syrup

½ medium onion, finely chopped
½ inch fresh ginger root, grated
¼ tsp nutmeg
¼-½ tsp hot pepper sauce

Combine all of the ingredients and store in a tightly sealed jar in refrigerator.

French-Style Marinade

3 medium cloves of garlic, minced
3 scallions, finely chopped
1 tbsp pure virgin olive oil
½ cup red wine vinegar
1 tsp Spicy Mrs. Dash
¼ cup water

2 tsp dried oregano
1 tbsp Dijon mustard
1 tbsp pure maple syrup
⅛ to ¼ tsp ground red pepper
⅛-¼ tsp sherry extract

Combine all of the ingredients and store in a tightly sealed jar in refrigerator.

Garlic-Tomato Marinade

½ cup low sodium tomato juice
Juice of 1 large fresh lemon
¼ cup water
4 medium cloves of garlic, chopped
½ medium onion, finely chopped

¼-½ tsp dry mustard powder
¼ cup fresh cilantro, chopped
⅛-¼ tsp ground red pepper
1 tbsp pure virgin olive oil (optional)

Combine all of the ingredients and store in a tightly sealed jar in refrigerator.

Herb Marinade

1 tbsp pure virgin olive oil
¼ cup balsamic vinegar
Juice of 1 large fresh lemon
1 tsp Spicy Mrs. Dash
3 medium cloves of garlic, chopped
½ medium onion, finely chopped

¼-½ tsp hot pepper sauce
¼ cup fresh parsley, chopped
1 tsp dried rosemary
1 tsp dried dill
1 tsp dried tarragon
2 tbsp hot water

1. Soak the dried herbs in hot water while preparing the rest of the marinade.
2. Combine the remaining ingredients.
3. Add the dried herbs and their soaking water to the combined ingredients.
4. Store in a tightly sealed jar in the refrigerator.

Minty Yogurt Marinade

¾ cup plain, low fat yogurt
Juice of 1 fresh lime
Rind of 1 lime, grated
3 medium cloves of garlic, minced
3 scallions, finely chopped

¼ cup fresh parsley, chopped
⅛-¼ tsp hot pepper sauce
½ tsp caraway seeds
1 tsp mint, finely chopped

Combine all of the ingredients and store in a tightly sealed jar in refrigerator. Use within 2-3 days.

Sweet and Sour Marinade

½ cup pineapple juice
½ cup organic cider vinegar
2 medium cloves of garlic, sliced
3 scallions, finely chopped
2 tbsp pure maple syrup

Rind of 1 lemon, grated
½ cup fresh parsley, chopped
½ tsp dry mustard powder
⅛-¼ tsp hot pepper sauce

Combine all of the ingredients and store in a tightly sealed jar in refrigerator.

Teriyaki Marinade

1 tbsp minced fresh ginger
3 medium cloves of garlic, minced
1 tbsp pure maple syrup
3 scallions, finely chopped
½ cup Bragg Liquid Aminos

Juice of 1 large fresh lemon
1 tbsp sesame oil
¼-½ tsp hot pepper sauce
¼ cup of white wine (optional)
¼ cup water

Combine all ingredients and keep in tightly sealed jar in refrigerator.

MAIN ENTREES

Baked Potato Wedges, Seasoned

These can be done from scratch, or using previously baked potatoes!

#1-The Quickie Version

Olive oil-based cooking spray
6 medium pre-baked potatoes,
   unpeeled*
All natural flavor spray

¼ cup fresh thyme, rosemary, dill,
   basil or parsley, chopped
Fresh ground black pepper, to taste

1. Cut the previously baked potatoes into ½" wedges.
2. Spray a baking sheet with nonstick cooking spray.
3. Arrange the potato wedges on the baking sheet, with space between the wedges.
4. Spray the surface of the wedges lightly with an all natural flavor spray of your choice.
5. Sprinkle the thyme, or other herbs, and black pepper over all of the potato pieces.
6. Grill briefly under the broiler, for about 4-5 minutes, or until wedges turn golden brown and slightly crispy on the outside, and are hot in the center.

* When I bake potatoes for a meal, I bake 5-10 potatoes at the same time. Saves energy! Fuel energy, as well as personal energy! Whatever is not eaten at the meal is covered and stored in the refrigerator for "near"-future meals. Some of the leftover potatoes may be used to make these potato wedges, others may be used to make a potato salad to carry to a potluck dinner, and others may simply be carried in the car for a nutritious emergency snack!

#2-The Scratch Version

Olive oil-based cooking spray
6 medium potatoes, scrubbed,
   unpeeled
All natural flavor spray, of choice

¼ cup fresh thyme, rosemary, dill,
   basil or parsley, chopped
Paprika

1. Preheat oven to 450°.
2. Cut potatoes into ½" wedges and arrange on lightly sprayed baking sheet.
3. Spray the surface of the wedges lightly with an all natural flavor spray of your choice.
4. Sprinkle the thyme, or other herbs, and paprika over all of the potato pieces.
5. Bake for 30-40 minutes, until the wedges are golden brown and crispy on the outside, and tender on the inside. Loosen the wedges from the pan once or twice during the baking period with a spatula.

Each recipe makes 4-6 servings

Bean Burritos with Salsa and Yogurt

One of the quickest meals I know!

1. Spoon some organic black beans (come in 16 ounce cans), slightly off center onto a corn or whole-wheat tortilla.
2. Sprinkle some grated nonfat or low fat cheese over the beans, and a spoonful each of chunky salsa, and of plain, low fat yogurt.
3. Fold the short sides of the tortilla over the filling. Then fold over the long sides, placing the seam side down on the plate.
4. They taste best when served warm. Serve with a salad of greens and tomatoes.

Beans and Vegetable Stew, Spicy

1 medium onion, chopped
4 medium cloves of garlic, minced
1 cup vegetable stock or water
1 carton (26 ounces) Pomi tomatoes
½ lb. fresh cauliflower, chopped
½ lb. fresh broccoli, chopped
2 stalks celery, chopped
1 large green pepper, chopped
3 medium zucchini, sliced
1 cup fresh mushrooms, halved

1 inch fresh ginger, grated
1 tsp paprika
1 tsp dried oregano
1 tsp dried thyme
1 tsp ground cumin
½ tsp fresh ground pepper
¼ tsp cayenne pepper
2 tbsp low sodium soy sauce
1 can (16 ounces) chickpeas, drained
1 can (16 ounces) black beans, drained

1. Put all ingredients, except zucchini, soy sauce and beans, into a Dutch oven. Bring to a boil.
2. Cover, reduce heat and simmer for 15-20 minutes.
3. Add zucchini, drained chickpeas and black beans to the stew.
4. Cover, and simmer, until zucchini is tender, but not soft. About 10 minutes.
5. Stir soy sauce into finished stew. Serve over steamed millet, or brown rice.

Variation: **Spicy Potatoes, Broccoli and Black-eyed Peas**: eliminate the tomatoes, cauliflower, celery and zucchini. Instead use 5 medium potatoes, unpeeled and chopped, and increase the broccoli to 1 lb. Substitute the chickpeas and black beans with 2 cans (16 ounces each) black-eyed peas, drained.

Note: This stew tastes even better the next day, after the flavors have had more time to blend together.

Makes 6-8 servings

Buckwheat Groats, Seasoned (also called Kasha)

1 cup whole buckwheat groats (kasha)   2 cups boiling water
1 small onion, diced   2 tbsp vegetable seasoning powder
2 medium cloves of garlic, minced   ¼ cup sun-dried tomatoes,
                                            chopped

1. In a fine mesh strainer, rinse kasha well under cool running water. Drain.
2. Put all ingredients into a medium-sized saucepan. Bring back to a boil.
3. Cover, reduce heat, and simmer until kasha is soft, about 12-15 minutes.
4. Remove from heat and let sit covered, and untouched, for 5 minutes.
5. Serve with **Baked Red Snapper**, or as is, topped with a serving of beans.

Makes 4 servings

Bulgur with Low fat Yogurt, Steamed

1 cup raw bulgur   1 cup plain, low fat yogurt
1 ¾ cups boiling water or vegetable broth

1. Place bulgur in a large bowl. Pour boiling liquid over bulgur.
2. Cover and let sit until grain has absorbed all of liquid, about 20-25 minutes.
3. Toughly blend yogurt throughout the bulgur, and serve.

Note: Any grain lends itself to preparation with vegetable broth and the addition of yogurt.

Makes 4 servings

Chicken Breast / Turkey Breast, Baked

3-4 skinless, boneless chicken
  or turkey breasts
¼ tsp black pepper
1 cup raw oatmeal, slightly ground
1 tsp minced garlic

1 tsp Mrs. Dash
¼-½ tsp Worcestershire sauce
1 egg white
¼ tsp hot pepper sauce

1. Whip together all of ingredients but chicken and oatmeal.
2. Roll chicken breast in egg white mixture and then coat with oatmeal.
3. Bake chicken breasts at 400° for 20-25 minutes; bake longer for turkey breasts.
4. Serve with brown rice, and a fresh green salad with nonfat, or low fat, dressing.
5. To toast the oatmeal, broil the chicken briefly, after actual baking is completed. It browns the coating nicely.

Note: If the oatmeal is initially ground slightly in a coffee mill, the consistency will be similar to bread crumbs and will therefore, more easily, become crispy during the baking period, eliminating the need to use the broiler.

Remember: always choose organic free range chicken and eggs whenever possible.

Makes 3-4 servings

Chicken Fajitas — Quick and Healthy!

Less cooking! More Crunch! Higher nutrition!

1 ½ lb. cooked skinless chicken breast
1 tbsp pure virgin olive oil
3 medium cloves of garlic, minced
1 large red onion, thinly sliced
1 large green pepper, in thin strips
1 large red pepper, in thin strips

¼ tsp cayenne pepper
½-1 cup fresh salsa
½ medium avocado, thinly sliced
½-1 cup low fat, plain yogurt
Cheddar cheese, low or nonfat, shredded
8 whole wheat tortillas, heated

1. Cut chicken into thin strips.
2. Place tortillas in covered Oven-safe dish in preheated 250° oven for about 10 minutes.
3. Heat oil in large skillet. Add garlic, onions, peppers, cayenne pepper and chicken.
4. Sauté over medium heat for about 5 minutes.
5. To assemble fajitas spoon the vegetable and chicken mixture down center of the tortilla. Top with a spoonful of salsa, a slice of avocado, a spoonful of yogurt, and a sprinkling of shredded cheese. Encase filling by folding like an envelope, leaving one end open.
6. Serve with **Mexican Brown Rice**.

Makes 8 servings

Curried Chickpeas and Onions

1 cup water
1 tbsp pure virgin olive oil
2 medium onions, sliced
2 medium cloves of garlic, minced
1 medium tomato, chopped
½ inch fresh ginger, grated
1 ½ tsp coriander
1 tsp cumin

1 bay leaf
½ tsp turmeric
1 tsp mustard seeds
¼ tsp cayenne pepper
½ tsp Real Salt
3 medium potatoes, chopped
2 cans (16 ounces each) chickpeas, drained
Juice of 1 fresh lemon

1. Heat oil in medium-sized saucepan. Add all of ingredients except water, potatoes, chickpeas and lemon juice.
2. Sauté mixture until mustard seeds begin to pop, about 3-5 minutes.
3. Add water, potatoes and chickpeas. Bring to a boil.
4. Cover, reduce heat, and simmer for about 20 minutes.
5. Remove from heat. Add lemon juice. Cover. Let sit for 10 minutes prior to serving.
6. Serve over steamed bulgur or brown rice.

Makes 4 servings

Curried Vegetables and Crabmeat

1 cup water, boiling
1 tbsp vegetable seasoning powder
1 medium onion, chopped
2 medium cloves of garlic, minced
4 medium potatoes, unpeeled, chopped
½ lb. fresh cauliflower, chopped
2 medium carrots, chopped

1 cup fresh or frozen green peas
2 tbsp curry powder
1 tsp dried basil
1 tsp sucanat
½ cup nonalcoholic,
    or dry, wine
½ cup plain, low fat yogurt
1 lb. crabmeat, flaked

1. Add the vegetable seasoning powder, e.g. brands by Gayelord Hauser or Bernard Jensen, to the boiling water. Mix thoroughly.
2. Place all but 2 tbsp of the broth into a Dutch oven. Add all of the vegetables to the broth.
3. Blend curry powder well with 2 tbsp broth. Mix with basil, sucanat, and wine.
4. Add the curry mixture to the vegetables and broth in the Dutch oven.
5. Bring to a boil. Cover, reduce heat and simmer about 20 minutes or until vegetables are tender, but not soft.
6. Stir the yogurt and flaked crabmeat throughout the vegetable mixture. Heat through, but do not bring to a boil.
7. Serve over steamed bulgur, plain, or mixed with yogurt. Also great with brown rice.

Variations:
1. Cooked, diced chicken, or turkey, breast can be substituted for the crabmeat
2. A mixture of steamed shrimps and lobster can be substituted.
3. Any whitefish can be substituted for the crabmeat. Either steam the fish and cut into 1" or 2" pieces, prior to adding it to the curried vegetables, or add raw fillets, cut into 1" or 2" pieces, 3-4 minutes prior to end of cooking time.

Makes 6-8 servings

Fettuccini Alfredo, Healthy

Whole grain or vegetable pasta noodles
½-1 tsp Spicy Mrs. Dash

1-2 tsp garlic, pressed
Fresh ground pepper

2-4 tbsp Parmesan cheese
¼-½ cup plain low
    fat yogurt
1-2 tsp butter sprinkles
Juice of ½ lemon

1. Cook enough pasta for 2-4 servings, according to directions on package.
2. Drain pasta, and add all ingredients except pepper
3. Toss pasta.
4. Serve with fresh ground pepper sprinkled on top, to taste. Excellent with a fresh green salad and steamed vegetables.

Makes 2-4 servings

Macaroni and Cheese, Light, Whole Grain

2 cups uncooked whole grain
   elbow macaroni
2 medium cloves of garlic, minced
1 tsp dry mustard
3 tbsp rolled oats, ground
½ tsp paprika

1-1 ½ tbsp butter sprinkles
½ cup low fat, plain yogurt
8 ounces shredded low or nonfat
   Cheddar cheese
1 tsp dried basil
2 tbsp fresh parsley, chopped

1. Cook macaroni to desired firmness as directed on the package. Drain.
2. Add garlic, seasonings, butter sprinkles, yogurt and cheese. Mix well.
3. Spoon into ungreased Oven-safe casserole dish. Top with oats, ground in coffee mill.
4. Bake at 350° for 25 minutes. Sprinkle with chopped parsley.

Variations: Tuna, salmon, crabmeat, shrimp, or other fish or shellfish, chopped skinless chicken or turkey breast, black beans or other legumes, cooked broccoli, snow peas or green beans, or any assortment of these ingredients can be added to the casserole prior to baking in the oven.

Makes 4-6 servings

Mexican Brown Rice

2 medium onions, chopped	3 cups boiling water
1 large green pepper, chopped	2 tbsp vegetable seasoning powder
2 large cloves of garlic, minced	2 cups uncooked brown rice
½ carton (13 ounces) Pomi tomatoes	2 tbsp fresh parsley, chopped

1. Put all ingredients into a heavy saucepan and bring to a boil.
2. Cover, reduce heat and simmer on low heat for about 40-45 minutes, or until all of the liquid is absorbed.

Makes 4-6 servings

Pasta and Vegetable Medley

A very simple dish for the end of a crazy work day, or for a community potluck dinner!

1 lb. wholegrain or vegetable pasta, elbows or bow ties	¼ cup Nayonnaise
	½ cup plain, low fat yogurt
1 lb. frozen mixed vegetables,	2 tbsp Dijon mustard
Mediterranean blend	½ tsp fresh ground pepper
4 scallions, finely chopped	1 tsp dried basil
2 large cloves of garlic, minced	¼ cup fresh parsley, chopped
½ cup pitted black olives, chopped	Hot pepper sauce, to taste
1 can (16 ounces) chickpeas, drained	

1. Cook pasta according to directions on package. Drain.
2. Cook frozen vegetables according to directions on package. Drain.
3. In a separate bowl, combine all of seasoning ingredients in the second column.
4. Combine pasta, vegetables, scallions, garlic, olives, chickpeas and seasoning mixture. Toss until thoroughly mixed.
5. Cover and refrigerate for at least 60 minutes prior to serving, to blend flavors.

Variations:
1. To increase protein, add marinated tofu chunks, tuna, salmon, or chunks of chicken breast or leftover cooked fish.
2. To serve hot, put mixture into a lightly sprayed oven safe glass casserole dish and bake at 350° for about 20 minutes.

Makes 6 servings

Pasta Marinara, Wholegrain/ High Protein

#1-The Quickie Version

1-26 ounce bottle natural, no fat or low fat, garlic and mushroom marinara
    sauce
8-10 ounces soft tofu

1. In a saucepan, heat the sauce until just beginning to bubble.
2. Using a potato masher, mash the tofu into the marinara sauce.
3. Remove saucepan from heat just as the mixture begins to form bubbles again. *Do not cook the tofu!*
4. Serve over wholegrain or vegetable pasta. Also good served over brown rice.

#2-From Scratch (Almost!)

¼ cup water	1 carton (26 ounces) Pomi tomatoes
1 tsp vegetable seasoning powder	1 tsp dried oregano
2 medium cloves of garlic, minced	⅓ cup fresh basil, chopped
1 medium onion, chopped	¼ tsp chili pepper flakes
¼ cup fresh parsley, chopped	8-10 ounces soft tofu
2 tbsp Parmesan cheese, optional	

1. Put all ingredients, except the tofu and Parmesan cheese, into a saucepan.
2. Simmer gently for 25-30 minutes.
3. Using a potato masher, mash the tofu into the marinara sauce.
4. Remove saucepan from heat just as mixture begins to form bubbles again. *Do not cook the tofu!*
5. Stir Parmesan into sauce until well combined. Serve over pasta or rice.

Variation: **Tofu-Mushroom Marinara Sauce,** prepare as for Marinara **#2-From Scratch,** adding 1 cup of sliced fresh mushrooms in the first step, and following as listed, steps #2 through #5.

Note: If you have a Vita-Mix machine, this recipe is a cinch! *Don't waste any time chopping or mincing!* Just throw all of the ingredients, except the tofu and Parmesan, into the Vita-Mix. Blend on high speed for about 1 minute. The action of the machine heats the food while it blends it. Then add the tofu and Parmesan and blend very briefly for about 5-10 seconds. Serve immediately.

Pasta Primavera, Wholegrain

Olive oil-based cooking spray
1 medium red onion, coarsely chopped
3 medium cloves of garlic, minced
2 medium zucchini, sliced
1 large green pepper, sliced
1 large red pepper, sliced
1 cup fresh snow peas
4 medium tomatoes, chopped
¼ cup water

2 tsp dried basil
1 tsp dried oregano
½ tsp dried thyme
¼ cup nonalcoholic or
   regular white wine
½ tsp Real Salt, optional
¼ tsp crushed red pepper flakes
6-8 ounces wholegrain linguine
Parmesan or Romano cheese

1. Prepare pasta according to directions on package.
2. Spray medium-sized saucepan with nonfat cooking spray.
3. Over medium-high heat, briefly sauté onions and garlic, about 3-4 minutes.
4. Add rest of ingredients, except linguine and cheese. Simmer uncovered for 5-8 minutes. Vegetables should remain very crisp.
5. Serve sauce over cooked linguine. Lightly sprinkle cheese over sauce.

Makes 6 servings

Red Snapper Baked with Gingery Pineapple Sauce

Olive oil-based cooking spray
1 ½ lb. skinless Red Snapper fillets
1 tsp sesame oil
1 medium onion, diced
2 medium cloves of garlic

1 cup fresh pineapple
1-2 tsp pure maple syrup
¾ inch fresh ginger, grated
⅛-¼ tsp hot pepper sauce
1 tbsp tamari sauce

1. Place the fillets in a shallow baking dish that has been sprayed.
2. Blend the rest of the ingredients together in a blender or Vita−mix machine. The Vita-Mix saves you the task of chopping and mincing!
3. Pour the sauce over the fillets. Cover and refrigerate for 30-60 minutes.
4. Bake fish, in marinade, in preheated oven at 450° for 8-10 minutes, or just until fish flakes easily.
5. Pour some of sauce from the baking dish, over each serving.

Makes 4-6 servings

Salmon Burger on Whole Grain Kaiser Roll

2 cans (7.5 ounces each) salmon,
    drained and rinsed
½ cup rolled oats, coarsely ground
½ large onion, chopped
1 egg, free range

¼ cup plain, low fat yogurt
1 ½ tsp dried dill weed
1 tsp dry mustard
½ tsp fresh ground pepper
Olive oil-based cooking spray

1. In a medium bowl, combine all ingredients. Mix well.
2. Shape mixture into 6 patties.
3. Spray large nonstick skillet with nonfat cooking spray.
4. Cook patties over medium heat for 6-8 minutes. Turn once during cooking.
5. Serve on whole grain Kaiser rolls, topped with any or all of the following:

red onion slices
zucchini slices
Dijon mustard
yogurt mustard dressing

tomato slices
cucumber slices
Nayonnaise
red and green peppers

lettuce
salsa
alfalfa sprouts
jalapenos

Makes 6 servings

Salmon Loaf with Mustard Sauce

1 can (15 ounces) water-packed
    salmon, drained and rinsed
1 egg, free range
½ cup plain, low fat yogurt
1 cup rolled oats, coarsely ground
½ large onion, diced
Olive oil-based cooking spray

1 medium tomato, chopped
1 ½ tsp curry powder
1 tsp tarragon
¼ cup fresh parsley, chopped
1 tsp Mrs. Dash
¼ tsp fresh ground pepper

1. Mix all ingredients together well, except spray.
2. Spray a nonstick loaf pan with nonfat cooking spray, and fill with salmon mixture.
3. Bake in preheated 400° oven for 20-25 minutes. Let sit for 10 minutes.
4. Serve with a mustard dressing of your choice. *See* **Dressings** chapter.

Makes 4-6 servings

Sweet Potato and Vegetable Casserole

3 medium sweet potatoes, unpeeled
cut into slices
1 medium onion, chopped
3 medium carrots, sliced
2 small zucchini, in chunks
2 stalks celery, chopped
1 carton (26 ounces) Pomi tomatoes
1 cup fresh green beans

1 can (16 ounces) red kidney beans
2 tbsp pure maple syrup
1 tsp dried oregano
1 tsp dried basil
½ tsp dried thyme
⅛-¼ tsp hot pepper sauce
Plain, low fat yogurt, optional
Parmesan or Romano cheese,
optional

1. In a large bowl, toss all ingredients to mix thoroughly.
2. Spoon into a Oven-safe casserole dish, sprayed with olive oil-based cooking spray.
3. Bake at 350° for about 30 minutes.
4. Can serve topped with plain, nonfat yogurt and a sprinkling of Parmesan cheese.

Makes 4 servings

Tofu-Vegetable Frittata

Olive oil-based cooking spray
1 large onion, thinly sliced
2 medium cloves of garlic, minced
1 large green pepper, thinly sliced
1 medium zucchini, sliced
1 large tomato, chopped
2 pre baked potatoes,
unpeeled, chopped

8 ounces soft tofu, mashed
2 eggs, free range
¼ tsp turmeric
1-2 tsp Mrs. Dash
1 tsp dried basil
⅛-¼ tsp hot pepper sauce
4 ounces nonfat cheddar cheese,
shredded

1. Spray large nonstick oven-proof skillet with nonfat cooking spray.
2. Add all of ingredients in the first column and sauté at medium heat for 3-4 minutes.
3. Mix together thoroughly all of ingredients in the second column. Pour over vegetable mixture.
4. Place skillet in preheated 350° oven. Bake 20-25 minutes, or until knife inserted in the center comes out clean.
5. Cut into pie-shaped wedges to serve.

Makes 4-6 servings

Trout with Lemon, Fresh Baked

1 ½ lb. boneless trout fillets
½ cup low sodium soy sauce
½ cup white wine

2 tbsp pure maple syrup
1-1 ½ inches fresh ginger, grated
1 medium onion, thinly sliced

1. Mix all ingredients except the trout together and pour into oven-safe baking dish.
2. Place trout in the mixture, cover and refrigerate.
3. Let marinate 30 minutes on each side before cooking.
4. Bake at 400° for 12-15 minutes, or until fish flakes easily when tested with a fork.
5. Pour marinade and baking juices over each serving. Serve with fresh lemon wedges and fresh ground black pepper.

Note: The alcohol content in the wine is cooked off during the baking of the fish.

Makes 4 servings

Turkey Chili

1 lb. ground turkey breast	1 tsp dried oregano
1 carton (26 ounces) Pomi tomatoes	½ tsp dried basil
2 medium unpeeled potatoes, diced	1 tsp Spicy Mrs. Dash
1 large onion, chopped	1-2 tbsp chili powder
3 large cloves of garlic, minced	¼ tsp fresh ground pepper
½ large green pepper, chopped	2 cans (16 ounces each) red kidney
1 or 2 fresh jalapenos, chopped	beans, drained and rinsed

1. Put all of the ingredients except kidney beans into a Dutch oven. Mix thoroughly.
2. Bring to a boil, then cover, reduce heat and simmer for about 20 minutes.
3. Add kidney beans and simmer for another 10 minutes.

Can be served in a variety of ways such as

♦ topped with plain, low fat yogurt
♦ with sprouted wholegrain bread or toast
♦ over brown rice, or other cooked grains
♦ as a dip for baked tortilla chips or nonfat wholegrain crackers
♦ as a topping on a tostada salad
♦ in a sprouted grain tortilla and topped with leafy greens, salsa and yogurt
♦ as a filling for a sprouted grain burrito wrap

Variation: **Vegan chili:** prepare as above without ground turkey

Makes 8-10 servings

Turkey Loaf

1 lb. ground turkey breast
1 medium onion, chopped
½ medium green pepper, chopped
½ medium red pepper, chopped
2 medium cloves of garlic, minced
1 free-range egg

¾ cup old fashioned oatmeal
¼ cup wheat germ
1 cup Pomi tomatoes, crushed*
1 tbsp Mrs. Dash or Spicy Mrs. Dash
1 tsp dried oregano
¼ tsp fresh ground pepper

1. Thoroughly combine all of the ingredients.
2. Form into a loaf shape, and then place in a loaf pan or dish.
3. Bake at 350° for 40-45 minutes. Let stand for 5 minutes before serving.
4. Serve with **Mustard Yogurt Dressing.**

* **Pomi tomatoes** come in a carton containing 26 ounces of tomatoes. They are vacuum packed fresh, with no salt, no preservatives, no water added, and no artificial flavoring. *This is the only way I will buy tomatoes, other than fresh!*

Pomi tomatoes are available in most grocery stores. See *Food Products* chapter.

Makes 4-6 servings

Vegetable and Bean Chili

1 medium onion, chopped
4 medium cloves of garlic, minced
1 carton (26 ounces) Pomi tomatoes
1 medium green pepper, chopped
1 medium red pepper, chopped
2 large carrots, sliced
1 can (16 ounces) red kidney
    beans, drained

2 fresh jalapenos, chopped
2 tbsp chili powder
1 tsp cumin
1-2 tsp Mrs. Dash
½ tsp fresh ground pepper
½ lb. fresh broccoli, chopped
¼ cup fresh cilantro, chopped

1. In a Dutch oven, put all ingredients except the cilantro.
2. Bring the chili to a simmer. Continue to simmer for 20-30 minutes.
3. Stir in the cilantro and serve.
4. Delicious served with fresh wholegrain cornbread. Also great over brown rice, or other grains.

Makes 4 servings

Vegetarian Chili

1 medium onion, chopped
2 large carrots, sliced
1 stalk celery, chopped
4 medium cloves of garlic, minced
1 medium green pepper, chopped
1 medium red pepper, chopped
2 fresh jalapenos, chopped**
1 cup water or vegetable stock*

2 tbsp chili powder**
1 carton (26 ounces) Pomi tomatoes
1 tsp cumin
2 tsp Spicy Mrs. Dash
½ tsp fresh ground pepper
1 can (16 ounces) pinto beans, drained
2 tbsp fresh cilantro, finely chopped

1. In a Dutch oven, combine all of the ingredients, except cilantro.
2. Bring the chili to a simmer. Cover and simmer for 20-30 minutes, or until vegetables are tender, but not mushy.
3. Stir in the cilantro and serve.

* For a healthy natural **Vegetable Stock,** to use in cooking, I collect all of the leftover liquid from steaming vegetables. I store it in an airtight glass jar in the refrigerator and use this instead of commercial canned stocks, which are generally loaded with sodium and often contain less than healthy fat sources. At the end of 1 week, whatever stock is still remaining, I throw out. After the jar is thoroughly washed, I begin collecting stock again.

Note: *There is rarely any stock left at the end of each week.*

** If you are not used to hot food, or rarely eat spicy foods, you may want to reduce the chili powder to 1 tbsp the first time you make this chili. You can always add more the next time you make it. *But you can't eliminate the heat after it has already been added!*

Note: *Experiment with the jalapeno peppers as well.* Start with only 1 pepper and then add more as you tolerate it. Make the recipe *work for you* and your taste buds!

Makes 4 servings

Vegetable-Tofu Medley

1 medium onion, sliced
2 medium cloves of garlic, minced
1 medium green pepper, sliced
1 medium red pepper, sliced
1 cup fresh mushrooms, sliced
1 fresh carrot, sliced

1 cup fresh broccoli, chopped
½ lb. extra firm tofu, diced
½ inch fresh ginger, grated
1-2 tbsp water or vegetable stock
1 tbsp low sodium soy sauce
1 tsp sesame oil

1. To a hot wok or large skillet, add the sesame oil, soy sauce, stock and ginger.
2. When mixture is steaming, add all of vegetables. Sauté briefly, just to heat vegetables, but not to cook them
3. Add tofu and toss quickly over the heat.
4. Serve over brown rice or wholegrain noodles. Great topped with a sprinkling of fresh ground pepper.

Makes 4 servings

4. THE LIBRARY

REFERENCES & RESOURCES

FOOD, NUTRITION AND FOOD SAFETY

Balch, J. & P. **Prescription for Nutritional Healing.** Avery Publishing Group, 2006

Barnard, N., M.D. **The Power of Your Plate, Eating Well For Better Health.** The Book Publishing Co., 1995.

Barnard, N., M.D. **Food for Life: How the New Four Food Groups Can Save Your Life.** Crown Trade Paperbacks, 1994.

Barnard, N., M.D. **Dr. Neal Barnard's Program for Reversing Diabetes.** Rodale Pr Books 2006

Batmanghelidj, F. M.D. **Your Body's Many Cries For Water, You Are Not Sick, You Are Thirsty.** Global Health Solutions, Inc., 1997

Brody, J. **Jane Brody's Nutrition Book.** Bantam Books, Inc., 1987.

Cousens, G., M.D. **Conscious Eating.** North Atlantic Books, 2000

David, M. **The Flow Down Diet.** Healing Arts Press, 2005

Deoul, K. **Cancer Cover-Up.** Cassandra Books, 2001

Esselstyn, Jr., C., M.D. Jr. **Prevent and Reverse Heart Disease.** The Penguin Group (USA) 2007

Frahm, A. & D. **Healthy Habits: 20 Simple Ways to Improve Your Health.** Penguin Group, 1998

Guest, J. **Extreme Health.** Instant Publisher.com, 2002

Haas, E., M.D. **Staying Healthy with Nutrition.** Ten Speed Press, 2006.

Havala, S., R.D. **Simple, Lowfat & Vegetarian.** The Vegetarian Resource Group, 1994.

Jacobson, M., Ph.D. **Safe Food: Eating Wisely in a Risky World.** Living Planet Press.

Jensen, B., M.D. **Foods That Heal.** Avery Publishing Group, Inc., 1993.

Joyce, M., Ph.D.,R.D. **I Can't Believe It's Tofu,** USA: 5 Minutes To Health, 1999

Knox, K. **Forget The Die-Its, Learn to Live-It.** Morgan James Publishing, 2007

Lappe, F. Moore. **Diet for a Small Planet.** Ballantine Books, 10th Ed. 1991.

Levin, J. & Cederquist, N. **A Celebration of Wellness.** GLO Inc., 1992

Levin, J. & Cederquist, N. **Vibrant Living.** GLO Inc., 2001

McAdoo, N. **Your Body Your Castle Your Kingdom Your Home.** Sunray Printing, 2007

McDougall, J. & M. **The McDougall Plan.** New Century Publishers, 1983.

Millers, D. Ph.D. **Simply DELicious.** Spiritwind Publications, 2003

Nestle, M. **What To Eat.** Farrar, Straus and Giroux, 2007

Nestle, M. **Food Politics.** University of California Press 2007

Null, G., Ph.D. **The 90's Healthy Body Book: How to Overcome the Effects of Pollution and Cleanse the Toxins from Your Body.** Health Communications, Inc., 1994.

Oelke, J., N.D., Ph.D **Natural Choices for Fibromyalgia**. Natural Choices, Inc. 2002

Ornish, D., M.D. **Eat More, Weigh Less.** HarperCollins Publishers, Inc., 2001.

Ornish, D., M.D. **Dr. Dean Ornish's Program for Reversing Heart Disease.** Random House Publishing Group, 1996

Petrini, C. **Slow Food Nation.** Rizzoli, 2007

Quillin, P., Ph.D. **Beating Cancer with Nutrition.** The Nutrition Times Press, Inc., 2005.

Robbins, J. **Diet for a New World: May All Be Fed.** Harper Perennial 1993.

Robbins, J. **Diet for a New America.** HJ Kramer, 1998

Robbins, J. **The Food Revolution.** Conari Press, 2001

Robertson, L. **The New Laurel's Kitchen.** Ten Speed Press, 1987.

Rose, S. **The Vegetarian Solution.** Healthy Living Publications 2007

Santillo, H. **Food Enzymes: The Missing Link to Radiant Health.** Lotus Press, 1993.

Schlosser, E. **Chew on This, Everything You Don't Want to Know About Fast Food.** Houghton Mifflin Company, 2006

Shelton, H. **Food Combining Made Easy.** : Willow Publishing, 1989.

Silberstein, S. **Hungry For Health**. Infinity Publishing, 2007

Simone, C. **Cancer and Nutrition.** Princeton Institute, 2005.

Spurlock, M. **Don't Eat This Book, Fast Food and the Supersizing of America.** Berkeley Trade, 2006

Spurlock, M. **Supersize Me** (DVD-Family Version) Hart Sharp Video, 2004

Wasserman, D. & Reed, M. **Simply Vegan.** The Vegetarian Resource Group, 1999.

Wigmore, A. **The Hippocrates Diet.** Avery Publishing Group, 1984.

Wolfe, D. **The Sunfood Diet Success System.** Maul Brothers Publishing, 2006

PSYCHONEUROIMMUNOLOGY, STRESS MANAGEMENT, ATTITUDE, RELAXATION, AND IMAGERY

Achterberg, J. **Imagery in Healing.** Shambhala Publications, 2002.

Anderson, G. **The Cancer Conqueror.** Andrews & McMeel, 1990.

Anderson, G. **The Triumphant Patient.** iUniverse, 2000

Benjamin, H., Ph.D. **From Victim to Victor.** Bantam Doubleday Dell Publishing Group, 1987.

Benson, H. **The Relaxation Response.** William Morrow & Co., 1975.

Benson, H. **Your Maximum Mind: Changing Your Life by Changing the Way You Think.** Avon Books, 1991

Borysenko, J. Ph.D. **Guilt is the Teacher, Love is the Lesson.** Grand Central Publishing, 1991

Borysenko, J., Ph.D. **Minding the Body, Mending the Mind.** Da Capo Press, 2007

Braden, G. **The Divine Matrix, Bridging Time, Space, Miracles and Belief.** Hay House, Inc., 2008

Byrne, Rhonda. **The Secret.** Beyond Words Publishing, 2006 **(DVD)** Primetime Productions 2006

Cohen, R., Flannery, C. & Biörn, K. **Take 10! How to Achieve Your 'Someday' Dreams in 10 Minutes a Day.** Entelekey, Inc., 2006

Castagnini, J. **Thank God I . . . Books.** 2008

Chopra, D., M.D. **Perfect Health — Revised and Updated.** Crown Publishing Group, 2001.

Cousins, N. **Anatomy of an Illness as Perceived by a Patient: Reflections on Healing and Regeneration.** W. W. Norton & Company, 2005

Cousins, N. **Head First: The Biology of Hope.** Smithmark Pub, 1992

Dooley, Mike. **Notes From The Universe, New Perspectives From An Old Friend.** Beyond Words Publishing, 2007

Dossey, L. **Recovering the Soul: A Scientific and Spiritual Search.** Bantam Books, 1990.

Dossey, L. **Meaning and Medicine.** New York: Bantam Books, 1992.

E, S. and Beard, L. **Wake Up Shape Up . . . Live The Life You Love.** Little Seed Publishing Inc. 2003

Eker, T.H. **Secrets of the Millionaire Mind.** HarperCollins, 2005

Epstein, G. **Healing Visualizations: Creating Health Through Imagery.** Bantam Books., 1989.

Forsythe, L. **Walking With the Wise.** Mentors Publishing House, Inc., 2003

Forsythe, L. **Walking With the Wise, For Health & Vitality.** Mentors Publishing House, Inc., 2004

Frenn, J. **Power To Change.** Summit Books, 2005

Harris, B. **Thresholds of the Mind,** Centerpointe Press, 2007

Hendricks, G. **Five Wishes.** New World Library, 2007

Hicks, E. & J. **Ask and It is Given.** (Book or CD) Hay House, Inc., 2004

Hicks, E. & J. **The Law of Attraction.** (Book or CD) Hay House, Inc., 2006

Kurek, A. **How Would Love Respond.** Benbella Books, 2008

LeShan, L. **How to Meditate.** Little, Brown and Company, 1999

LeShan, L. **Cancer as a Turning Point.** Plume, 1994.

Lipton, B. **The Biology of Belief.** Mountain of Love/Elite Books, 2005

Morrison, T. **Settle for Excellence.** Topher Morrison, Inc., 2006

Moyers, B. **Healing and The Mind.** Main Street Books, 1995

Myss, C. **Anatomy of the Spirit.** 3 Rivers Press, 1997

Myss, C. **Energy Anatomy, The Science of Personal Power, Spirituality and Health.** Sounds True, 2001 (9 CD's)

O'Toole, M. & Peterson, S. **(The Gift) Becoming a Better You!** O'Toole, Peterson, Coots Publishing, 2005

Northrup, C., M.D. **Women's Bodies, Women's Wisdom, Creating Physical and Emotional Health and Healing,** Bantam Books, 2002

Pelletier, K. **Mind as a Healer, Mind as a Slayer.** Peter Smith Publisher Inc., 1984

Seligman, M., Ph.D. **Learned Optimism: How to Change Your Mind and Your Life.** Knopf Publishing Group, 2006

Selye, H. **The Stress of Life.** McGraw-Hill, 1978

Shimoff, M. **Happy For No Reason**. Simon & Schuster, 2008

Siegel, B., M.D. **Love, Medicine and Miracles.** HarperPerennial, 1998.

Siegel, B., M.D. **Peace, Love and Healing.** BDD Promotional Books Company, 1992

Simonton, O.C. & S. **Getting Well Again.** : Bantam Books, 1992.

Simonton, O.C. & Henson, R. **The Healing Journey.** Authors Choice Press, 2002

Stricker, P., M.D. **Sports Success Rx! Your Child's Prescription for the Best Experience.** American Academy of Pediatrics, 2006

Tolle, E. **A New Earth, Awakening Your Life's Purpose.** Penguin Group, 2008

Tolle, E. **The Power of Now.** New World Library, 1999

Ward, Susan Winter, **Yoga For The Young At Heart.** CD and DVD

Williamson, M. **A Return to Love,** HarperCollins, 1996

Williamson, M. **The Age of Miracles, Embracing the New Midlife.** Hay House, Inc. 2008

Notes: This is by no means an exhaustive list. But it will assist you on the road to wellness. There is enough of a selection here that everyone should be able to find something from the list which is in line with his or her interest, or concern.

CD and DVD RENTALS

Apart from the books listed, many of the authors also offer recorded versions of their books or programs, or of meditations for specific conditions. So if books are just not your thing, have no fear! Simply inquire about the availability of CDs and DVDs by an author whose book title appeals to you.

Something that I have found to be of great value for more than 15 years, has been a membership with a company which sells and rents CDs and DVDs by a mail order system. Instead of spending huge amounts of money buying every taped program that interests me, I simply rent it and *"try it before I buy it"*, at the rate of approximately one program per month. I get what I need from the program, playing it in the car, or at home when I'm relaxing, and then return it, and wait for the next program I have ordered to arrive. It has saved me tremendous amounts of money and has been a great way to avoid the clutter of a lot of programs taking up valuable shelf space. **After all, how many times have we bought an expensive CD or DVD, listened to it, or viewed it, only once, and then left it sitting on a shelf to collect dust until we gave it away or threw it away?**

The company I'm speaking of always has an up-to-date listing of programs available. And if you decide you want to buy a copy of a particular program you have listened to, members receive excellent discounts. For further information contact:

The Motivational Tape Company,
(800) 735-3660
www.achievementlibrary.com
Contact: Paul Arroyo
www.achievementlibrary.com

MAGAZINES, JOURNALS & NEWSLETTERS

American Fitness Magazine
www.americanfitness.com
(877) Your Body

Berkeley Wellness Letter
www.wellnessletter.com
(800) 829-9170

Changes Magazine
www.changemagazine.net
(281) 486-0064

Consumer Reports on Health
www.consumerreports.org
(914) 378-2000

Coping Magazine
www.copingmag.com
(615)790-2400

Eating Well Magazine
www.eatingwell.com
(802) 425-5700

Evolution Catalog of Music
www.evolutioncatalog.com
(800) 562-8283

The Green Guide
www.TheGreenGuide.com
(800) 647-5463

Health Freedom Watch
www.forhealthfreedom.org
(202) 429-6610

Health Magazine
www.health.com
(800) 274-2522

HerbalGram
www.herbalgram.com
(512) 926-4900

Natural Health Magazine
www.naturalhealthmag.com
(212) 743-6614

New Perspectives Magazine
new.perspectives@verizon.net
(951) 925-6117

Nutrition Action Health Letter
www.SCPInet.org
(202) 332-9110

Taste for Life
www.tasteforlife.com
(603) 924-7271

Tufts University Health & Nutrition Letter
www.healthletter.tufts.edu
(800) 274-7581

Vegetarian Journal
www.vrg.org
(410) 366-8343

Vegetarian Nutrition
www.vegetariannutrition.net
(800) 877-1600

Vegetarian Times
www.vegetariantimes.com
(800) 793-9161

Veggie Life
www.veggielife.com

Yoga Journal
www.yogajournal.com
(415) 591-0555

Notes: Because a magazine or journal is listed here, does not mean that everything in the content of each will agree with the information contained within **INSTANT *E.N.E.R.G.Y.*™**. There is simply enough good information that warrants the magazine or journal being listed. It is up to you, as a discerning reader, to evaluate what is written and use only what will benefit your health to the maximum. For example, where recipes list ingredients, such as sweeteners and fats, not recommended, substitute with those included in your **INSTANT *E.N.E.R.G.Y.*™** Shopping list.

ORGANIZATIONS & CENTERS FOR NUTRITION AND HEALTH

American Botanical Council
www.herbalgram.org
(512) 926-4900

Ann Wigmore Foundation
www.wigmore.org
(505) 552-0595

The Cancer Project
www.cancerproject.org
(202) 244-5038

Center For Science in the Public Interest
www.CSPInet.org
(202) 332-9110

Consumers Union
www.consumersunion.org
(914) 378-2000

Creative Health Institute
www.creativehealthinstitute.com
(517) 278-6260

Food & Water Watch
www.foodandwaterwatch.org
(202) 797-6550

Herb Research Foundation
www.herbs.org
(303) 449-2265

Hippocrates Health Institute
www.hippocratesinst.com
(561) 471-8876

Optimum Health Institute of San Diego
www.optimumhealth.org
(619) 464-3346

Organic Consumers Association
www.organicconsumers.org
(218)-226-4164

Physicians Committee for Responsible Medicine
www.pcrm.org
(202) 686-2210

Simonton Cancer Centers
www.simontoncenter.com
(800) 338-2360

Society of Nutrition Education
www.sne.org
(317) 328-4627

Slow Food USA
www.slowfoodusa.org
(718) 260-8000 or 877-SlowFoo(d)

Soy Foods of North America
www.soyfoods.org
(202) 659-3520

Vegetarian Nutrition Dietetic Practice Group
www.ada.org
(800) 877-1600

The Vegetarian Resource Group
www.vrg.org
(410) 366-8343

Vegetarians of Washington
www.vegofwa.org
(206) 706-2635

INFORMATION, REFERRALS, DIRECTORIES

The American Association of Naturopathic Physicians
www.naturopathic.org
(206) 323-7610

American Biologics
www.americanbiologics.com
(800) 227-4473

American Cancer Society
www.cancer.org
(800) 227-2345

American Dietetic Association
www.eatright.org
(800) 877-1600

American Heart Association
www.americanheart.org
(800) 242-8721

American Holistic Medical Association
(425) 987-0737

The American Institute for Cancer Research
www.aicr.org
(800) 843-8114

The American Massage Therapy Association
www.amtamssage.org
(877) 905-2700

American Stroke Association
www.strokeassociation.org
(800) 787-8984

The Animal Rights Foundation
Pocket Compassionate Shopping Guide
www.arff.org
(954) 727-ARFF

Association for Research of Childhood Cancer
www.arocc.org
(716) 681-4433

Cancer Control Society
www.cancercontrolsociety.com
(323) 663-7801

Committee for Freedom of Choice in Medicine
www.forhealthfreedom.org
(202) 429-6610

Environmental Health Strategy Center
www.preventharm.org
(207) 827-6331

The Health Resource
www.thehealthresource.com
(800) 949-0090

Intl. Academy of Nutrition & Preventative Medicine
www.iapm.org
(800) 296-3651

International Holistic Center, Inc.
www.holisticresources.org
(928) 771-1742 or(602) 287-0605

National Center for Homeopathy
www.homeopathy.org
(206) 720-7000

National Self-Help Clearinghouse
www.selfhelpweb.org
(212) 817-1822

National Women's Health Network
www.nwhn.org
(202) 347-1140 or (202) 628-7814

Vegetarian Restaurant Guide
www.vegdining.org

Wellness Community National Headquarters:
www.thewellnesscommunity.org
(888) 793-WELL or (202) 659-9709

World Research Foundation
www.wrf.org
(928) 284-3300

Notes: Some of the above organizations, institutes, centers, and services charge a nominal fee for their services and information. It is wise to inquire as to the cost, if any, prior to receiving what they have to offer. This saves confusion and prevents embarrassment later.

GOVERNMENT CONTACTS

Cancer Information Service National Cancer Institute:
www.cis.nih.gov
(800) 422-6237

Community Nutrition Institute
www.ars.usda.gov
(301)504-0610

Consumer Information Center
www.pueblo.gsa.gov
(800) 888-8PUEBLO or (800) FED INFO

Department of Agriculture Human Nutrition Info Service
www.fnic.nal.usda.gov/nai
(301) 436-8617

www.marilynjoyce.com

Department of Agriculture Food and Nutrition Service
www.fns.usda.gov
(303) 504-5414

Environmental Protection Agency (EPA)
www.epa.gov
www.epa.gov/safewater
(800) 426-4791

Food and Drug Administration (FDA)
www.fda.gov
(888) 468-6332

National Food Safety Information Network
www.foodsafety.gov
www.fsis.usda.gov/food_safety_education/USDA_meat_&_poultry_hotline
www.cfsan.fda.gov/

National Marine Fisheries Service
www.nmfs.noaa.gov
(301) 301-713-2334

United States Department of Agriculture (USDA)
www.usda.gov

USDA Food Safety and Inspection Service (FSIS)
www.fsis.usda.gov
(402) 344-5000
Meat and Poultry Hotline: (888) 674-6854

ORGANIC RESOURCES/ORGANIC FARMERS

For more information about ways to keep "organic" organic, contact:

Let's Keep "Organic" Organic at their website at: www.saveorganic.org

Go Organic for Earth Day is another great resource packed with organic information at: www.organicearthday.org

Organic Trade Association (OTA): For information about the organic products industry: farmers, certifiers, manufacturers, processors, distributors, retailers, organic: visit their website at www.ota.com, or call (413) 774-7511, or fax (413) 774-6432; or write to: P.O. Box 1078, Greenfield, MA 01302

Environmental Nutrition: This is a monthly newsletter, which encompasses diet, nutrition and health. Though I do not endorse everything contained on their pages wholeheartedly, it is one of the best newsletters I have come across addressing these matters from a somewhat holistic perspective while referring to the scientific data available. For subscription information call (800) 829-5384.

E, The Environmental Magazine: A real treasure, this magazine acts as a clearinghouse of information, news and commentary on environmental issues for the general public, as well as the dedicated environmentalist. It informs and inspires individuals to make the changes necessary for the improvement of our water, air and earth. Call (203) 854-5559; or write to E Magazine at Subscription Dept., P.O. Box 2047, Marion, OH 43306; or check out their website at www.emagazine.com

EarthSave: This organization is committed to educating people about the profound impact our food choices have on our environment. The resources, educational materials and programs are extensive and versatile, addressing every aspect of a safe and healthy environment and what we need to do to achieve such. For information about the organization and their products and educational materials contact EarthSave at 706 Frederick Street, Santa Cruz, CA 95062-2205 or call (408) 423-4069.

The Campaign to Label Genetically Engineered Foods: Their name speaks for itself. P.O. Box 55699, Seattle, WA 98155; Ph: 425-771-4049; Fax: 603-825-5841; Website: www.thecampaign.org; Email: label@thecampaign.org

Safe Food: Eating Wisely in a Risky World:
> A book written by Jacobson, M.F., Lefferts, L.Y., and Garland, A.W. For this book and a list of other valuable resources, contact the **Center for Science in the Public Interest,** 1875 Connecticut Ave., N.W., Suite 300, Washington, D.C. 20009-5728, or call (202) 332-9110. www.cspinet.org

Organic Farmers: Mail Order Services

Though many stores in large cities carry certified organic produce and grains, these products may be very difficult to find in smaller centers and remote areas. As there are several sources for listings of organic farmers who mail order to the general public, I am not including a long list here. However, to assist you in this search I will include some sources of such listings.

Charan Springs Farm:
> Owned by Michael Limacher. For some of the most flavorful organic produce available overnight by mail order, at very reasonable prices, write to **Charan Springs Farm,** Route #1, Box 521, Cambria, CA 93428, or call (805) 927-8289 or www.charansprings.com. And for anyone who wants a magical break from their daily routine, stay at one of the farm's secluded, well-equipped cabins. The combination of the all-natural food and the peaceful, unspoiled environment promotes the total rejuvenation of both body and mind!

Certified Organic Food Directory:
> Natural Food Network creates magazines, newsletters, directories and business intelligence that help the natural and organic food industry operate with greater insight. Their goal is to inform and connect buyers and sellers and others who collaborate in bringing wholesome products to market. Contact: NaturalFoodNet 309 8th Avenue, San Mateo, CA 94401
> 1-877-236-5633 www.naturalfoodnet.com

Earl's Organic Produce:
> Located on the San Francisco Wholesale Produce Market, Earl's Organic Produce is the sole 100% organic operation on the market. They are a Bay Area wholesaler of certified organic produce, and work with customers of all sizes — from the natural foods co-op to the independent grocery to the national chain store. 2101 Jerrold Ave, Ste. 100, San Francisco, CA 94124 (415) 824-7419 www.earlsorganic.com

National Organic Directory:

Though not specifically targeted to the general public, it is an excellent and comprehensive resource, listing farmers and wholesalers who actually do mail order to such an audience. For information on how to order this directory, contact the **Community Alliance with Family Farmers,** P.O. Box 464, Davis, CA 95617, or call (800) 852-3832. www. caff.org

FOOD PRODUCTS

The following is by no means an exhaustive list of healthy and/or alternative food products. It is simply a summation of some of the items which have been mentioned throughout this book, some of which may be, at this time, unavailable or difficult to find, in the regular marketplace. The sources, accompanying each of the items listed, will provide you with information on how to order the products, or guide you to the retail locations nearest you that carry the specific products.

Note: Because a company's products are mentioned here, does not indicate that **INSTANT E.N.E.R.G.Y.™** *exclusively endorses that specific brand of that particular product. It is simply a base from which to begin your own research.*

REMEMBER! Be adventurous! Try new foods, seasonings and condiments!

Coffee Substitute

Cafix
www.internaturalfoods.com

InterNatural Foods, LLC
300 Broadacres Dr.
Bloomfield, NJ 07003
(973) 338-1499

Raja's Cup
www.mapi.com

MAPI
1068 Elkton Dr.
Colorado Springs, CO 80907
(800) 255-8332

Teeccino
www.teeccino.com

Teeccino
1720 Las Canos Rd.
Santa Barbara, CA 93105
(800) 498-3434

Dairy & Dairy Alternatives

Almond, Hazelnut, Oat & Rice Milks
www.pacificfoods.com

Pacific Natural Foods
19480 SW 97th Ave.
Tualatin, OR 97062
(503) 692-9666 x1124

www.marilynjoyce.com

Cheese Substitutes:
Vegan Rella, Tofu Rella,

300 Broadacres Dr.
Bloomfield, NJ 07663
(973) 338-0300

Kefir
www.lifeway.net

Lifeway
6431 West Oakton Ave.
Morton Grove, IL 60053
(847) 967-1010

Milk, Butter & Half 'n Half
www.horizonorganic.com

Horizon Organic
P.O. Box 17577
Boulder, CO 80308
(888) 494-3020

Organic Farmers Co-op
Dairy, eggs, snacks, meats
www.organicvalley.com

Organic Valley Family of Farms
CROPP Cooperative
One Organic Way
La Farge, WI 54639
(888) 444-6455

Parmesan Cheese
www.alpinelace.com

Alpine Lace
4001 Lexington Ave. N
Arden Hills, MN 55126
(651) 481-2222

Yogurt, Ice Cream, Milk, organic
www.stonyfield.com

Stonyfield Farm
10 Burton Drive
Londonderry, NH 03053
(800) PRO-COWS (776-2697)

** also see Soymilk

Fat Replacements & Healthier Fats & Oils

Dried Plums in Baking
(Dried Plum Puree)
www.californiadriedplums.org

California Dried Plum Board
3841 N. Freeway Blvd., Suite 120
Sacramento, CA 95834
(916) 565-6232

Nayonaise
www.vitasoy-usa.com

Vitasoy USA, Inc.
Ayer, MA 01432
(800) VITASOY (848-2769)

Oils
www.spectrumorganics.com

Spectrum Organic Products, Inc.
5341 Old Redwood Hwy., Suite 400
Petaluma, CA 94954

Udo's Oils
www.florahealth.com

Flora, Inc.
Post Office Box 73
805 E. Badger Road
Lynden, Washington, USA 98264
(800) 446-2110

Vegan Gourmet
www.followyourheart.com

Follow Your Heart Natural
Foods/Earth Island
P.O. Box 9400
Canoga Park, CA 91309-0400
(818) 725-2820

Vegenaise
www.followyourheart.com

Follow Your Heart Natural
Foods/Earth Island
P.O. Box 9400
Canoga Park, CA 91309-0400
(818) 725-2820

Healthy Snack Bars & Cookies

Clif Bar
www.clifbar.com

Clif Bar, Inc.
Berkeley, CA 94710
(800) CLIFBAR (254-3227)

Dagoba Organic Chocolate
www.dagobachocolate.com

Dagoba Organic Chocolate
1105 Benson Way
Ashland, OR 97520
(541) 482-2001

Lara Bar and Jocalat Bar
www.larabar.com

LÄRABAR
PO Box 18932
Denver, Colorado 80218
(720) 945-1155

Maca Bar
www.potentfoods.com

Potent Foods, Inc.
4000 Kruse Way Place, Bldg 3, Suite 255
Lake Oswego, OR 97035
(877) 4 POTENT (476-8368)

Organic Food Bar
www.organicfoodbar.com

Organic Food Bar, Inc.
215 E. Orangethorpe Ave. Suite 284
Fullerton, CA 92832
(800) 246-4685

Soy Pal Cookie Diet
Meal Replacement & Snack Food
www.soy4healthyweight.com

Vibrant Health Academy Unlimited
450 Hillside Dr., Bldg. B, Suite 200
Mesquite, NV 89027
(800) 352-3443

Think Green & Think Organic Bar
www.thinkproducts.com

Prime Health
Ventura, CA
(866) 98THINK (988-4465)

Ultra Lean Gluco-Support Bar
www.bio-genesis.com

Biogenesis
Mill Creek, WA 98012
(425) 487-0788

Meat & Meat Alternatives

All American Veggie Burger
www.amys.com

Amy's Kitchen, Inc.
P.O. Box 449
Petaluma, CA 94953
(707) 578-7270

Boca Burgers-Organic
www.bocaburger.com

Boca Foods Company
PO Box 8995
Madison, WI 53708
(877) 966-8769

Hormel Natural Choice Deli Meats
(no preservatives, or nitrates)
www.hormel.com

Hormel Foods Sales, LLC
1 Hormel Place
Austin, MN 55912
(800) 523-4635

Poultry, Beef
www.colemannatural.com
Email: coleman@colemannatural.com

Coleman Natural Foods
1767 Denver West Marriott Road
Suite 200
Golden CO 80401
(800) 442-8666

Sunshine Burgers–Organic
www.sunshineburger.com

Sunshine Burger Corp
92 Center St.
Ellenville, NY 12428

Smart Bacon, other "Smart" Choices
www.lightlife.com

Light Life
153 Industrial Blvd.
Turner Falls, MA 01376
(800) Soy-Easy (769-3279)

The Excellent Chicken
www.bellandevans.com

Bell & Evans
154 W. Main St.
Fredericksburg, PA 17026
(717) 865-6626

The Great Organic Hot Dog
Deli Meats, no nitrates
www.applegatefarms.com
E-mail: help@applegatefarms.com

Applegate Farms, Inc.
750 Rte 202, Suite 300
Bridgewater, NJ 08807-5530
(866) 587-5858

Veggie Turkey or Ham
www.yvesveggie.com

Yves Veggie Cuisine
Consumer Relations
4600 Sleepytime Dr.
Boulder, CO 80301
(800) 667-YVES

Protein Powders, Green Foods, & Spirulina

Juice Plus+® Complete
Identity Preserved Soy Protein Powder
www.DrJoyce4Nutrition.com

Vibrant Health Academy Unlimited
450 Hillside Dr., Bldg. B, Suite 200
Mesquite NV 89027
(800) 352-3443

Perfect Food
Super Green Formula
www.gardenoflife.com

Garden of Life
5500 Village Blvd., Suite 202
West Palm Beach, FL 33407
(866) 465-0051

Spirulina Powder
www.nutrex-hawaii.com

Nutrex Hawaiian Inc.
73-4460 Queen Kaahamanu Hwy
Kailua-Kona, HI 96740
(800) 453-1187

Super-Green Pro-96 Protein Powder
www.natlife.com

Nature's Life
900 Larkspur Landing Circle, Suite 105
Larkspur, CA 94939
(800) 247-6997 or (435) 655-6790

Seasonings

Bac'Uns
www.frontierherb.com

Frontier Natural Products
P.O. Box 299
3021 78th St.
Norway, IA 52318
(800) 669-3275

Bragg Liquid Aminos
www.bragg.com

Bragg Live Foods
Box 7
Santa Barbara, CA 93102
(800) 446-1990

Celtic Sea Salt
www.celticseasalt.com

Celtic Sea Salt
4 Celtic Dr.
Arden, NC 28704
(800) 867-7258

Dr. Bronner's Mineral Bouillon

All-One-God-Faith, Inc.
Box 28, Escondido, CA 92033
(760) 743-2211

Garlic Juice
www.garlicvalleyfarms.com

Garlic Valley Farms
624 Ruberta Ave.
Glendale, CA 91201
(800) 424-7990

**Gayelord Hauser's All Natural
Vegetable Broth Powder**
www.modernfearn.com

Gayelord Hauser Products
6425 W. Executive Dr.
Mequon, WI 53092

Mrs. Dash Spices
www.mrsdash.com

Alberto Culver Co.
(800) 622-DASH (622-3274)

NOH of Hawaii Seasoning Mixes
www.nohfoods.com

NOH Foods of Hawaii
1402 W 178 St.
Gardena, CA 90248
(310) 324-6770

Real Salt (Natural Mineral Salt)
www.realsalt.com

Redmond Trading Company, L.C.
475 W. 910 South
Heber City, UT 84032
(800) For-Salt or (800) 367-7258

The Spice Hunter
www.spicehunter.com

The Spice Hunter, Inc.
San Luis Obispo, CA 93401
(800) 444-3061

Vegetable Seasoning Powder

Bernard Jensen's
(available on Amazon.com)

Yamaka All Purpose Sauce
www.realfreshcookin.com

Real Fresh Cookin'
P.O. Box 1950
Honokaa, HI 96737
(808) 775-8100

Snacks

Baked Rice Krisps
www.mrkrispers.com

TH Foods
2154 Harlem Rd.
Loves Park, IL 61111
(888) Krispers (574-7737)

Corn Thins
www.cornthins.com

Real Foods PTY, Ltd
47 Campbell Road
St. Peters NSW 2044 Australia
+61 2 8595 6600

Flax Crackers
www.foodsalive.com

Foods Alive
4840 County Rd. #4
Waterloo, IN 46793
(260) 488-4497

Multi Grain Crisps
www.soycrisps.com

World Gourmet Marketing LLC
P.O. Box 753
Wayne, NJ 07474
(800) 913-6637

Rice Cakes & Rice Chips, organic
www.lundberg.com
Email: info@lundberg.com

Lundberg Family Farms
5370 Church Street
Richvale, CA 95974
(530) 882-4551

Soy Jerky
www.tastyeats.com
Email: info@tastyeats.com

Tasty Eats
Lewes, DE 19958
(302) 236-7503

Soup or Meal-in-a-Cup or Pouch or Carton

Soups and Meals, in a Cup
Dehydrated, Natural
www.pacificfoods.com

Pacific Natural Foods
19480 SW 97th Ave.
Tualatin, OR 97062
(503) 692-9666 x1124

Soups and Meals, in a Cup
Dehydrated, Natural
www.fantasticfoods.com

Fantastic Foods, Inc.
Consumer Relations
564 Gateway Dr.
Napa, CA 94558
(800) 288-1089

Miso-Cup (organic, reduced sodium)
www.edwardandsons.com

Edward&SonsTradingCompany,Inc.
Box 1326
Carpenteria, CA 93014
(805) 684-8500

Organic, Instant Miso Soup
www.greenol.co.uk

Greenline
Chulmleigh,
Devon EX18 7YU

Trader Joe's Instant Miso Soup
www.traderjoes.com

Trader Joe's
Monrovia, CA 91016

Soymilk & Soy Yogurt

Endensoy
www.edenfoods.com

Eden Foods
701 Tecumseh Road
Clinton, MI 49236
(800) 424-3336

Vitasoy
www.vitasoy-usa.com

Vitasoy, Inc.
1 New England Way
Ayer, MA 01432
(800) VITASOY (848-2769)

Silk Soymilk
www.silksoymilk.com

White Wave Foods Co.
Consumer Affairs
12002 Airport Way
Bromfield, CO 80021
(888) 820-9283

SoyTreat
www.lifeway.net

Lifeway
6431 West Oakton Ave.
Morton Grove, IL 60053
(847) 967-1010

Soy Yogurt
www.stonyfield.com

Stonyfield Farm
10 Burton Drive
Londonderry, NH 03053
(800) PRO-COWS (776-2697)

Westsoy
www.westsoy.biz

West Soy Consumer Relations
The Hain Celestial Group
4600 Sleepytime Dr.
Boulder, CO 80301
(800) 434-4246

Sweeteners

Date Sugar, Unsulphured Molasses, Agave Syrup
www.auntpattys.com

Aunt Patty's Natural Foods &
Ingredients/ GloryBee Foods, Inc.
120 N. Seneca Rd
Eugene, OR 97402
(800) 456-7923

Demerara Cane Sugar
www.floridacrystals.com

Florida Crystals Food Corp
P.O. Box 4671
West Palm Beach, FL 33402
(877) 835-2828

Stevia
www.steviva.com

Stevia Brands, Inc.
818 SW 3rd Ave., Suite 1340
Portland, OR 97204
(800) 851-6314

Sweetleaf Stevia
www.wisdomnaturalbrands.com

Wisdom Natural Brands
1203 W. San Pedro St.
Gilbert, AZ 85233
(800) 899-9908

Sucanat
www.wholesomesweeteners.com

Wholesome Sweeteners
8016 Hwy 90-A
Sugar Land, TX 77478
(800) 680-1896

Turbinado
www.sugarintheraw.com

Sugar In The Raw
Cumberland Packing Corp.
2 Cumberland St.
Brooklyn, NY 11205

Xylitol
www.xylitolforyou.com
Email: sales@XylitolForYou.com

Xylitol For You
Polyresins International Corporation
7335 Orangethorpe Avenue
Buena Park, CA 90621
(877) 224-7496

Teas

Celestial Seasonings Herb Teas
www.celestialseasonings.com

Celestial Seasonings
4600 Sleepytime Dr.
Boulder, CO 80301
(800) 434-4246

Gods' Herbs' Teas
www.godsherbs.com
Email: info@godsherbs.com

God's Herbs Company
730-C Tamiami Trail
Port Charlotte, FL 33953
(941) 766-8068

Good Earth Natural Herb Teas
www.goodearthteas.com

Good Earth Teas
831 Almar Avenue
Santa Cruz, CA 95060

Traditional Medicinals Teas
www.traditionalmedicinals.com

Traditional Medicinals
4515 Ross Road
Sebastopol, CA 95472
(800) 543-4372

Tofu

Silken Tofu, Mori-Nu Brand
www.morinu.com

Morinaga Nutritional Foods, Inc.
2441 205th St., Suite C102
Torrance, CA 90501
(310) 787-0200
(831) 423-7913

Wholegrain Products

All Natural Baked Granola

Margi G's Bowl 'A Granola
St. Petersburg, FL
(727) 251-7137

Alpen Muesli & Weetabix
www.wheetabixusa.com

The Weetabix Company, Inc.
20 Cameron St,
Clinton, MA 01510
(978) 368-0991

**Barbara's Nature's Choice Organic
Whole Grain Products and Snacks**
www.barbarasbakery.com

World Pantry / Barbara's Bakery, Inc.
601 22nd St.
San Francisco, CA 94107
(866) 972-6879

**Brown Jasmine Rice, Risotto
Wild Rice, organic**
www.lundberg.com

Lundberg Family Farms
5370 Church Street
Richvale, CA 95974
(530) 882-4551

Brown Rice Pasta
www.traderjoes.com

Trader Joe's Organic Pasta
Monrovia, CA 91016

**Health Valley Cereals, Cookies,
Crackers, Snacks, Soups, Meals**
www.healthvalley.com

Health Valley Consumer Relations
4600 Sleepytime Dr.
Boulder, CO 80301
(800) 434-4246

Manna Breads
www.naturespath.com

Nature's Path Organic
available in most grocery store and
health food stores

**Natural Stone Ground Wholegrains,
Bulk Grains, Cereals, Meals, Seeds,
Seasoning Mixes and Beans**
www.bobsredmill.com

Bob's Red Mill Natural Foods, Inc.
5209 S.E. International Way
Milwaukee, OR 97222
(800) 349-2173

Nine Grain Wholewheat Bread
www.greatharvest.com

Great Harvest Bread Co.
28 S. Montana St.
Dillon, Mt 59725
(800) 442-0424

Sprouted Corn Tortillas
www.foodforlife.com

Food For Life Baking Co., Inc.
P.O. Box 1434
Corona, CA 92878
(800) 797-5090

Organic Pastas and Cereals
www.annies.com

Annie's Homegrown
564 Gateway Drive
Napa, CA 94558
(800) 288-1089

Spelt Pasta
www.purityfoods.com

VitaSpelt
2871 W. Jolly Rd.
Okemos, MI 48864
(800) 99 SPELT (997-7358)

Sprouted Wheat Tortillas
www.organicbread.com

French Meadow Bakery
2610 Lyndale Ave. South
Minneapolis, MN 55408
(877) NO-YEAST (669-3278)

Other

BB536 Bifidus Probiotic
www.morinu.com

Morinaga Nutritional Foods, Inc.
P.O. Box 7969
Torrance, CA 90504
(310) 787-0200

Juice Plus+®
Encapsulated concentrated fruits
& veggies
www.DrJoyce4Nutrition.com

Vibrant Health Academy Unlimited
450 Hillside Dr., Bldg. B, Suite 200
Mesquite NV 89027
(800) 352-3443

Nut Butters, organic
www.worldpantry.com
E-mail: info@worldpantry.com

Maranatha Nut Butters
c/o WorldPantry.com, Inc.
601 22nd Street
San Francisco, CA 94107
(866) 972-6879 or (415) 401-0080

Marinara Sauce
www.muirglen.com

Muir Glen Organics
(800) 832-6345

Pomi Chopped Tomatoes
Only ingredient: **Tomatoes**
www.farmlanddairies.com

Parmalat S.P.A. Italy
Distributed by: Farmland Dairies LLC
520 Main Ave.
Wallington, NJ 07057
(888) 727-6252

EQUIPMENT

Cell Phone EMF/RF Exposure
The Aulterra Neutralizer
www.aulterra.com

Aulterra
560 W. Canfield Ave., Suite 400
Coeur d'Alene, ID 83815

Fit 10 Exercise Program
www.fit10.com

Fitex Solutions, LLC
1558 Anna Ruby Lane, Suite A
Kennesaw, GA 30152
(800) 576-3067

ReboundAIR
www.healthbounce.com

American Institute of Reboundology
520 S. Commerce Dr.
Orem, UT 84058
(888) 464 – JUMP (5867)

Vita-Mix and Total
Nutrition Center
www.marilynjoyce.com
NOTE:

Vita Mix Corporation
8615 Usher Road
Cleveland, OH 44138
(800) VITAMIX (848-2649)

If you contact Vitamix directly, be sure to mention my special code for . . .
Free shipping when you order.
Special Code: 06-001182

PERSONAL PRODUCTS

SkinLift Light
www.gloriamartel.com

Gloria Martel Products
Los Angeles, CA 90049
(866) 411-0033
(310) 471-7901

Organic Cotton Personal Care Products
www.organicessentials.com

Organic Essentials
822 Baldridge Street
O'Donnell, TX 79351
(800) 765-6491

INDEX OF RECIPES

C

D

E

F

G

H

www.marilynjoyce.com

T

V

W

Y

Z

SPECIAL BONUS OFFER

The Vitality Doctor's 4-week
INSTANT *E.N.E.R.G.Y.*™ & VITALITY FOR LIFE
Teleseminar Series *FREE!*

As a thank you for purchasing **INSTANT *E.N.E.R.G.Y.*™: The 5 Keys to Unlimited Energy & Vitality,** Dr Marilyn Joyce is offering a scholarship for you and a loved one to attend the 4-week **INSTANT *E.N.E.R.G.Y.*™ & VITALITY FOR LIFE** Teleseminar series as her complimentary guests.

These guest passes are available only to purchasers of Dr Joyce's book, **INSTANT *E.N.E.R.G.Y.*™: The 5 Keys to Unlimited Energy & Vitality!** The course must be completed by December 31, 2009, and this offer is made on a space-available only basis. Every attempt will be made to insure that you get into the program as quickly as possible. All attendance is on a first-come, first-serve basis. To insure your spot, please register immediately at www. InstantEnergyToday.com.

The teleseminar series will expand on your understanding of the insights, strategies, and techniques provided throughout this book. You will learn:

➢ The 5 universal keys for absolute health & longevity, physically, mentally, emotionally and spiritually

➢ The world's easiest and most effective health-management system

➢ The underlying cause of almost all health challenges and how to change it in an instant

➢ A step-by-step process for winning the *E.N.E.R.G.Y.*™ game, so that you never have to struggle again to get, and stay, healthy

➢ How to permanently create a lifestyle that will give you energy on command

➢ A step-by-step approach to fitting in fitness no matter where you are or how busy your day is

> ➤ The world's easiest, and most effective, nutritional system that can be achieved by anyone, anywhere

> ➤ The simple habits of truly healthy people

> ➤ 10 secrets to outstanding health that can be done by even the laziest person on the planet

> ➤ How to release the hidden blocks to vibrant health & longevity

> ➤ How to recognize your "health personality" so that you can build on your strengths and overcome your weaknesses

> ➤ Miraculous tips that will result in the most relaxing deep sleep, filled with wonderful dreams, that you will ever have experienced

And so much more!!!

By the end of the course, you will have an inner sense of what real health truly feels like, and more importantly, how to automatically keep it expanding and improving. The best part is that every area of your life will be positively enhanced by all of the strategies, techniques and insights you learn, implement, and embody. Peace, joy, happiness, and an overwhelming experience of abundance in every aspect of your life will be emanating from you to such a degree that people will want to be in your presence as much as possible. Talk about becoming popular easily and effortlessly!

If you're not currently 100% satisfied with your level of health, in every area of your life — physically, mentally, emotionally and spiritually — and you know you have the potential for outstanding health greater than the results you are presently experiencing, then don't wait another minute. Regardless of whether you are currently at a level of seeming optimum health, a world-class athlete, a fitness buff, a health food advocate, or a fatigued, often sick burned out shell of your former self, or perhaps you are even overcome with some form of dis-ease; whatever your situation, there is always room for improvement. Register immediately for the program that will change your life forever at www.InstantEnergyToday.com.

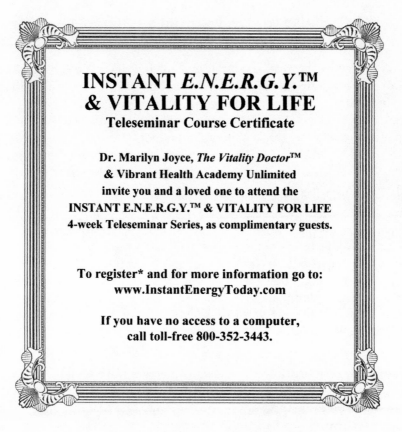

INSTANT *E.N.E.R.G.Y.*™ & VITALITY FOR LIFE
Teleseminar Course Certificate

Dr. Marilyn Joyce, *The Vitality Doctor*™
& Vibrant Health Academy Unlimited
invite you and a loved one to attend the
INSTANT E.N.E.R.G.Y.™ & VITALITY FOR LIFE
4-week Teleseminar Series, as complimentary guests.

To register* and for more information go to:
www.InstantEnergyToday.com

If you have no access to a computer,
call toll-free 800-352-3443.

* This offer is open to all purchasers of **INSTANT *E.N.E.R.G.Y.*™: The 5 Keys to Unlimited Energy & Vitality!** by Dr Marilyn Joyce, The Vitality Doctor™. Original proof of purchase is required. The offer is limited to the 4-week **INSTANT *E.N.E.R.G.Y.*™ & VITALITY FOR LIFE** Teleseminar series only, and your registration is subject to availability of space on the call lines, and/or changes to the program schedule. The course must be completed by December 31, 2009. The value for this free admission for you and a loved one is $398.00 as of June 2008. Corporate and organizational purchasers may not use one book to invite more than two people. Though there may be a long distance charge for the call-in line, depending on the long distance carrier and service that you have, admission to the actual program is complimentary. Participants on the teleseminar calls are under no additional financial obligations whatsoever to Vibrant Health Academy Unlimited or to Dr Marilyn Joyce. Vibrant Health Academy Unlimited reserves the right to refuse admission to anyone it believes may disrupt the seminars, and to block/deny access to anyone who it believes is disrupting the calls.

Praise for Dr. Marilyn's Programs

You were able to accomplish something for me that no other nutritionist, book or diet program had ever been able to do. You changed my eating and lifestyle habits for good. And one of the things that really helped was the regular phone consultations. You were able to answer my questions and motivate me to stay on track. You really know how to get lasting results!
— **Stephen Harrison, Publisher, Radio-TV Interview Report, Pennsylvania**

Working with Dr. Marilyn has taught me how to be joyous as I walk my journey. I've always found that what she says is very impactful because it's from her heart, it's real, and it's from her experience. The program was totally customized to me. I felt personally seen. I always felt heard. I felt that I have someone in my corner. She is so full of compassion. She's not just doing a job. Most people wait until they have a serious illness to seek help. It's unfortunate because we have people like Dr. Marilyn who are there to help us prevent disease in the first place. But for those who already have health challenges, Dr. Marilyn should be the first call they make.
— **Judy Cole, Teacher, California**

Last year after serious surgery, I knew my lifestyle and eating habits required major change. I listened to a CD by Dr. Marilyn Joyce, and I knew she was the right person to instruct and encourage me. I've incorporated all of her personalized eating and lifestyle strategies. The results: My high blood pressure is resolved, my cholesterol, glucose and HDL are all normal, and I remain cancer free. I've lost 85lbs and I'm joyfully moving toward my goal weight. I can't believe how easy it's been. Our phone conferences are fun, encouraging, informative and instructive. Following her suggestions has been the easiest and best way to my healthy new life!!!!!!
— **Sharon Hirsch, RN, Wisconsin**

If it weren't for Marilyn's outstanding counsel, I don't think I would have survived. She's a life saver! I highly recommend her services because she really delivers more than money can buy.
— **Jenny Redding, Language Professor, California**

I began working with Marilyn in an effort to lower my cholesterol—and I did! She gave me a great deal of information about food in general and specific, customized information that pertained to my personal goals. I noticed that the more closely I worked with Marilyn the better I felt. My energy increased dramatically and my problems with indigestion completely disappeared. Regular phone coaching with Marilyn has helped me fine tune my entire lifestyle.
— **Joyann Gongaware, Choir and Music Teacher, California**

Special Bonus — Save a whopping 50+%

(with original proof of purchase of this book, INSTANT *E.N.E.R.G.Y.*™)
You will not believe how little you pay for how much you get!

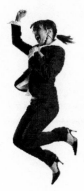

<u>The Only One-On-One Extreme Health (Mind-Body-Spirit)
Make-Over Coaching Package You Will Ever Need!</u>
<u>Your Healthy Tomorrow Starts Today!</u>
<u>The One of a Kind E.N.E.R.G.Y.™ Boost & Complete Personal
Renewal *Everyone* Needs NOW — Today!</u>

Only a very limited number of spots are available for this special coaching program, so <u>DO NOT WAIT</u> to sign up! Dr Joyce can only accommodate 10 to 12 of these intense sessions per year due to her hectic speaking and training schedule.

You can fully experience three exclusive days with Dr. Marilyn Joyce, *The Vitality Doctor*™, just you (and perhaps your partner*), in the privacy of her beautifully appointed home, situated in the exquisite setting of Southern California's robust wine country. Here you will be comfortably and lovingly cared for as you enjoy complete one-on-one, hands on, coaching and counseling sessions that will help you jump-start your health back to maximum energy, vitality and overall health. And whether your goal is to simply jump-start your energy and vitality back to where it used to be — or to where you wish it used to be — or to completely transform your health — maybe you have a serious illness you want to conquer so you can become whole again — this program is definitely for you!

Who better than someone who has a wealth of both, personal experience, having conquered a major life-threatening illness — *not once but 5 times* — as well as more than 25 years of professional expertise gained from fulfilling her life's mission as a nutrition and whole person health educator, speaker, writer and coach to thousands of people around the world? Dr Joyce is *The Vitality Doctor*™, and <u>*the expert in creating maximum energy using amazingly effective 5-minute strategies anyone can do anywhere, anytime.*</u>

Just a few of the many things you will learn and practice over approximately 30 hours that you spend with Marilyn in her beautiful private environment:

> *You will rev your energy into high gear with easy and effortless 5-minute Food & Lifestyle strategies!*

> ➢ *You will detox and energize the 5-minute way every day!*
> ➢ *You will change your health and jump from victim to victor by using this magical, mind-shifting 5-minute strategy!*
> ➢ *You will close your eyes and breathe your way to sanity in just 5 minutes!*
> ➢ *You will heal your body and maintain maximum health from deep within each one of the trillions of cells in your body*
> ➢ *You will protect your health & prevent disease the proven way in just 2 easy one-minute steps every day!*
> ➢ *You will shop like a hawk for only those things that will add to the health of your body, your home, your community, and the planet: physically, mentally, emotionally, spiritually and environmentally.*
> ➢ *You will go home with all of the tools and bonus items that will jump-start your journey, and keep you on track.*
> ➢ *You will tap Marilyn's knowledge and experience base for all of the answers to the questions that are specific to your health goals.*

SO, WHAT DO YOU GET? A LOT MORE THAN YOU EVER BARGAINED FOR!

This is the beginning of the rest of your life, and one of the most important steps *you will take today to save your life tomorrow.* Dr. Joyce has put together one of the most comprehensive packages you will ever have an opportunity to participate in. It literally includes everything that she teaches her individual clients over years of coaching — all yours over 3 days. This program can literally change your life!

And another reminder: Please be aware that Dr. Joyce sincerely has only a limited number of spots available each year for this extremely personalized program. Due to her very demanding speaking and training schedule, involving extensive global travel, *she can only take 10-12 clients* in a given calendar year. SO DON'T WAIT TO RESERVE YOUR SPOT! They fill up *very* quickly.

WHAT DO YOU GET?	VALUE
3 days of one-on-one coaching	$10,500.00 (approx. @ $350.00/hr)
Private guest room, with private bathroom (2 nights)	$300.00
Meals-2 each breakfast, lunch and dinner, plus snacks, beverages (Second dinner will be a field trip to a nice restaurant)	$400.00
Private phone consultation with Music Therapist	$200.00
Vita-Mix Machine (shipped upon receipt of payment)	$500.00
Ultimate Rebounder with Safety Bar (shipped as with V-M)	$500.00
Starter Kit (of foods and nutrients recommended by Dr Joyce)	$650.00 (approximate value)
Starter Kit (of books, CD's, DVD's and other printed materials)	$300.00 (approximate value)
Several Additional Bonuses (TBA):	$1200.00 (approximate value)
Travel from and to our local airports (details upon registration)	$300.00
Six 30-minute Follow-Up Telephone Sessions over 6 months	$1050.00
Total value for everything:	**$15,900.00**
Your Price only (more than 50% discount):	**$7,897.00**

Note: Support partner/spouse for an additional cost of ONLY: $495.00 (Includes all of above listed meals, lodging, and consultation with Music Therapist)

* The participants will be responsible for their air travel and personal expenses. All other costs for the program are inclusive in the fee to attend.

And of course, you will get lots and lots of TLC from both, Dr Joyce, and her caring assistant, Laurie. Heart-centered love and heart-centered listening form the foundation of the entire program. And we are very happy to work out a payment plan if necessary.

Contact Vibrant Health Academy Unlimited right now at: 800-352-3443. Email us at info@marilynjoyce.com

So what are you waiting for?
This may well be the absolute best investment of your entire life!
It may be the very step that you take today, that saves your life tomorrow!

"Hugging"

No movable parts
No batteries to wear out
No monthly payments
No insurance requirements
Non-taxable
Non-polluting
Low energy consumption
High energy yield
Inflation proof
Hugging is healthy
It relieves tension
It combats depression
It reduces stress
It improves blood circulation
It is invigorating
It is rejuvenating
It elevates self-esteem
It generates good will
\It has no unpleasant side effects
It is nothing less that a miracle drug
It will cure whatever ails you
And, of course, Fully Returnable.

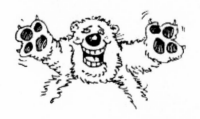